Medicine and Paradoxography in the Ancient World

Edited by
George Kazantzidis

DE GRUYTER

ISBN 978-3-11-066037-1
e-ISBN (PDF) 978-3-11-066177-4
e-ISBN (EPUB) 978-3-11-066047-0
ISSN 1868-4785

Bibliographic information published by the Deutsche Nationalbibliothek
The Deutsche Nationalbibliothek lists this publication in the Deutsche Nationalbibliografie; detailed bibliographic data are available on the Internet at http://dnb.dnb.de.

Editorial Office: Alessia Ferreccio and Katerina Zianna
Logo: Christopher Schneider, Laufen
Printing and binding: CPI books GmbH, Leck

www.degruyter.com

Preface

The present volume arose from a colloquium held at the University of Patras on the 15th of December 2016 on the topic of 'Medicine and Paradoxography in the Ancient World'. Its aim is to bring together two strands of literature, which for a long time have been kept apart in scholarship: on the one hand, ancient medicine has been traditionally treated as a 'high' genre, committed to a scientific, 'rational' understanding of human *phusis*; paradoxography, on the other hand, has been mostly discussed as representing some sort of 'low fiction' which appeals to lay imagination and whose main objective is to entertain its audience with marvellous stories which contest people's established notion of reality

On the face of it, there is little that would seem to invite a dialogue between these two domains. And yet, a closer comparative reading of the primary sources yields some rather rewarding results. Ancient medical literature allows considerable space for paradoxical elements which effectively obscure the boundaries between science and folklore. A commitment to finding solutions by means of careful observation and logical deduction often goes hand in hand with absurd claims about the (unseen) interior of the human body, lines of treatment which clearly put a patient's life at risk and a systematic reproduction of cultural stereotypes – especially with regard to female patients – which form a regressive movement within an epistemic field that is otherwise aspiring to be forward-looking and revolutionary. On the other hand, it would be a mistake to see paradoxography as being simply a compilation of mumbo-jumbo stories. What lies beneath the surface of its 'frivolous' material is a sustained, critical and often subversive engagement with scientific literature, aiming at placing *thauma* at the centre of a serious debate about what constitutes reality and how our notion of it can be continuously questioned and expanded. As part of this engagement, we often see a paradoxographer reproducing claims and notions which, absurd though they may sound, can be ultimately traced back to serious scientific sources, including medical literature. The point here is not necessarily that of deconstructing and exposing a medical notion as false; the paradoxographer may rather be interested in fleshing out that much of what is considered paradoxical is closely aligned with a normative scientific idiom and that *thauma*, by implication, lies at the centre of nature rather than at its margins. Thus, while the present volume brings out the tensions which undoubtedly exist between medicine and paradoxography, it is also intensely focused on the symbiotic relationship between the two, by paying particular attention on how wonder unites within its conceptual and affective space conflicting discourses of rational and non-rational understandings of the world.

https://doi.org/10.1515/9783110661774-202

Preface

[illegible]

Contents

George Kazantzidis

Introduction: Medicine and Paradoxography in Dialogue

Approaching *thauma* across science and fiction

Most of the evidence we have about disease in the ancient world has been transmitted to us by medical literature; this means that our sources are largely embedded in scientific contexts which set out to rationalize the various pathologies that affect the body and the mind by explaining their symptoms as following fixed patterns of cause and effect – similar to the natural laws that permeate the world around us. Yet, by virtue of the fact that disease is conceived in essence as a disruption of norms, suddenly incurring changes which often lie beyond our control, it never ceases to look odd and to alienate us from our bodies,[1] revealing the latter's intrinsic capacity to transform into something that is entirely foreign to us.[2] As Ellaine Scarry observes, "the person in great pain experiences his own body as the agent of his agony. The ceaseless, self-announcing signal of the body in pain, at once so empty and undifferentiated and so full of blaring adversity, contains not only the feeling 'my body hurts' but the feeling 'my body hurts me".[3] It is at this crucial moment of fracture, when one's own perception of the self has been altered, that a person enters the strange territories of disease, at once hostile and profoundly mystifying. The intricate links between medicine and paradoxography in antiquity attest, in fact, to an ongoing dialogue between disease and the marvellous, which shapes an understanding of the (sick) body as a terrain

1 As well as from our external environment. According to Carel 2016, 212, "illness may cause a sudden and often disturbing sense of the contingency of the meanings and uses we assign to things .... The changes brought about by illness are not localized to a specific object, but modify one's entire interaction with objects and the environment, i.e. their being in the world. For a wheelchair-user it is not just this shop or that doorway that are inaccessible, but the environment as a whole becomes less inviting or even hostile".

2 Cf. Napier 1992, 148: "Diseases, like foreigners, are things different from ourselves ... Even our mostly highly trained scientists cannot avoid the vocabulary of the foreign when discussing how diseases take hold of a person. Moreover, the tendency is so deeply rooted that learned discussions of immunology inevitably make use of a vocabulary that can only be described as animistic. Note, for example, how we conceive of allergic reactions, of how "one cell fails to recognize another cell for what it is"."

3 Scarry 1985, 47.

https://doi.org/10.1515/9783110661774-001

inhabited by forces that cannot always be explained rationally and verge on the realm of paradox.

Let us start with two brief accounts of peculiar manifestations of mental illness, as found in the Hippocratic *Epidemics* and in one of the earliest surviving paradoxographical collections, the ps.-Aristotelian Περὶ θαυμασίων ἀκουσμάτων.[4] First comes the story of Nicanor, a patient with a strange fear for the sound of the flute ([Hipp.] *Epid.* 5.81 = 5.250 L.):

> Τὸ Νικάνορος πάθος, ὁπότε ἐς ποτὸν ὥρμητο, φόβος τῆς αὐλητρίδος· ὁκότε φωνῆς αὐλοῦ ἀρχομένης ἀκούσειεν αὐλεῖν ἐν ξυμποσίῳ, ὑπὸ δειμάτων ὄχλοι· μόλις ὑπομένειν ἔφη, ὅτε εἴη νύξ· ἡμέρης δὲ ἀκούων, οὐδὲν διετρέπετο· τοιαῦτα παρείπετό οἱ συχνὸν χρόνον.
>
> Nicanor's affection, whenever he went out drinking, was terror of the flute girl. Whenever he heard one starting to play at the symposium, masses of terror rose up. He said that he could hardly bear it when it was at night. But when he heard it in the daytime he was not affected. This continued over a long period of time.[5]

Then comes the bizarre story of a wine-seller in Tarentum ([Arist.] *Mir. ausc.* 32):

> Καὶ ἐν Τάραντι δέ φασιν οἰνοπώλην τινὰ τὴν μὲν νύκτα μαίνεσθαι, τὴν δ' ἡμέραν οἰνοπωλεῖν. καὶ γὰρ τὸ κλειδίον τοῦ οἰκήματος πρὸς τῷ ζωνίῳ διεφύλαττε, πολλῶν δ' ἐπιχειρούντων παρελέσθαι καὶ λαβεῖν οὐδέποτε ἀπώλεσεν.
>
> In Tarentum they say that a seller of wine went mad at night, but sold wine by day. For he kept the key of his room at his girdle, and, though many tried to get it from him and take it, he never lost it.[6]

There are several points, both stylistic but also in terms of content, on which these two accounts converge.[7] Although we must assume that the intended audi-

---

4 The title of the collection is alternatively transmitted in the manuscript tradition as: Περὶ παραδόξων ἀκουσμάτων, Θαυμάσια, Συναγωγὴ ἀκουσμάτων. The largest part of the collection may be dated to the first half of the 3rd century BCE; see Flashar 1972, 39–50; Geus/King 2018, 435.

5 Translation in Smith 1994, 387.

6 Translation in Hett 1936, 251.

7 Note, especially, the fact that both patients display symptoms of insanity during the night and then recover during the day. Neither of the accounts gives the slightest indication as to what may be causing these peculiar conditions, focusing instead on intricate details which concern the patients' habits and everyday life activities. One main point of divergence regards the fact that while in the first case autopsy is implied – the doctor must have seen and treated Nicanor as a personal patient – in the second case the paradoxographer relies on hearsay (καὶ ἐν Τάραντι δέ

ence is different in each case, as well as that each account has a different objective, the fact of the matter is that both stories could have easily switched places without being noticeably 'out of context': the story of the wine-seller who suffers from madness during the night but is perfectly functional during the day[8] could have featured in the Hippocratic collection as an instance of insanity worthy of consideration.[9] Nicanor's strange affection,[10] on the other hand, presents us precisely with the kind of material that a paradoxographer would have seen as fit to leave his readers perplexed and in a state of amazement. The points of contact between these two stories bring out well the conceptual overlap of medicine and paradoxography in the ancient world: to the extent that disease remains something profoundly alien to us,[11] it requires explication, but it also retains a power to instill wonder and to energize our imagination in ways that extend far and beyond the boundaries of scientific speculation.

For a long time, the relationship between medicine and paradoxography in antiquity has been assumed to be virtually non-existent.[12] Being broadly situated

---

φασιν). That said, the Hippocratic author draws his information from an experience that is being reported to him (μόλις ὑπομένειν ἔφη), rather than witnessing it himself.

8 For this and similar stories of insanity in ancient paradoxography, see Kazantzidis 2018a; cf. Vanotti 2007, 151.

9 The wine-seller's case, along with that of the man in Abydus ([Arist.] *Mir. ausc.* 31) who visits the empty theatre and is hallucinating performances that only he can watch, foreground another story of insanity, which is significantly placed at the very end of the ps.-Aristotelian collection. As we read in the concluding ch. 178: Δημάρατον ... νοσήσαντα ἄφωνόν φασιν ἐπὶ δέκα γενέσθαι ἡμέρας· ἐν δὲ τῇ ἑνδεκάτῃ ἀνανήψας βραδέως ἐκ τῆς παρακοπῆς ἔφησεν ἐκεῖνον τὸν χρόνον ἥδιστα αὑτῷ βεβιῶσθαι. Compare Demaratus' nosological profile with e.g. the medical case of Parmeniscus in [Hipp.] *Epid.* 7.89 [5.446 L.]: Τῷ Παρμενίσκῳ καὶ πρότερον ἐνέπιπτον ἀθυμίαι καὶ ἵμερος τῆς ἀπαλλαγῆς βίου, ὁτὲ δὲ πάλιν εὐθυμίη. Ἐν Ὀλύνθῳ δέ ποτε φθινοπώρου ἄφωνος κατείχετο, ἡσυχίην ἔχων, βραχύ τι ὅσον ἄρχεσθαι ἐπιχειρέων προσειπεῖν· εἰ δὲ δή τι καὶ διαλεχθείη, καὶ πάλιν ἄφωνος ... Περὶ δὲ τὴν τεσσαρεσκαιδεκάτην ἀνῆκεν. On *aphonia* and its puzzling nature as a clinical condition in antiquity, see Gourevitch 1983; Montiglio 2000, 228–233.

10 For some recent discussions of Nicanor's exceptional case, see King 2013; Thumiger 2016, 118; 2017, 354–355.

11 See Sontag 1989, 48: "there is a link between imagining disease and imagining foreignness. It lies perhaps in the very concept of the wrong, which is archaically with the non-us, the alien".

12 Strangely so, considering, for instance, that Ctesias of Cnidus (5th cent. BCE), acknowledged by later sources, such as Lucian, as a seminal figure in the history of paradoxography (see Leigh 2013, 93–94; ní Mheallaigh 2014, 174), was himself a physician. In fact, it is very probable that Ctesias' medical concerns had a direct impact on his ethnographic discourse and, more generally, on his view of 'otherness' and what constitutes a 'wonder'; see Tuplin 2004 and Llewellyn-Jones/Robson 2010, 10–11. McKeown 2017 has recently produced a volume which collects 'strange tales' and 'surprising facts' from Greek and Roman medical texts; this is an extremely

within the realm, or more accurately in the margins of what we would call today 'natural sciences', ancient paradoxography[13] is primarily concerned with disclosing a world full of marvels and wondrous occurrences (including odd animal behaviour, springs that taste like wine, color-changing stones, etc.), though without providing an answer as to how these phenomena can be explained: "the key to the genre", as Nita Krevans points out, "is the objective and rational presentation of an item which appears to break the laws of nature"; its "aim is not the satisfied 'aha!' of understanding but the round-eyed 'oh!' of wonder".[14] In this sense, paradoxography seems to operate at the opposite side of what Aristotle sees as true knowledge. Philosophy, according to *Metaph.* 983a12–21,[15] begins in

---

welcome contribution to the field, although – for what concerns us here – the book pays no particular attention to paradoxography as such, and to how the notion of *thauma* harboured in that genre infiltrates medical discourse. See also Bondeson 1997.

13 On ancient paradoxography, see Giannini 1963; 1964; Jacob 1983; Sassi 1993; Schepens and Delcroix 1996; Petsalis-Diomidis 2010, 151–167; Pajón-Leyra 2011; Geus and King 2018. See also Bianchi/Thévenaz 2004 and the recent, rich volume edited by Gerolemou 2018, especially the essays by Dellatre, Nichols and Pajón-Leyra.

14 Krevans 2005, 91. Cf. Cameron 2004, 268. Key phenomenological discussions of Greek wonder, *thauma*, are: Llewelyn 1988; Prier 1989; Heidegger 1994, ch.5; Sallis 1995; Neer 2010, 20–69.

15 983a12–21: ἄρχονται μὲν γάρ … ἀπὸ τοῦ θαυμάζειν πάντες εἰ οὕτως ἔχει, καθάπερ <περὶ> τῶν θαυμάτων ταὐτόματα ἢ περὶ τὰς τοῦ ἡλίου τροπὰς ἢ τὴν τῆς διαμέτρου ἀσυμμετρίαν (θαυμαστὸν γὰρ εἶναι δοκεῖ πᾶσι <τοῖς μήπω τεθεωρηκόσι τὴν αἰτίαν> εἴ τι τῷ ἐλαχίστῳ μὴ μετρεῖται)· δεῖ δὲ εἰς τοὐναντίον καὶ τὸ ἄμεινον κατὰ τὴν παροιμίαν ἀποτελευτῆσαι, καθάπερ καὶ ἐν τούτοις ὅταν μάθωσιν· οὐθὲν γὰρ ἂν οὕτως θαυμάσειεν ἀνὴρ γεωμετρικὸς ὡς εἰ γένοιτο ἡ διάμετρος μετρητή, "all begin … by wondering that things should be as they are, e.g. with regard to marionettes, or the solstices, or the incommensurability of the diagonal of a square; because it seems wonderful to everyone who has not yet perceived the cause that a thing should not be measurable by the smallest unit. But we must end with the contrary and (according to the proverb) the better view, as men do even in these cases when they understand them; for a geometrician would wonder at nothing so much as if the diagonal were to become measurable" (transl. in Tredennick 1933, 17). On wonder in Aristotle, see Nightingale 2004, 254; 261–265. As the philosopher has explained a few lines above, we begin to wonder about 'unusual' (*atopa*) things which are close at hand, before we gradually move to matters of greater significance (*Metaph.* 982b13–15): ἐξ ἀρχῆς μὲν τὰ πρόχειρα τῶν ἀτόπων θαυμάσαντες, εἶτα κατὰ μικρὸν οὕτω προϊόντες καὶ περὶ τῶν μειζόνων διαπορήσαντες, see Warren 2014, 71. One may argue that what is implicitly dismissed by Aristotle in this passage as a trivial kind of oddity (useful only to the extent that it subsequently makes us wonder about more significant issues) constitutes the prime material of paradoxography, which often lingers on wondrous trivialities without aiming at any kind of resolution. This kind of wonder constitutes an impediment to knowledge; see Rubenstein 2008, 202: properly experienced, "wonder is self-destructive" and should act only as a provocation for the knowledge of increasingly complex ideas; cf. George 1995.

wonder, *thaumazein*;[16] once we have started to properly examine whatever it is that initially puzzled us, wonder is gradually substituted with knowledge, until in the end it becomes eradicated. As **Katerina Oikonomopoulou** argues in her contribution to this volume ('Paradoxography and the pseudo-Aristotelian *Problemata*') the ps.-Aristotelian *Problems*, a considerable part of which are devoted to 'medical matters' that pertain the human body and its functions, follow in this tradition: "far from being collected for their own sake (as in the pseudo-Aristotelian collection *De Mirabilibus Auscultationibus*), wondrous phenomena function within this work as propellers of scientific inquiry, serving to categorise empirical reality and helping to discover the full range and complexity of the mechanisms that govern physical bodies' interior workings and interaction with the natural environment".[17] By way of a reversal, paradoxography presents us with 'factual' information whose main aim is to astonish and leave us bewildered and confused;[18] even if we assume that *thauma* is implicitly functioning in that case as an impulse to further mental inquiry, the latter remains a process which the text declines to actualize, creating instead a sense of suspense that has no obvious closure (it would be useful to think here of paradoxography in general as the kind of literature which consists of 'open-ended' lists, catalogues of strange events which are open to 'inifinity', as Umberto Eco would have it:[19] given that our horizon of expectations is constantly liable to expansion, *thauma* is intrinsically linked to nature's endless reserve of wonders, some of which have not yet been revealed, but which are bound to be).[20]

---

16 Cf. Plato, *Theaetetus* 155d: μάλα γὰρ φιλοσόφου τοῦτο τὸ πάθος, τὸ θαυμάζειν· οὐ γὰρ ἄλλη ἀρχὴ φιλοσοφίας ἢ αὕτη.

17 Cf. Menn 2015, 28.

18 As I have argued in Kazantzidis 2018b, in early paradoxography, this astonishment derives mainly from the weirdness of the natural world which surrounds humans; by contrast, human beings are relatively rarely considered a cause of wonder per se. Interestingly enough, as Oikonomopoulou observes, "the *Problemata* appears to foreground the investigation of humans over that of the other animals"; humans appear in that case "as an anomaly or a notable exception in the animal world".

19 Eco 2009.

20 In some cases, paradoxographers explicitly claim that they have no interest in providing an explanation for the bizarre phenomena collected in their writings; see Romm 1992, 92. See Schepens/Delcroix 1996, 391: "θαῦμα" in these texts "is no match for 'explanation'; the sense of the marvellous cannot survive on a rational basis. It is imperative for the paradoxographer to concentrate on… the establishment and the recording of facts without explaining them."

In contrast to paradoxography, medicine is committed to rational explanation[21] in ways that make it incompatible with *thauma*. As I have argued elsewhere, "the vast majority of *thauma*- occurrences in the Hippocratic Corpus is generated precisely at points of the narrative which hint at how impressionable people can be, as opposed to sober technical expertise which intervenes and helps to explain away the mystifying and 'wonderful' aspects of the human body... [T]he high frequency with which doctors feel the need to stress that what they are dealing with can be accounted for rationally – and should by no means cause 'wonder' or 'surprise' (θαῦμα δὲ οὐδὲν/ οὐδὲν θαυμαστόν/ οὐ θαῦμά ἐστι/ οὐ θαυμάσαιμι δ' ἂν)[22] – suggests that, to some degree at least, they are alert, and perhaps even self-consciously opposed to 'alternative' practices and explanations"[23] circulating among a lay audience which sees disease as being inherently marvellous. This tension between true knowledge and wonder is best fleshed out in a discussion of epilepsy, the so-called 'sacred disease', which the medical author explains as the result of a malfunction in the brain and an excess of phlegm, thereby disproving the widespread belief that the condition is divinely inflicted (*Morb. sacr.* 1, 6.352–4 L.):

> Περὶ τῆς ἱερῆς νούσου καλεομένης ὧδ' ἔχει. οὐδέν τί μοι δοκεῖ τῶν ἄλλων θειοτέρη εἶναι νούσων οὐδὲ ἱερωτέρη, ἀλλὰ φύσιν μὲν ἔχει καὶ πρόφασιν, οἱ δ' ἄνθρωποι ἐνόμισαν θεῖόν τι πρῆγμα εἶναι ὑπὸ ἀπορίης καὶ θαυμασιότητος, ὅτι οὐδὲν ἔοικεν ἑτέροισι ... εἰ δὲ διὰ τὸ θαυμάσιον θεῖον νομιεῖται, πολλὰ τὰ ἱερὰ νοσήματα ἔσται καὶ οὐχὶ ἓν, ὡς ἐγὼ ἀποδείξω ἕτερα οὐδὲν ἧσσον ἐόντα θαυμάσια οὐδὲ τερατώδεα,[24] ἃ οὐδεὶς νομίζει ἱερὰ εἶναι.

> I am about to discuss the disease called 'sacred'. It is not in my opinion any more divine or more sacred than other diseases, but has a nature and a cause. But humans have considered it a divine thing because of their inexperience and their wonder at its peculiar character, since it looks quite different from other diseases ... But if it is to be considered divine just because it is wonderful, there will be not one sacred disease but many, for I will show that

21 As Holmes 2010, 38 observes, "[h]owever wary scholars have become about using labels like 'secular' and 'rational' to describe Greek medicine in the fifth and fourth centuries, a shift from personal, daemonic explanation to natularizing explanations remains basic to our understanding of learned medicine in this period and the medical tradition that unfolds from it". Geoffrey Lloyd's work remains essential for appreciating the rationalising agenda on which early Greek medicine operates; see, especially, Lloyd 1979; 1983; 1987 and, for a concise discussion, Lloyd 2003, 40–60. Cf. Good 1994.

22 For these formulae, see e.g. [Hipp.] *Coac.* 80 (5.600 L.); *Cord.* 3 (9.84 L.); *Prorrh.* 1.116 (5.548 L.).

23 See Kazantzidis 2018b, 39.

24 On the link between wonder and dread (with special reference to early paradoxography), see Gutzwiller 2007, 166.

other diseases are no less wonderful and portentous, and yet nobody considers them sacred. [25]

The author goes on to mention 'tertian' and 'quartan' fevers and 'sudden fits of delirium' as equally remarkable with epilepsy, the underlying assumption being that their peculiar manifestation and symptomatology should make these conditions look no less astonishing. Yet, as he states, no one 'wonders at them' (ὧν οὐ θαυμασίως γ' ἔχουσιν). His aim is not, of course, to claim that one has to, but to suggest instead that people should likewise refrain from attributing to epilepsy any 'wonderful' qualities.[26] The disease, as the author implies throughout the treatise, may be regarded as 'divine', but only in the sense that "it shares in the divine character of nature in showing a fixed pattern of cause and effect and in being subordinated to what may perhaps be called … a natural 'law' of regularity"[27] – in this respect, all diseases are divine. Such knowledge is premised upon careful scientific inquiry and is strongly opposed to the bewildering effect that the disease continues to have on lay people's imagination.

But there are always exceptions to prove the rule. In one instance, a doctor warns against excessive theatricality during anatomical demonstrations performed in public. Tying a patient on a ladder – sometimes with his head pointing downwards – and shaking him violently to straighten a humpback or relocate a fracture, as we read at [Hipp.] *De articulis* 42 (4.182 L.), is of no help at all; in fact, it can put the patient's life at grave risk.[28] However, the text continues, one can find many physicians who adopt this method, "mainly because they wish to make the crowd gape and stare (ἐκχαυνοῦν τὸν πολὺν ὄχλον), for to such people it seems marvellous to see a man suspended or shaken or treated in such ways (τοῖσι γὰρ τοιούτοισι ταῦτα θαυμάσιά ἐστιν, ἢν ἢ κρεμάμενον ἴδωσιν, ἢ ῥιπτεόμενον, ἢ ὅσα τοῖσι τοιούτοισιν ἔοικε); and they always applaud these performances, never troubling themselves about the result of the operation, whether good or bad".[29] The epideictic nature of anatomical performances reaches its climax during the Second Sophistic, at which point the boundaries between *thaumatopoiia* and actual medical practice are often blurred.[30] The passage cited

25 Text and translation (modified at points) in Jones 1923.
26 For the treatise's rhetorical strategies, see Laskaris 2002.
27 Van der Eijk 2005, 45.
28 See Nutton 2004, 352 n.62; cf. Laes 2018, 157.
29 Translation in Withington 1928, modified at points.
30 See, e.g., how Dio Chrysostom (*Or.* 33.6) compares medical displays (*epideikseis*) to public spectacles and processions: Ἡ μὲν οὖν τοιάδε ἀκρόασις θεωρία τις οὖσα καὶ πομπὴ παραπλήσιον ἔχει τι ταῖς ἐπιδείξεσι τῶν καλουμένων ἰατρῶν, οἳ προκαθίζοντες ἐν τῷ μέσῳ ξυμβολὰς ἄρθρων

above indicates that already in classical Greek medicine doctors indulged in 'wonder-making' practices, even to the detriment of their clients' health. And while the tone at *De articulis* 42 is without a doubt dismissive, in *Progn.* 1 (2.110–112 L.) *thauma* seems to be positively endorsed as a quality that is essential in shaping the authoritative relationship between a physician and his patients:[31] "To restore every patient to health is impossible. To do so indeed would have been better even than forecasting the future (τοῦτο γὰρ τοῦ προγιγνώσκειν τὰ μέλλοντα ἀποβήσεσθαι κρέσσον ἂν ἦν). But as a matter of fact men do die, some owing to the severity of the disease before they summon the physician, others expiring immediately after calling him in ... It is necessary, therefore, to learn the natures of such diseases, how much they exceed the strength of men's bodies, and to learn how to forecast them (τὴν πρόνοιαν ἐκμανθάνειν). For in this way you will justly be admired (οὕτω γὰρ ἂν θαυμάζοιτό τε δικαίως) and be an efficient physician".[32] Overall, while the Hippocratic doctors insist that there is nothing particularly marvellous about disease per se, the way medicine was practiced seems to have occasionally invited wonder/admiration/awe as the medium through which lay people were expected to engage with – what must have remained for them, for its most part – an incomprehensible world of pain and sickness.[33]

καὶ ὀστέων συνθέσεις καὶ παραθέσεις καὶ τοιαῦθ' ἕτερα ἐπεξίασι, πόρους καὶ πνεύματα καὶ διηθήσεις. οἱ δὲ πολλοὶ κεχήνασι καὶ κεκήληνται τῶν παιδίων μᾶλλον, "Well then, the sort of recitation of which I speak, being a kind of spectacle or parade, has some resemblance to the exhibitions of the so-called physicians, who seat themselves conspicuously before us and give a detailed account of the union of joints, the combination and juxtaposition of bones, and other topics of that sort, such as pores and respirations and excretions. And the crowd is all agape with admiration and more enchanted than a swarm of children" (transl. in Cohoon/Lamar Crosby 1940, 279). Cf. Aelius Aristides, *Regarding the Well in the Temple of Asclepius* 39.14: ὥσπερ γὰρ οἱ παῖδες οἱ τῶν ἰατρῶν τε καὶ τῶν θαυματοποιῶν γεγυμνασμένοι πρὸς τὰς διακονίας εἰσὶ καὶ συμπράττοντες ἐκπλήττουσι τοὺς θεωμένους καὶ χρωμένους, οὕτω τοῦ μεγάλου θαυματοποιοῦ καὶ πάντα ἐπὶ σωτηρίᾳ πράττοντος ἀνθρώπων εὕρημα τοῦτο καὶ κτῆμά ἐστι, "For just as the sons of doctors and of marvel-makers have been trained to help out and aid in astonishing spectators and those making use of their services, so this well is the discovery and possession of the great 'marvel-maker' [i.e. Asclepius] who does everything for the salvation of men" (transl. by Lightfoot, who discusses the passage in her contribution to this volume).

31 On issues of authority in the Hippocratic Corpus, see Holmes 2013.

32 Translation in Jones 1923 (slightly modified). See Jouanna 2013, 3.

33 The phrase οὕτω γὰρ ἂν θαυμάζοιτό τε δικαίως in [Hipp.] *Progn.* 1 does not indicate the kind of appreciation that a doctor would have enjoyed from an informed and learned audience. Rather, it seems to allude to an audience (the patient's family, friends etc.) who see in him a person with the power to 'forecast the future'. While prognostication was based on a fixed set of scientific rules, to those who were not aware of these they must have seemed as astonishing as a

On a broader level, though subject to scrutiny and careful examination, the body remains in many ways an uncharted territory – more so, if we consider the fact that in classical Greek medicine dissection of human bodies was prohibited by powerful taboos.[34] In Brooke Holmes' words:

> Physicians face a number of obstacles in their attempts to bind effects to causes: the opacity of the *sōma*, the infinite variability of bodily constitutions, the fluid dynamics of the humors, and so on. Each body contains factors (existing levels of a humor, a patient's constitution) that help or hinder the disease. Interposed between catalyst and symptom, physical bodies are spaces of multiple possibilities that exceed what medicine can map. The *sōma* is, then, not simply an object of rational control but also something that evades control.[35]

A terrain of hidden and unseen forces that cannot be fully mapped, the body retains the power to instill wonder – even if, as we have seen above, Hippocratic doctors refrain from explicitly admitting this fact. At the same time, the way that the external environment intervenes and causes illness and death can sometimes take extraordinary forms ([Hipp.] *Epid.* 5.86, 5.252 L.):

> Νεηνίσκος δέ τις πολὺν ἄκρητον πεπωκὼς ὕπτιος ἐκάθευδεν ἔν τινι σκηνῇ· τούτῳ ὄφις ἐς τὸ στόμα παρεισεδύετο ἀργής. καὶ δὴ ὅτε ᾔσθετο, οὐ δυνάμενος φράσασθαι, ἔβρυξε τοὺς ὀδόντας, καὶ παρέτραγε τοῦ ὄφιος, καὶ ἀλγηδόνι μεγάλῃ εἴχετο, καὶ τὰς χεῖρας προσέφερεν ὡς ἀγχόμενος, καὶ ἐρρίπτει ἑωυτόν, καὶ σπασθεὶς ἔθανεν.

> A youth who had drunk much undiluted wine was sleeping on his back in a tent. A shining snake went into his mouth. When he felt it, unable to consider what to do, he ground his teeth together and bit off part of the snake. He was seized by a great pain and brought up his hands as though choking, tossed himself about, and died in convulsions.[36]

The mention of sleep and the snake in this story could be an allusion to Asclepian medicine. One way of interpreting the text is by reading it as a critique of the sensational, miraculous stories reported in temple inscriptions dedicated to Asclepius (the correspondences between these inscriptions and the wondrous healings found in Greek epigrams are explored by **Lucia Floridi** in this volume, 'Wondrous

---

prophecy come true. On the intricate dialectics between prognosis and divination, see Langholf 1990, 232–254.

34 See Witt 2018, 223. Aristotle, writing after the Hippocratics, notes that "the internal parts of the body, especially those of man, are unknown. We must as a result refer to the parts of other creatures with a nature similar to that of humans" (*Hist. an.* 494b). For the appearance of human dissection during the first half of the 3rd cent. BCE, see von Staden 1992a.

35 Holmes 2010, 26.

36 Transl. in Smith 1994, 137.

Healings in Greek Epigrams – and their Parodic Counterparts'):[37] while sleep in those cases is essential for the recovery of the patient's health,[38] in the Hippocratic account it turns out to be fatal. More to the point, death is caused by a snake – which, in the context of temple medicine, is believed to have sacred, healing associations (Asclepius is typically depicted as holding a staff around which a serpent is coiled).[39] Recent studies, however, have shown that the imposition of a dividing line between rational and temple medicine runs the risk of anachronism.[40] As the argument goes, the evidence of explicit attacks against temple medicine in the Hippocratic Corpus is too limited to support the hypothesis of a widely circulating skepticism against the divine among medical circles;[41] what is more, the relationship between the two domains seems to have been symbiotic both in terms of shared disease terminology and, more importantly, at the level of therapy (involving the same pharmaceutical means, healing plants, etc.).[42] Physicians themselves might even have allowed their patients to visit temples for additional help.[43] In this interactive environment, rather than being intended as a criticism, the story of the man swallowing a snake could be read as a doctor's attempt to claim his own share in the marvellous by incorporating a bizarre narrative in what otherwise remains, for the most part, a collection of realistic case studies of patients.[44]

---

37 For the importance of *thauma* in the healing inscriptions of Epidaurus, see Kazantzidis 2018b, 35–36. The first story that is inscribed at the top of Stele A significantly draws attention to the 'wonderful' healing act of the god (…τυχοῦσα δὲ τούτων ἐπὶ τὸ ἄνθεμα ἐπεγράψατο· "οὐ μέγε/[θο]ς πίνακος θαυμαστέον, ἀλλὰ τὸ θεῖον").

38 For the ritual of incubation and dream healing in Asclepius' temples, see Cilliers/Pieter Retief 2013 and Petridou 2015, 186–191.

39 See Pearcy 2013, 105–106, who contrasts [Hipp.] *Epid.* 5.86 to *IG* IV², 1, no.121: "A man had his toe healed by a serpent. He, suffering dreadfully from a malignant sore in his toe, during the daytime was taken outside by the servants of the Temple and set upon a seat. When sleep came upon him, then a snake issued from the Abaton and healed the toe with its tongue, and thereafter went back again to the Abaton" (transl. by Pearcy).

40 As Parker 1996, 184 puts it, "the truest explanation for the rise of Asclepius may be that he was, as it were, in partnership with Hippocrates".

41 See especially King 1998, 99–113; 2006. Cf. Nutton 1985, 46.

42 For bibliography on the symbiosis between 'secular' and 'religious' medicine, see Holmes 2008, 84 n.10.

43 See Gorrini 1995, 143–145, with the objections in Harris 2009, 249 n.17.

44 [Hipp.] *Epid.* 5.86 is in many ways exceptional. After noting its unusual mention of a snake (suggestive of a healing cult), Craik 2015, 80 observes: "The story is told in jerky clauses or sentences, linked by the conjunction 'and' (καί). There is a rhythmic, part hexametric pattern in the cadences. It seems that a passage of quite alien origin has crept into *Epidemics* 5". Hughes 2017, 77 and n.28 associates the story with votive body parts in which internal organs are modeled into

If classical medicine allows some space for *thauma*, paradoxography in its turn keeps a close eye on medical discourse. To begin with, in early paradoxographical collections the marvelous is often generated by the way in which nature interacts with humans either to cause or to cure specific types of sickness. In most of those cases, and considering that paradoxography presents us with what remains in principle an unsettling and hostile world,[45] sickness is produced as the result of an unfortunate encounter with nature's wondrous aspects. In [Arist.] *Mir. ausc.* 152, for instance, we read about a spring at Tyana whose bubbling water "leaps at the eyes, hands and feet of perjurers, causing them to suffer from dropsy and consumption" (ἁλίσκονταί τε ὑδέροις καὶ φθόαις).[46] In ch. 167 of the same collection, a stone at the river Maeander in Asia is said to cause madness (ἐμμανὴς γίνεται), and a crave for killing, to those who hold it on their lap. Occasionally, though, nature can also cure ([Arist.] *Mir. ausc.* 66):

> Τὸν δὲ γαλεώτην, ὅταν ἐκδύσηται τὸ δέρμα, καθάπερ οἱ ὄφεις, ἐπιστραφέντα καταπίνειν· τηρεῖσθαι γὰρ ὑπὸ τῶν ἰατρῶν διὰ τὸ χρήσιμον εἶναι τοῖς ἐπιληπτικοῖς.
>
> The spotted lizard, when it has sloughed its skin like a snake, is said to turn round and devour it; for it is watched for by physicians because of its value for epileptics.[47]

The reference to epilepsy is not without its significance, especially if we consider that the author mentions as a fact that doctors (ὑπὸ τῶν ἰατρῶν) recognise the therapeutic qualities of the lizard's skin. None of the medical sources prior to the ps.-Aristotelian collection confirm such a statement. It may be the case that the

---

the form of the snake; these textual and material sources, as she argues, "confirm that patients did sometimes see themselves as occupied by animals".

45 The paradoxographical world could be read as a reverse image of the utopian, idyllic landscapes which are dominant in bucolic poetry, e.g. in Theocritus. For a reading of Nicander's *Theriaca* along these lines, see Overduin 2014. For Nicander and paradoxography, see the contribution by Overduin in this volume. Cf. Holmes 2017, 248 (on Pliny's books on medicine in his encyclopaedia): "the human condition must be defined by a lack of intuitive knowledge about where the human belongs in the network of sympathies and antipathies underlying the natural world". In contrast with Pliny's, early paradoxography's nature is less friendly and less generous with providing help to humans.

46 As the text concludes, "it is impossible for the perjurers to get away before it happens, but they are rooted to the spot lamenting by the water, and confessing their perjuries" (transl. in Hett 1936, 317). One assumes that medical intervention would be thought as useless in this case; the only cure is to confess.

47 Translation in Hett 1936, 263.

original source has been lost to us,[48] but there is also a good chance that the point here is one of irony: given that epilepsy is known to be discussed among medical circles as a condition that is falsely assigned with marvelous qualities, it is tempting to assume that the paradoxographer deliberately implicates it in a wondrous story. Paradoxography, in this instance, would turn out to 're-enchant' a condition which medical discourse had previously demystified.[49]

The way paradoxography is crossing paths with medicine is by no means accidental. Unlike its male counterpart, the female body in the Hippocratic Corpus preserves the capacity to generate wonder,[50] especially in connection with its reproductive functions and its imagined internal anatomy: the fact, for instance, that doctors agree on the existence of the so-called 'wandering womb' – the uterus acts as an entity of its own and travels throughout the body seeking moisture, sometimes causing delirium and suffocation[51] – is indicative of their tendency to view the female gender as biologically weird and abnormal, deviating from the norms that define the ideal male body.[52] In [Hipp.] *De natura pueri* 13

---

48 Vanotti 2007, 160 argues that the original source in this case is Theophrastus. See also Sharples 1988, 42.

49 Cf. [Arist.] *Mir. ausc.* 166, about a stone in Nile which is said to cure insanity by "driving off wild spirits". Again, this is a claim that a medical writer would have unequivocally dismissed.

50 For a detailed discussion, see Kazantzidis 2018b, 44–55.

51 For some illuminating discussions, see Manuli 1983, 147–192; Hanson 1990, esp. 319–321 and Dean-Jones 1994, 69–77. Cf. Faraone 2011 (for a comparative reading of the wandering womb in magic and medicine) and Mattern 2015.

52 Cf. Arist. *Gen. an.* 775a14–17: ἀσθενέστερα γάρ ἐστι καὶ ψυχρότερα τὰ θήλεα τὴν φύσιν, καὶ δεῖ ὑπολαμβάνειν ὥσπερ ἀναπηρίαν εἶναι τὴν θηλύτητα φυσικήν, "because females are weaker and colder in their nature; and we should look upon the female state as being as it were a deformity, though one which occurs in the ordinary course of nature" (transl. in Peck 1942, 459–461). The use of the term ἀναπηρία in this context is very pointed: it qualifies the female body as being by constitution a (wondrous?) 'freak of nature'. The notion of deformity leads us straight into the paradoxical realm of monstrosities (*Gen. an.* 769b 31: καὶ γὰρ τὸ τέρας ἀναπηρία τίς ἐστιν). What is more, there are cases where the production of females is explicitly said to resemble that of monsters, considering that, according to Aristotle at least, the process of generation is teleologically ordered towards the production of a male offspring in the likeness of the father: when this fails to happen, nature has 'in some way, departed from the type'; see *Gen. an.* 767b5ff.: καὶ γὰρ ὁ μὴ ἐοικὼς τοῖς γονεῦσιν ἤδη τρόπον τινὰ τέρας ἐστίν. παρεκβέβηκε γὰρ ἡ φύσις ἐν τούτοις ἐκ τοῦ γένους τρόπον τινά. ἀρχὴ δὲ πρώτη τὸ θῆλυ γίγνεσθαι καὶ μὴ ἄρρεν. That females are not in accordance with nature (they are παρά φύσιν) is evident also in *Gen. an.* 728a17–20 and 738b19–22 (the language used in these passages lies rather close to Aristotle's remarks on 'freaks' in *Phys.* II 8 and *Metaph.* 1034a34–b4). See Witt 2012, 86 and Nielsen 2008. On the close association between *pêrôma* and *teras*, see Stavrianeas 2018, 67. And for a general discussion of the female in Aristotle, see Connell 2015.

(7.490 L.) the medical author reports his personal involvement in a peculiar case of abortion:

> ὡς δὲ εἶδον τὴν γονὴν ἑκταίην ἐοῦσαν ἐγὼ διηγήσομαι. Γυναικὸς οἰκείης μουσοεργὸς ἦν πολύτιμος, παρ’ ἄνδρας φοιτέουσα, ἣν οὐκ ἔδει λαβεῖν ἐν γαστρὶ, ὅκως μὴ ἀτιμοτέρη ἔῃ· ἠκηκόει δὲ ἡ μουσοεργὸς, ὁκοῖα αἱ γυναῖκες λέγουσι πρὸς ἀλλήλας· ἐπὴν γυνὴ μέλλῃ λήψεσθαι ἐν γαστρὶ, οὐκ ἐξέρχεται ἡ γονὴ, ἀλλ’ ἔνδον μένει· ταῦτα ἀκούσασα ξυνῆκε καὶ ἐφύλασσεν αἰεὶ, καί κως ᾔσθετο οὐκ ἐξιοῦσαν τὴν γονὴν, καὶ ἔφρασε τῇ δεσποίνῃ, καὶ ὁ λόγος ἦλθεν ἕως ἐμέ· καὶ ἐγὼ ἀκούσας ἐκελευσάμην αὐτὴν πρὸς πυγὴν πηδῆσαι, καὶ ἑπτάκις ἤδη ἐπεπήδητο, καὶ ἡ γονὴ κατεῤῥύη ἐπὶ τὴν γῆν, καὶ ψόφος ἐγένετο, κἀκείνη δὲ ἰδοῦσα ἐθεῆτο <u>καὶ ἐθαύμασεν</u>.
>
> And I will now recount how I came to see the form that a seed has on the sixth day. A female relative of mine once owned a very valuable singing girl who had relations with men but who was not to become pregnant lest she lose her value. The singing girl had heard what women say to one another, that when a woman is about to conceive, the seed does not run out of her, but remains inside. She understood what she heard and always paid attention, and when she one time noticed that the seed did not run out of her, she told her mistress and the case came to me. When I heard what had happened, I told her to jump up and down so as to kick her heels against her buttocks, and when she did this for the seventh time the seed ran out onto the ground with a noise, and then on seeing it gazed at it and was amazed.[53]

Crucially placed at the end of the narrative we find the verb ἐθαύμασεν. It may be argued that the one experiencing *thauma* on this occasion is the female patient, but not the doctor himself. Still, the narrative contains several details which effectively invite the reader to react in the same way as the patient (e.g., the fact that the seed is visible on the sixth day is itself astonishing, all the more so since it is said to produce a distinct noise, *psofos*, when it hits the ground).[54] While

53 Translation in Potter 2012, 35–37 (with slight modifications).

54 Compare the case reported in [Hipp.] *Carn.* 19 (8.608–10 L.). In this case, the medical author claims to have produced the abortion of a seven-day embryo not once but several times; and in each case, he says, the embryo was already fully formed. He claims to have seen, by immersing the embryo in water, the facial features, the limbs including fingers and toes, and the genitals. The Greek text reads as follows: πρῶτον μὲν ἐπὴν ἐς τὰς μήτρας ἔλθῃ ὁ γόνος, ἐν ἑπτὰ ἡμέρῃσιν ἔχει ὁκόσα περ ἐστὶν ἔχειν τοῦ σώματος· <u>τοῦτο δέ τις ἂν θαυμάσειεν ὅκως ἐγὼ οἶδα</u> ... αἱ ἑταῖραι αἱ δημόσιαι, αἵτινες αὐτέων πεπείρηνται πολλάκις, ὁκόταν παρὰ ἄνδρα ἔλθῃ, γινώσκουσιν ὁκόταν λάβωσιν ἐν γαστρί· κἄπειτ’ ἐνδιαφθείρουσιν· ἐπειδὰν δὲ ἤδη διαφθαρῇ, ἐκπίπτει ὥσπερ σάρξ· ταύτην τὴν σάρκα ἐς ὕδωρ ἐμβαλὼν, σκεπτόμενος ἐν τῷ ὕδατι, εὑρήσεις ἔχειν πάντα μέλεα καὶ τῶν ὀφθαλμῶν τὰς χώρας καὶ τὰ οὔατα καὶ τὰ γυῖα. The doctor’s statement, ‘one may wonder how I know this’ (τοῦτο δέ τις ἂν θαυμάσειεν ὅκως ἐγὼ οἶδα), implies that the author is aware that his claim is lacking in realism; nonetheless, he proceeds to substantiate it with what remains in many ways an incredible story. See Lonie 1981, 160; cf. Dean-Jones 1995, 45–46.

commenting on this text in *De semine* 1.4 (4.525 K.), Galen places emphasis on Hippocrates' ability to combine in his writings the virtues of solid scientific observation with a story-telling that induces 'pleasure' (παιδεύσει τε γὰρ ἡμᾶς τῷ τῆς θεωρίας ἀκριβεῖ καὶ τέρψει κεράσας οἵᾳ δὴ λέξει τὴν διήγησιν). For Galen, *terpsis* is mostly connected to non-scientific, literary works. In *De anatomicis administrationibus* 3.9 (2.393 K.), he warns his addressee against reading medical texts 'as if they were Herodotus'; the point, as he says, is not to derive pleasure from them but to stick to the hard facts of science (σὲ δ' οὐχ ὡς Ἡροδότου τὴν ἱστορίαν ἕνεκα τέρψεως ἀναγνῶναι προσήκει, ἀλλὰ τῇ μνήμῃ παραθέσθαι τῶν ὀφθέντων ἕκαστον, ὅπως εἰδῇς ἁπάντων τῶν μερῶν αὐτῆς ἀκριβῶς τὴν φύσιν).[55] And yet, insofar as *De natura pueri* 13 is concerned, Galen does not dismiss its sensational details: in part, this has to do with the fact that Hippocrates, being the best of all physicians, can combine both pleasure and instruction; at the same time, it is also linked to Galen's underlying belief that the female body has the capacity to create stories which, even when reported in the context of a clinical διήγησις, remain intrinsically 'wonderful' by their very nature.

Early paradoxographers invest, time and again, in this 'breach of rationality' already evident in the Hippocratic Corpus with regard to the female body. Conceptually, this is facilitated by the fact that, as a genre, paradoxography has a deep fascination with images of fertility, procreation, and abundance – this is a feminine world, strange precisely because it is inhabited by too many things that mother-nature gives birth to. As Pliny the Elder observes in a passage concerned with human oddities (*HN* 7.32): "Nature has cleverly contrived these and similar species of the human race to amuse herself and to amaze us (*ludibria sibi, nobis miracula ingeniosa fecit natura*). As for the individual creations she produces every day, and almost every hour, who could possibly reckon them up (*quis enumerare valeat*)? Let it be a sufficient revelation of her power to have placed entire races among her miracles".[56]

---

55 *In Hippocratis librum vi Epidemiarum* 3.13, 17B.33 K. On pleasure and the satisfaction of intellectual curiosity in paradoxography, see Vanotti 2007, 22; cf. Jacob/Polignac 2000, 93. Elsewhere, Herodotus is associated by Galen with Ctesias of Cnidus – a seminal figure in early paradoxography; see Tuplin 2004, 345–347 and Nutton 2009, 25.

56 Translation in Beagon 2005, 65–66. The Latin text reads as follows: 'Haec atque talia ex hominum genere ludibria sibi, nobis miracula ingeniosa fecit natura. ex singulis quidem quae facit in dies ac prope horas, quis enumerare valeat? ad detegendam eius potentiam satis sit inter prodigia posuisse gentes'. For the importance of *mirabilia*, and paradoxography in general, in Pliny's encyclopaedia, see Healy 1999, 63–70; Beagon 2005, 17–21; 2011; 2014; Naas 2011.

Individual marvelous stories confirm that in this thriving and, in a number of significant ways, oddly shaped universe, women occupy a special place. A couple of examples will help to illustrate this point. Antigonus of Carystus (3rd cent. BCE), whose book of marvels has been transmitted with the title Ἱστοριῶν παραδόξων συναγωγή, reports at one point the story of the Lemnian women who, after Medea's arrival on their island, became affected with "a dreadful smell so that nobody could approach them": δυσώδεις αὐτὰς οὕτως γίνεσθαι, ὥστε μηδένα προσιέναι (ch.118).[57] Antigonus' account has been read by some as containing allusions to menstruation and its potentially polluting effects.[58] Although menstrual blood is never explicitly discussed by medical writers as a miasma,[59] filth seems to be a peculiar characteristic of the female gender. In a seminal article published in 1992 entitled 'Women and Dirt', Heinrich von Staden was the first to observe that animal excrement occurs in the Hippocratic Corpus as a pharmacological ingredient exclusively in the gynaecological treatises. According to his explanation, the underlying notion of combating female filth with animal filth resonates with the widespread belief across Greek ritual, magic, and religion that women, unlike men, are excessively susceptible to impurity and pollution.[60] Whether it alludes to menstruation or not, the 'dreadful smell' mentioned by Antigonus would thus appear to converge with rather than deviate from the 'scientific norm' insofar as medical discourse sanctions the uncleanness of the female body as one of its constitutional elements.

---

57 The full text reads as follows: τὰς δὲ Λημνίας δυσόσμους γενέσθαι Μηδείας ἀφικομένης μετ' Ἰάσονος καὶ φάρμακα ἐμβαλούσης εἰς τὴν νῆσον· κατὰ δή τινα χρόνον καὶ μάλιστα ἐν ταύταις ταῖς ἡμέραις, ἐν αἷς ἱστοροῦσιν τὴν Μήδειαν παραγενέσθαι, δυσώδεις αὐτὰς οὕτως γίνεσθαι, ὥστε μηδένα προσιέναι. On the links between mythography and paradoxography, see Higbie 2007.

58 See Jackson 1990. Cf. Plin. *HN* 7.63–4: "Woman is the only creature to have monthly periods ... It would be difficult to find anything more bizarre than a woman's menstrual flow. Proximity to it turns new wine sour; crops tainted with it are barren, grafts die, garden seedlings shrivel, fruit falls from the tree on which it is growing, mirrors are clouded by its very reflection, knife blades are blunted, the gleam of ivory dulled, hives of bees die, even bronze and iron are instantly corroded by rust and a dreadful smell contaminates bronze" (transl. in Beagon 2005, 72–73).

59 Still, the menstrual flux brings out the 'bestial', as it were, nature of woman; see [Hipp.] *De mulierum affectibus* 1.6 (8.30 L.): "if a woman is healthy, then during menstruation the blood flows like that of a sacrificed victim and it clots quickly", χωρέει δὲ αἷμα οἷον ἀπὸ ἱερείου, καὶ ταχὺ πήγνυται, ἢν ὑγιαίνῃ ἡ γυνή. Aristotle agrees that a young girl's menstrual blood is οἷον νεόσφακτον, "like that of a freshly-slaughtered beast" (*Hist. an.* 581b1–2).

60 von Staden 1992b. See also von Staden 2008 and, for a different interpretation of the 'filthy medicaments' prescribed for women, Hanson 1998.

In another instance, found in [Arist.] *Mir. ausc.* 174, women are reported to interact with their external environment in strange ways:

> ἐν ὄρει δὲ Τμώλῳ γεννᾶσθαι λίθον παρόμοιον κισσήρει, ὃς τετράκις τῆς ἡμέρας ἀλλάσσει τὴν χρόαν· βλέπεσθαι δὲ ὑπὸ παρθένων τῶν μὴ τῷ χρόνῳ φρονήσεως μετεχουσῶν.
>
> On Mount Tmolus they say that there is a stone like ivy which changes its colour four times a day; it is seen by girls who have not yet reached the age of discretion.[61]

What is especially intriguing about this account is the specification that this odd phenomenon is witnessed (apparently only) by virgins[62] who have not yet reached the age of *phronēsis*. The transition from virginity to womanhood is described by Hippocratic doctors as a critical stage in a female's life. As we read at [Hipp.] *De virginum morbis* (8.466–71 L.),[63] if protracted for a long period of time – that is, if it extends beyond the point that the girl should have got married – virginity can have extremely detrimental effects on health: being trapped inside the body, menstrual blood moves upwards and collects itself around the heart,[64] thus affecting the seat of reasoning and intelligence (ὥστε παραφρονέειν): as a result, the virgin experiences intense mental agony, 'apoplexies', sudden seizures and – for what concerns us here – unnatural visions.[65] What lies at the basis of [Arist.] *Mir. ausc.* 174 could thus be approached as deriving its origin from a 'medical fact', namely that virginity, being a stressful period in a woman's life, makes one see (or, more precisely, makes one think that she sees) 'strange' things.[66] At the

---

61 Translation in Hett 1936, 323.

62 For the meaning of *parthenos*, 'young girl'/'virgin', see King 1998, 75–80.

63 The Greek title is Περὶ παρθενίων.

64 The medical author could be referring to a virginal hymen which has not yet been ruptured through intercourse and therefore does not let the blood flow out of the body; see Hanson 1990, 324–330. But since we have no concrete evidence in Hippocratic gynaecology to suggest the existence of an imperforate membrane in the vagina (Sissa 1990; 2013), the passage is generally interpreted as referring to the constricted nature of the female body and the narrowness of a young girl's veins: on this interpretation, first intercourse should not be imagined as removing some sort of closing device but extending a pre-existing, yet protected, fissure.

65 More specifically, unnatural visions take the form of dreadful hallucinations: ὥστε παραφρονέειν καὶ ὁρῆν δοκέειν δαίμονας τινας ἐφ' ἑωυτῶν δυσμενέας, ὁκότε μὲν νυκτὸς, ὁκότε δὲ ἡμέρης, ὁκότε δὲ ἀμφοτέρησι τῇσιν ὥρῃσι.

66 The phrase τῶν μὴ τῷ χρόνῳ φρονήσεως μετεχουσῶν could be suggestive of some sort of mental instability. For the Hippocratic vocabulary of insanity, and specifically for terms which indicate a suspension/malfunction of *phronesis* (*aphron*, *paraphronesis*, *upokataphroneo*, *allophroneo*, *aphrosune* etc.), see Thumiger 2013, 61.

same time, the mention of the stone which changes its color brings to mind a passage from Aristotle's *De somniis* 459b–460a, which tells us that when a menstruating woman looks at herself in a bronze mirror, the object's surface becomes stained with blood. Significantly, Aristotle speaks of the menstrual flux as a 'disturbance' and 'bloody inflammation' (διὸ γινομένων τῶν καταμηνίων διὰ ταραχὴν καὶ φλεγμασίαν αἱματικὴν, 460a6–7), using language similar to that of the Hippocratic text when it refers to the trapped menses in the virgin's body (ὑπὸ μὲν τῆς ὀξυφλεγμασίης μαίνεται). In line with the medical author, Aristotle implies that menstrual blood has the power to deform vision and perception more generally.[67] In light of this evidence, it might be argued that the color-changing stones on Mount Tmolus do not really exist except in the affected imagination of young girls. The paradox in this case is explained away – or, rather, by way of a transference, it is substituted by the female body's marvelous capacity to (re)shape the external environment in accordance with what is taking place inside it.

As we move from the Hippocratic Corpus to Hellenistic medicine, anatomy takes over. The fact that Hellenistic physicians can have direct access to the inner life of the human body, either through dissection or vivisection,[68] naturally entails that the space for fanciful assumptions as to what is taking place beneath the skin and the flesh of the body is substantially reduced.[69] Surprisingly, however, what we witness is a new, crucial shift in the dialogue between medicine and paradoxography. As Rebecca Flemming has argued, the groundbreaking anatomical discoveries of Herophilus and Erasistratus appear generally to have had little effect "on the understanding of how the body worked, fell ill and was cured"; "the practical ramifications", for instance, of identifying the nerves as distinct entities, separate from the arteries and veins, "are hard to detect", and, though the body's interior is mapped in unprecedented ways, there seems to be limited "therapeutic response to the new conceptualization".[70] More to the point, there is no evidence to show that either dissection or vivisection – the hallmark of Alexandrian medicine – continued after the lifetimes of Herophilus and Erasistratus. The reason why this happens may have been due to the fact that the

---

67 Is the mirror actually stained with blood or is this just what the menstruating woman thinks she is seeing? See Cole 2004, 109 discussing Hippocratic texts in which doctors 'claimed to be able to predict a heavy menstrual flow by detecting a mist hovering before a woman's eyes'. On Aristotle's remarkable passage, see Sprague 1985; Mayhew 2004, 89–91; Berthold 2016.

68 See von Staden 1992a.

69 See Flemming 2003, 451 on "the rather loosely conceived, and imaginative, approach to the human interior which characterizes the writings of the Hippocratic Corpus". Cf. Holmes 2018.

70 Flemming 2003, 451–452.

main drive behind these anatomical discoveries was to 'colonize' the human body with knowledge that had been previously inaccessible. In Flemming's words:

> Conquest is not something that needs to be repeated. It is, by definition, a one-off occurrence, though often the platform for further developments. Once the knowledge of the body has been won – the territory mapped and named – then that is the end of it.[71]

Situating Hellenistic medicine within a broader imperialist agenda of 'mapping' and 'discovering' helps to bring out the existing links with paradoxography, a genre which is principally concerned with collecting a body of 'strange' knowledge that becomes available from previously uncharted – and now conquered – territories of the external world.[72] "This expansion in occult knowledge about nature", as Flemming points out, "is often seen as being in contrast with, if not in opposition to the more rationalistic medical developments" that take place in early Alexandria:

> Indeed it is possible that an overwhelming rationalism will inevitably produce its opposite ... Overall, however, these contrasts seem too sharply drawn, the picture constructed seems too simple given the many factors involved ... Certainly the development of bodies of occult knowledge about nature can be seen as the extension of methods of organization, of systematization, established in more 'rational' areas of natural knowledge, rather than their contradiction.[73]

The discursive continuity between medicine and paradoxography does not mean, of course, that we should assume an unproblematic relationship between the two. The Herophilean Andreas (c. 244–205 BCE), one of the most renowned pharmacologists during the early Hellenistic period, is known to have written an entire treatise, entitled 'On False Beliefs' (Περὶ τῶν ψευδῶς πεπιστευμένων), which was directed – among other things – against folk medicine as this could be found forming the substrate of various marvels recorded by paradoxographers.[74] But in

71 Flemming 2003, 455.

72 The standard account of 'wonder' as a dominant trope in ethnographic, imperialist discourse is Greenblatt 1991. On the ideological implications of paradoxography and its crucial place in discourse of the empire's expanding horizons, see especially Naas 2002, ch. 5; 2011 and Murphy 2004 (with a focus on the presence and function of *mirabilia* in Pliny the Elder's *Natural History*).

73 Flemming 2003, 460.

74 See von Staden 1989, 473; 1999, 157–158. 'Popular medicine', and 'folk medicine', as Harris 2016, 2–3 observes, "are problematic categories, especially in societies such as those of the classical Greeks and Romans in which there were professional healers but no 'professions' in a mod-

other instances, the two domains appear to interact with each other in more productive ways. As Floris Overduin's chapter in this volume aptly illustrates ('In the Realm of the Two-Headed Snake: Pragmatics and Aesthetics of *Mirabilia* in Nicander's *Theriaca* and *Alexipharmaka*') medical knowledge, accurate observation and diagnosis, and a fascination with the paradox coexist side by side in Nicander's poetry, in a pure Hellenistic vein. Before Nicander, a characteristic example is provided by Bolus of Mendes,[75] a shadowy figure writing under the pseudonym 'Democritus' and working at the crossroads of natural philosophy, paradoxography, and learned magic. Bolus appears to have been mainly preoccupied with identifying the vital powers or properties (*dunameis*) naturally inherent in things as well as with unveiling the marvelous web through which everything in the world was linked through networks of sympathy or antipathy. Scholars have noted how the concept of *dunamis*, interpreted as the vital energy of various bodily organs or of the body itself, is also extremely significant in Herophilus' work;[76] further to the point, the idea of disease arising from 'sympathetic' connections through various body parts is common in medical lore[77] (in the ps.-Aristotelian *Problems* 886a25–887b7, a chapter headed εκ συμπαθείας mentions as an instance of 'sympathy' the passing of diseases from one to another). By virtue of his attraction to the 'weird' aspects of nature, Bolus may even have contributed to the exploration of specific medical conditions that appeared more bizzare than others: for instance, he is credited with one of the earliest discussions of 'hydrophobia', a strange disease during which patients were simultaneously tortured by thirst and, as the name indicates, by dread of water.[78] The condition appears to have also attracted the attention of the Hellenistic physician Andreas[79] whom later sources present as a doctor with a special interest for extreme paranoias of

ern sense... 'Popular medicine' is however an indispensable category if we are going to understand the way in which healthcare really worked in antiquity. This for the obvious reason that when people had to deal with physical ailments or wanted to ward them off, they very frequently turned to the gods and their representatives, or to healers whose 'knowledge' and techniques, handed down to a large extent by word of mouth, were mostly – though with many exceptions – rejected or marginalized by the elite/learned/rationalistic doctors".

75 Active during the first half of the second century BCE; see Dickie 2001, 113–114; Gaillard-Seux 2010.

76 For the connection between Herophilus and Bolus, see Flemming 2003, 460; cf. von Staden 2000, 89.

77 See Struck 2016, 182–184; cf. Holmes 2013.

78 See von Staden 1989, 568 n.14; and, on hydrophobia, see Thumiger 2018, 263–266.

79 See von Staden 1989, 568 n.14.

that sort. Caelius Aurelianus (*On Acute Diseases* 3.108) links his name with a condition labelled 'pantophobia': the content and details of Andreas' discussion of this particular disease remain entirely subject to speculation; in sum, however, it looks as if mental illness and its strange manifestations presented a common point of interest for physicians and paradoxographers alike – presumably more so when compared to less intriguing, as it were, conditions of the body. As we can easily imagine, being paranoid about water and avoiding it for no apparent reason would have been perceived by external observers as being far more perplexing – and, potentially, wondrous – than getting a simple cold or having a cough.[80]

The emphasis on anatomy in Hellenistic medicine and the increasing conceptualisation of bodily organs and their functions in direct analogy to artificial devices discussed in the contemporary fields of mechanics and pneumatics[81] opens up the space for *thauma* during this period in yet another, crucial way. The beauty of the human body in ancient Greek thought and the aesthetic pleasure one derives from it are primarily matters of its exterior appearance; when it comes to its interior, the body yields instead a messy picture consisting of fluids and organs that can occasionally elicit strong emotions of repulsion and disgust. As Aristotle points out in *De partibus animalium* 645a29–30, "it is not possible to look upon the blood, flesh, bones, blood-vessels, and suchlike parts of which the human body is constructed without considerable disgust" (ἄνευ πολλῆς δυσχερείας).[82] For Aristotle, it is only when we understand how even the tiniest and humblest part in the body serves a specific purpose that we can overcome our feelings of repugnance: once we grasp, for instance, the reason why the liver is there, we are no more concerned with how it 'looks' and we end up being amazed by its function and its smooth interaction with other bodily organs. The realization that seemingly 'ugly things' do not stand in isolation, but occupy a place in a larger, patterned system suffices to make us find beauty in them.[83]

Although teleology and mechanics should by no means be confused with each other (many, in fact, see them as being mutually exclusive), recent research

---

80 For the intricate links between insanity and paradoxography, see Kazantzidis 2018a.

81 A much-cited example concerns the structural and functional parallels between the heart, as discussed by Erasistratus, and the water pump designed by Ctesibius (fl. 285–222 BCE): both thinkers rely on the theory that continuous void does not exist, but interstitial void does. Von Staden 1996, 91–95 speaks of a 'cross-fertilization' between the two domains; see also von Staden 1998; Webster 2014, 71–92. Cf. Schiefsky 2007; Rihl 2018.

82 Translation in Peck and Forster 1937, 101.

83 *Part. an.* 645a25–7: Τὸ γὰρ μὴ τυχόντως ἀλλ' ἕνεκά τινος ἐν τοῖς τῆς φύσεως ἔργοις ἐστὶ καὶ μάλιστα· οὗ δ' ἕνεκα συνέστηκεν ἢ γέγονε τέλους, τὴν τοῦ καλοῦ χώραν εἴληφεν. See Kazantzidis 2017, 55.

has shown that the two models are not as incompatible as they appear at first sight. Aristotle, for example, explains respiration in different parts of his work either by invoking a teleological model of natural necessity (*Part. an.* 642a31–b4) or by analogy with the 'bellows in a smithy' (*Resp.* 21), and there is no pressing reason to doubt that the two modes of thinking can be combined.[84] What is more, the 'mechanical hypothesis',[85] when applied to the human body, helps Hellenistic physicians to appreciate it aesthetically – just as for Aristotle teleology works towards unveiling the human interior's innate beauty. *Thauma* plays a crucial role in this process. The ps.-Aristotelian *Mechanical Problems*, considered to be the earliest surviving Greek text on mechanics and dated by some to the early third century BCE,[86] opens with a statement which brings into contrast two different kinds of 'remarkable' things in the world, those which are produced naturally and those which are produced artificially (*Mech.* 847a11–13):

> Θαυμάζεται τῶν μὲν κατὰ φύσιν συμβαινόντων, ὅσων ἀγνοεῖται τὸ αἴτιον, τῶν δὲ παρὰ φύσιν, ὅσα γίνεται διὰ τέχνην πρὸς τὸ συμφέρον τοῖς ἀνθρώποις.

> Remarkable things occur in accordance with nature, the cause of which is unknown, and others occur contrary to nature, which are produced by skill for the benefit of mankind.[87]

Paradoxical as it may sound, it is precisely when the interior of the human body is assimilated to the 'non-natural' beauty of artificial mechanisms that medical scientists, during the Hellenistic period, discover its aesthetic potential; as a parallel to this concept one may think of Herodotus' language of marvel, which is often applied to the human body after the latter has been 'technologically' improved by means of medicine, regulated diet, and artificial enhancements – this is the main argument of **Maria Gerolemou**'s chapter in this volume, 'Technological Wonder in Herodotus' *Histories*'. As Gerolemou observes, "while on the face of it several 'marvels' in Herodotus are presented as natural, they turn out in the course of the narrative to be the product of an artificial intervention grounded in *techne*". To mention one example from Hellenistic medicine, Erasistratus is reported by Galen (*On Venesection against Erasistratus* 4, 11.158 K.) as 'marveling' (*thaumazein*) at nature "for being at once capable of expert craftmanship and of

84 See Johnson 2017, 132–133; cf. von Staden 1997.
85 The standard account of the 'mechanic hypothesis' in ancient Greek thought is Berryman 2009.
86 See Berryman 2009, 55 and 106; cf. Bodnár 2011.
87 Translation in Hett 1936, 331.

forethought for living beings": while the metaphorical language of craftsmanship, *technikê*, has obvious philosophical connotations (ranging from Plato and Aristotle to the Stoics),[88] it can also be an allusion to contemporary material culture and, more specifically, to the actual possibility of viewing bodily organs as operating in ways similar to artificial devices of remarkably complex and astonishing designs. On this reading, the machine, in combination with anatomy which lays bare previously unseen parts of the body, allows doctors to 'marvel' at human *phusis* in an unprecedented, analogical fashion.

But what kind of marvel would that be and, more crucially, how can it be connected with paradoxography's elusive world? One possible objection is that the marvelous capacities of the human body in Hellenistic medicine are brought out in an epistemic context which relies on a thorough and exhaustive understanding of the human organism; this is a body that holds no secrets, its functions and causes have been fully accounted for, and therefore it can only be an object of *thaumazein* in the sense of admiration, without implicating, that is, feelings of perplexed wonder. Still, wonder persists in at least two significant ways: on the one hand, as Richard Dawkins has argued, scientific reductionism is not by itself enough to eliminate our feelings of astonishment in our encounters with nature; on the contrary, the 'poetry of science' – to use Dawkins' term – opens up new ways of looking at things and leads to new discoveries and understandings which enhance the 'stunning' element of the world that surrounds us.[89] On the other hand, though explained in mechanical and purely rational terms, the body in Hellenistic medicine is simultaneously remystified since it is revealed to occupy a liminal, hybrid space, combining the attributes of both biological entity and machine in the same conceptual continuum. Whether we are dealing with evidence attesting to the new conceptualization of the body as a technological artifact or we take into account sources about complex surgical devices designed by Hellenistic physicians to operate automatically and with 'a life of their own',[90] the case remains that medicine in this period is deeply embedded in a culture of wonder – a wonder that results from the body's fluid nature and its paradoxical alignment and interaction with the realm of machines. At the same time, it is worth

88 See von Staden 2007, 38–39. Cf. the seminal discussion by Solmsen 1963.

89 Dawkins 1998; cf. Porter 2007, 168 (on the 'defamiliarising' function of ancient atomism and of philosophical explanation in general): "Indeed, atomism seems practically designed to elicit feelings of sublimity, of fear and awe, again with the aim of realigning in a radical way one's view of oneself and the world, well beyond the mere replacement of mythological and theological awe with secular or scientific awe".

90 For the use of such devices in Hellenistic medicine, in performative contexts which aimed at producing *thauma*, see Berrey 2017, 182–188.

considering that though developed according to strict scientific principles and mathematical rules, the machine involves a considerable degree of trickery. At the opening of his treatise, the author of the ps.-Aristotelian *Mechanical Problems* places particular emphasis on practical skill, *technê*, and how it can help people gain control over things which nature has created to be bigger and stronger than humans: for instance, using a small mechanical device that possesses little weight to move successfully heavy weights is essentially a way of "making the lesser master the greater".[91] As Jean-Pierre Vernant has argued, the idea recalls the sophistic knack for 'making the worse argument seem the better'; significantly, according to the author, it also shows that wonder is at play:

> Wherever the machines described by the engineers have a utilitarian purpose, they are used and conceived of as instruments for multiplying human strength, on which – despite their complexity – they depend for their only motive principle. When they call upon other sources of energy and, instead of amplifying a force given at the outset act as automata producing their own movement, they turn out to be constructions that follow a whole tradition concerned with objects to be marveled at, and, as such, they are marginally relevant to technology in the strict sense. They are *thaumata* made to astonish people. Their value and interest lie not so much in their usefulness as in the admiration and pleasure they arouse in the spectator.[92]

Later evidence from Hero of Alexandria (1st cent. CE) confirms that 'wonder-making' is essential in the construction of mechanical devices.[93] As we read in *Pneumatics* 2.18–20: "For through the combination of air, fire, water, and earth and combining three or four principles, varied (*poikilai*) arrangements can be actualized; these on the one hand provide the most necessary needs (*anankaiotatai chreiai*) of this life and, on the other, display some stunning wonder (*ekplêktikos thaumasmos*)".[94] All in all, though relying on firm scientific principles, machines

91 [Arist.] *Mech.* 847a18–24: διὸ καὶ καλοῦμεν τῆς τέχνης τὸ πρὸς τὰς τοιαύτας ἀπορίας βοηθοῦν μέρος μηχανήν. καθάπερ γὰρ ἐποίησεν Ἀντιφῶν ὁ ποιητής, οὕτω καὶ ἔχει· τέχνῃ γὰρ κρατοῦμεν, ὧν φύσει νικώμεθα. τοιαῦτα δέ ἐστιν ἐν οἷς τά τε ἐλάττονα κρατεῖ τῶν μειζόνων, καὶ τὰ ῥοπὴν ἔχοντα μικρὰν κινεῖ βάρη μεγάλα, καὶ πάντα σχεδὸν ὅσα τῶν προβλημάτων μηχανικὰ προσαγορεύομεν.

92 Vernant 2006, 304. See also the discussion in Berryman 2009, 50–53, with Close 1969. Cf. Asper 2017, 43: sometimes, extremely complicated machines had no practical use; they were merely intended to be presented as marvels in the Ptolemaic court.

93 See the discussion in Tybjerg 2003.

94 Translation in Tybjerg 2003, 447. On the association of marvel and *ekplêxis*, indicating a violent state of shock and terror, see Porter 2016, 227.

do not cease to baffle the audience, especially in the performative context of Hellenistic mechanics and medicine.[95] In light of this evidence, it is tempting to conclude that the assimilation of a bodily organ to an artificial device with 'wonderful' aspects, would have had a double effect: while it certainly helped to elucidate the function of the body by means of the analogy, at the same time it ended up associating it with complex objects that would have looked, without a doubt, odd and confusing: rather than eliminate the paradox, this association seems rather to enhance the body's mystifying aspects.

As we move from the Hellenistic period to the Imperial age, and to the writings of Phlegon of Tralles, Galen, and Aelius Aristides, paradoxography and medicine merge in unprecedented ways. The increased dialogue between the two domains is in part owing to the fact that the human body (which is relatively absent from the early instances of the genre)[96] occupies a more central place as a *source* of wonder in later paradoxographical collections.[97] In one of the stories reported by Phlegon of Tralles (2nd cent. CE), a young girl is taken ill with excruciating pains just before her wedding (*Mirabilia* 6.2–4):

> παρθένος γὰρ γονέων ἐπισήμων τρισκαιδεκαέτις ὑπάρχουσα ὑπὸ πολλῶν ἐμνηστεύετο, οὖσα εὐπρεπής. ὡς δ' ἐνεγυήθη ᾧ οἱ γονεῖς ἐβούλοντο, ἐνστάσης τῆς ἡμέρας τοῦ γάμου προϊέναι τοῦ οἴκου μέλλουσα αἰφνιδίως πόνου ἐμπεσόντος αὐτῇ σφοδροτάτου ἐξεβόησεν. ἀναλαβόντες δ' αὐτὴν οἱ προσήκοντες ἐθεράπευον ὡς ἀλγήματα ἔχουσαν κοιλίας καὶ στρόφους τῶν ἐντός· τῆς δὲ ἀλγηδόνος ἐπιμενούσης τρισὶν ἡμέραις ἑξῆς ἀπορίαν τε πᾶσι τοῦ πάθους ποιοῦντος, τῶν πόνων οὔτε νυκτὸς οὔτε ἡμέρας ἔνδοσιν λαμβανόντων, <u>καίτοι πᾶσαν μὲν θεραπείαν αὐτῇ προσφερόντων ἐν τῇ πόλει ἰατρῶν, μηδεμίαν δὲ τοῦ πάθους δυναμένων αἰτίαν εὑρεῖν</u>, τῇ τετάρτῃ τῶν ἡμερῶν περὶ τὸν ὄρθρον μείζονα τῶν πόνων ἐπίδοσιν λαμβανόντων, σὺν μεγάλῃ οἰμωγῇ ἀνακραγούσης, ἄφνω αὐτῇ <u>ἀρσενικὰ μόρια προέπεσεν</u>, καὶ ἡ κόρη ἀνὴρ ἐγένετο.

> A maiden from prominent family, thirteen years of age, was good-looking and had many suitors. She was betrothed to the man whom her parents wished, the day of the wedding was at hand, and she was about to go forth from her house when suddenly she experienced an excruciating pain and cried out. Her relations took charge of her, treating her for stomach pains and colic, but her suffering continued for three days without a break, perplexing everyone about the nature of her illness. Her pains let up neither during the night nor during the day, and although the doctors in the city tried every kind of treatment they were unable to discover the cause of her illness. At around daybreak of the fourth day her pains

95 See Berrey 2017.
96 See Kazantzidis 2018b.
97 On Phlegon's almost exclusive interest in human oddities, see Doroszewska in this volume. For a systematic treatment of Phlegon's paradoxography and the place occupied by humans in his strange world, see Doroszewska 2016.

> became stronger, and she cried out with a great wailing. Suddenly male genitals burst forth from her, and the girl became a man.[98]

The story follows in the tradition which presents the female body as a matrix of wonders.[99] While its details and eventual outcome sound incredible (in fact, the girl's 'pathology' is explicitly said to leave the doctors, *iatroi*, who visit her in a state of confusion), closer investigation of medical sources reveals that spontaneous sex-changes of this kind would have been accepted by contemporary physicians as feasible. In *De usu partium* 14 (4.164–5 K.), Galen explains in detail that the female genitalia are morphologically identical to the male ones, the only difference being that, due to lack of heat, they stay inside her body in a state of inverse position, instead of 'popping out' – as happens with men (cf. Phlegon's ἀρσενικὰ μόρια προέπεσεν).[100] The notion derives originally from classical sources. In [Arist.] *Hist. an.* 637a23–25[101] we even read that women posses something like a penis: "The path along which the semen passes in women is of the following nature: they [women] possess a tube (*kaulos*) – like the penis of the male, but inside the body – and they breathe through this by a small duct which is placed above the place through which women urinate. This is why, when they are eager to make love, this place is not in the same state as it was before they were excited".[102] It is indeed highly plausible that Phlegon is toying with these medical and biological theories: to an informed audience the story of the sex-changing maiden would appear to rely on medical lore and, more precisely, to allude to a woman's 'hidden' male nature. Gender, it should be remembered, is not always a fixed category in ancient Greek medicine; rather, in many cases it seems to be defined according to a scale of heat and cold, dryness and moisture, across which the human body slides and acquires different attributes depending

98 Translation in Hansen 1996, 38–39.

99 For sex-changes in Phlegon, see Doroszewska 2013; cf. Brisson 2002.

100 Roughly speaking, for Galen the cervix and vagina correspond to the penis, the uterus to the scrotum, the ovaries to the testes. See Hanson 1991, 103 n.54, who discusses how "male sexual apparatus ... offered medical writers a model from which to deduce ... a vocabulary with which to name female organs". Long before Galen, we can spot this tendency already in Hellenistic medicine; for instance, Herophilus calls the woman's ovaries 'testicles' (see Galen, *De sem.* 2.1, 4.596–7 K.). See also Soranus, *Gyn.* 1.16: "The inner part of the vagina grows around the neck of the uterus like the prepuce in males around the glans ... [T]he neck of the uterus, elongating like the male genital, occupies a certain part of the vagina"; translation in Temkin 1956, 14–15.

101 The passage comes from the spurious book 10 of the treatise.

102 Transl. in Laqueur 1990, 33, who discusses this passage in detail at pp.33–35.

on its temperature, age and the dynamics of liquids which define it from the inside.[103] Thus, in the case of Phaethousa, the female patient in [Hipp.] *Epid.* 6.8.32 (5.356 L.), we read that after she stopped menstruating, "her body was masculinized and grew hairy all over; she grew a beard and her voice became harsh (τό τε σῶμα ἠνδρώθη καὶ ἐδασύνθη πάντα, καὶ πώγωνα ἔφυσε, καὶ φωνὴ τρηχέη ἐγενήθη)". "The same thing", as the report continues, "happened to Nanno, Gorgippos' wife, in Thasos".[104] The fact that 'sexual transformations' have a long history in Greek science makes us think twice of Phlegon's 'paradox'. What at first sight appears to be an incredible story may be explained by the peculiatiries of the female body; that these peculiarities are systematically discussed, and endorsed, by medical authors additionally suggests that what underlies a world of marvels can occasionally transpire to be a world of reason and science. This is the main argument of **Julia Doroszewska's** contribution to this volume ('Beyond the Limits of the Human Body: Phlegon of Tralles' Medical Curiosities'). As she concludes, however marvelous they may sound and look, the vast majority of the human oddities reported by Phlegon are "potentially explicable on the grounds of contemporary medicine". Furthermore, they corroborate the hierarchies and polarities established in the 'rational' realms of philosophy and science: with the exception of Tiresias, as Doroszewska notes, all cases of sex-change reported by Phlegon involve a metamorphosis from female to male. Behind this, one may detect an allusion to the female gender's inferiority, common in Aristotle and Galen:[105] "the female gives way to the male, just as the imperfect, when bettered, leads to perfection. This in turn allows us to appreciate the sex-changing marvels ... not as random tricks of nature, but as cultural phenomena, endowed with a profound (if disturbing to modern sensibilities) teleological sense". One case that is worthy of attention is Phlegon's discussion of a centaur at *Mir.* 34–5. **Kelly Shannon-Henderson**, in her chapter entitled 'Phlegon's Paradoxical Physiology: Centaurs in the *Peri Thaumasion*', provides a review of the ancient evidence (especially Galen), which objects to the hybrid creature's existence. As the author argues, a close reading of Phlegon's account in this case shows that the paradoxographer is aware of and reacts to pre-existing medical-scientific discussions which dismiss centaurs as a mere fantasy. In her words, "this reveals Phlegon to be aiming at an educated readership whose recognition of the medical-scientific background to the creature he describes will deepen their appreciation of the *thauma* it represents".

103 See Holmes 2012.
104 Translation in Smith 1994, 275.
105 See Flemming 2000, 306.

Galen, in his turn, is by no means dismissive of *thauma*. Unlike what we find in the Hippocratic Corpus, he insists, time and again, in pointing out that the human body (especially the facts revealed about it through dissection) works in 'wonderful' ways; at certain points, he even compares the study of the human body to being initiated into the Eleusinian or Samothracian mysteries, whereas often he remarks how certain functions and parts of the body have to be seen first, before one believes in them.[106] Here is what Galen has to say on the resemblance between water circulation in gardens and the circulation of blood through conduits in the body (*De naturalibus facultatibus* 3.15, 2.210–11 K.):

> ἐκ τούτων γὰρ [sc. τῶν ἐν τοῖς κήποις ὀχετῶν] εἰς μὲν τὰ παρακείμενα καὶ πλησίον ἅπαντα διαδίδοταί τις ἰκμάς, εἰς δὲ τὰ πορρωτέρω προσελθεῖν οὐκέτι δύναται καὶ διὰ τοῦτ' ἀναγκάζονται πολλοῖς ὀχετοῖς μικροῖς ἀπὸ τοῦ μεγάλου τετμημένοις εἰς ἕκαστον μέρος τοῦ κήπου τὴν ἐπίρρυσιν τοῦ ὕδατος ἐπιτεχνᾶσθαι· καὶ τηλικαῦτά γε τὰ μεταξὺ διαστήματα τούτων τῶν μικρῶν ὀχετῶν ποιοῦσιν, ἡλίκα μάλιστα νομίζουσιν ἀρκεῖν εἰς τὸ ἱκανῶς ἀπολαύειν ἕλκοντα τῆς ἑκατέρωθεν αὐτοῖς ἐπιρρεούσης ὑγρότητος. οὕτως οὖν ἔχει κἀν τοῖς τῶν ζῴων σώμασιν. ὀχετοὶ πολλοὶ κατὰ πάντα τὰ μέλη διεσπαρμένοι παράγουσιν αὐτοῖς αἷμα καθάπερ ἐν κήποις ὑδρείαν τινά. καὶ τούτων τῶν ὀχετῶν τὰ μεταξὺ διαστήματα θαυμαστῶς ὑπὸ τῆς φύσεως εὐθὺς ἐξ ἀρχῆς διατέτακται πρὸς τὸ μήτ' ἐνδεῶς χορηγεῖσθαι τοῖς μεταξὺ μορίοις ἕλκουσιν εἰς ἑαυτὰ τὸ αἷμα μήτε κατακλύζεσθαί ποτ' αὐτὰ πλήθει περιττῆς ὑγρότητος ἀκαίρως ἐπιρρεούσης.

> For a certain amount of moisture is distributed from the garden conduits into every part lying close at hand but it cannot reach those lying further off: therefore one has to arrange the flow of water into all parts of the garden by cutting a number of small channels leading from the large one. The intervening spaces between these small channels are made of such a size as will, presumably, best allow them [the spaces] to satisfy their needs by drawing from the liquid which flows to them from every side. So also is it in the bodies of animals. Numerous conduits distributed through the various limbs bring them pure blood, much like the garden water-supply, and, further, the intervals between these conduits have been wonderfully arranged by Nature from the outset so that the intervening parts should be plentifully provided for when absorbing blood, and that they should never be deluged by a quantity of superfluous fluid running in at unsuitable times.[107]

Just like in the passage above, the language of wonder, *thaumasion/ thaumaston*, is for its most part embraced by Galen in contexts which maintain that every part of the body has been manufactured by nature (or the divine 'Demiurge')[108] so as

106 See Tieleman 2013, 104–105 with the passages cited at n.10. Cf. Grant 1952, 13.

107 Translation in Brock 1916, 325–327.

108 Nature for Galen is often just another word to speak of the divine 'demiurge' who is responsible for the world's design; see Kovačić 2001, 210–247. On Galen's 'divine craftsman', see Flemming 2009; and on his religious feelings, see Pietrobelli 2017.

to serve a specific purpose in the best possible way.[109] Conceptually, this leads us back to the teleologies of both Plato and Aristotle.[110] Thus, while Aristotle (*Metaph.* 983a12–21), as we have seen, considers *thauma* a cognitive and affective state which betrays one's lack of knowledge, on other occasions he endorses it as a positive concept: the word can also designate a kind of 'admiration' that only those who have contemplated and have come to understand the true nature of the world are able to enjoy. This is precisely what lies behind Aristotle's statement in *De partibus animalium* 645a17, that "in all natural things, there is something wonderful" (θαυμαστόν).[111] To appreciate the 'wonder' in this case, one first has to grasp how every tiny part in the body serves a purpose and is there for a reason: in other words, ascribing a function and a meaning to it suffices to qualify it as 'beautiful' (*Part. an.* 645a25–27: Τὸ γὰρ μὴ τυχόντως ἀλλ' ἕνεκά τινος ἐν τοῖς τῆς φύσεως ἔργοις ἐστὶ καὶ μάλιστα· οὗ δ' ἕνεκα συνέστηκεν ἢ γέγονε τέλους, τὴν τοῦ καλοῦ χώραν εἴληφεν, "in the works of nature purpose and not accident is predominant; and the purpose or end for the sake of which those works have been constructed or formed has its place among the beautiful").[112] Galen's 'wonderful' human body should be placed in this intellectual tradition: *thauma* is used by the physician to indicate his firm understanding of the human organism and, more broadly, of the divinely inspired, beautiful order of things – rather than any kind of perplexed amazement – and to maintain an aesthetic relationship with what would have otherwise remained a mere object of clinical inquiry. As **Michiel Meeusen** argues in his contribution to the volume ('Unknowable Questions and Paradoxography in ps.-Alexander of Aphrodisias' *Medical Puzzles and Natural Problems*'), in contrast with Galen, who "repeatedly claims to admire the wonderful organization of the human body and the artful way in which the Demiurge arranged it", ps.-Alexander of Aphrodisias refrains from exploring what he calls "the ἀπόρρητα of nature. By emphatically excluding paradoxical phenomena from his research on the basis that they produce unknowable questions known only to the prime cosmic τεχνίτης, ps.-Alexander seems to place himself more in

---

109 See the discussion in Hankinson 1989. The language of *thauma* is especially prominent in Galen's *De usu partium*. See e.g. 3.134K, 3.225K, 3.252K, 3.254K, 3.288K, 3.335K, 3.426K, 3.508K, 3.530K, 3.545K, 3.566K, 3.589K, 3.601K, 3.792K, 3.883K, 3.884K, 3.885, 3.939K, 4.5K, 4.15K, 4.58K, 4.61K, 4.197K, 4.243K.

110 Galen's teleology has been linked to both Plato (especially the *Timaeus*) and Aristotle; see Chiaradonna 2009 and van der Eijk 2009 respectively.

111 Even in the study of the lowest, most inconspicuous and initially repulsive animal; see Tipton 2014, 68–69.

112 Translation in Peck/Forster 1937, 101.

the camp of irrational marvel writers (like Aelian), who assume that there are certain things in the world that cannot be fully accounted for, than in that of the rational admirers of divine providence in nature (like Galen)".

But this is not the whole picture. Often, the language of 'marvel' and 'astonishment' occurs in the context of Galen's public anatomical demonstrations: conducting an anatomical experiment successfully leaves the audience (which consists of both experts and laymen, but mostly laymen) dumbfounded, so much so that doctors, as Galen himself tells us, are believed by some to be 'wonder-workers'.[113] In *De anatomicis administrationibus* 7.4 (2.669 K.), for example, Galen sets out to explain how the vocal mechanism works by rendering a pig voiceless, *aphonon*:[114] after applying pressure to its intercostal nerves, he would strike the animal and it would remain silent. "This", as Galen reports, "shocks the spectators (τούς θεατάς ἐκπλήττει), for its seems marvelous (θαυμαστόν) that the voice is destroyed by small nerves being tied along the torso".[115] Then he would stop exerting pressure and the animal would resume its voice: when the pig cried out, the audience "would marvel even more" (οὕτω γὰρ μᾶλλον οἱ θεαταί θαυμάζουσιν). As Maud Gleason has illustrated in a brilliant discussion of the subject, although Galen believes strongly that there is a perfectly rational explanation for everything that happens in the body, he nonetheless flirts with his emerging self-image as a wonder-worker: "indeed, once his opponents have been effectively silenced, Galen's anatomical performances look less and less like an intellectual debate and more and more like a magic show".[116] Though executed according to strict scientific principles, his performances "tapped into the realm of unreason. What most spectators experienced most may have been what Galen's texts discuss least: blood, pain, fear, and scopophilia itself".[117] The spectacle that Galen is staging is simultaneously scientific and mystifying. Assuming that,

---

113 *De Placitis Hippocratis et Platonis* 2.4.29, 5.233 K.: ... κἄπειτα θαυμάζουσιν ἐξαίφνης ἀκούσαντες ἐξ ἐγκεφάλου γίγνεσθαι τὴν φωνήν. ἔτι δὲ μᾶλλον, ἐπειδὰν ἀκούσωσιν ὡς αἱ κατὰ προαίρεσιν ἅπασαι κινήσεις ὑπὸ μυῶν ἐπιτελοῦνται, θαυμάζουσί τε καὶ παραδοξολόγους ἡμᾶς ἀποκαλοῦσι. Cf. *Praen.* 8.1 (14.641 K.): ἓν οὖν ὄντως θαυμάσιον πραχθὲν ὃ οὐ μόνον με παραδοξολόγον ὡς ἔμπροσθεν οἱ πολλοὶ τῶν ἰατρῶν ὠνόμαζον ἀλλὰ καὶ παραδοξοποιὸν ἐποίησε κληθῆναι. See Rothschild 2013.

114 This passage is also discussed by Lightfoot in the present volume.

115 Translation in Gleason 2009, 100.

116 Gleason 2009, 100. Cf. Mattern 2008, 85–86 and King 2018, 90. On the similar responses elicited by public declamation and public dissection in this period, see von Staden 1995, 59 and 1997, 51. For a general discussion of Galen's place within the context of contemporary Second Sophistic culture, see Bowersock 1969, 59–75, Kollesch 1981, 1–12 and Swain 1996, 357–379.

117 Gleason 2009, 114.

for the most part, his audiences consisted of laymen who would not have been in a position to understand what they were seeing, we can infer that *thauma* is primarily evoked by Galen in these contexts as a means of conveying sensational astonishment. In his treatise on *polupragmosunê*, Plutarch speaks of those who, instead of enjoying the beautiful statues and paintings at Rome, "haunt the monster-market (περὶ τὴν τῶν τεράτων ἀγορὰν ἀναστρέφονται), examining those which have no calves, or are weaselarmed, or have three eyes, or ostrich heads" and "search to learn whether there has been born some commingled shape and misformed prodigy" (*Mor.* 520C).[118] There is no doubt that among the malformed human beings displayed in the *teratôn agora*, one would have also found cases of diseased people, incapacitated by chronic illnesses and congenital conditions.[119] Plutarch's account offers a painful glimple into how disease in antiquity entered the realm of paradox and was exploited as such. What is impressive is how close Galen's anatomical demonstrations can bring us to this sub-culture of voyeurism: a considerable part of Galen's audience would have had no interest in medicine as such or in discovering and marveling at nature's wonderful workings; instead, the kind of *thauma* that attracted them must have consisted in pure thrill and excitement, emerging as it did from spectacles which, to them, remained incomprehensible or elusive at best. In her contribution to this volume ('Galen's Language of Wonder: *Thauma*, Medicine and Philosophy in *On Prognosis* and *On Affected Parts*'), **Jessica Lightfoot** focuses on cases in which *thauma* is elicited in direct connection with Galen's 'wonderful' prognostic abilities as a doctor. Rather than deal with it as a superficial, sensationalist aspect of Galen's medical art, Lightfoot argues that the "evocation of *thauma* confirms medicine's essential compatibility with philosophical inquiry", in the sense that it turns out to be firmly grounded on a series of strict logical deductions and effectively reveals the "fundamental wonder which lies at the heart of the natural order itself".

The writings of the sophist Aelius Aristides, a contemporary of Galen's, yield a picture in which medicine and the marvelous blend with each other even more intensely.[120] Being himself a fervent devotee of Asclepius and having spent a considerable part of his life as a resident in the healing temple at Pergamum, Aelius

---

118 Transl. in Helmbold 1939, 501. Plutarch's text reads as follows: περὶ τὴν τῶν τεράτων ἀγορὰν ἀναστρέφονται, τοὺς ἀκνήμους καὶ τοὺς γαλεάγκωνας καὶ τοὺς τριοφθάλμους καὶ τοὺς στρουθοκεφάλους καταμανθάνοντες καὶ ζητοῦντες εἴ τι γεγένηται σύμμικτον εἶδος καὶ ἀποφώλιον τέρας.

119 For Plutarch's 'monster market', see Barton 1995, 85–86; Garland 1995, 47; Felton 2012, 128–129.

120 See especially Petsalis-Diomidis 2010. For some recent discussions of Aelius Aristides, see the collections of essay in Harris/Holmes 2008 and Israelowich 2012; 2015.

follows blindly the god's medical advice, even in cases in which the suggested prescriptions, revealed through dreams, look odd. As we read in one of the sophist's orations, entitled 'An Address Regarding Asclepius' (*Or.* 42): "Indeed, there is plenty of paradox in the remedies prescribed by the god, for example one man drinking gypsum, another hemlock, and another undressing and bathing in cold water with no need of warmth, as one would have expected", καὶ μὴν τό γε παράδοξον πλεῖστον ἐν τοῖς ἰάμασι τοῦ θεοῦ, οἷον τὸν μὲν γύψου πίνειν, τὸν δὲ κωνείου, τὸν δὲ γυμνοῦσθαι καὶ λούειν ψυχρῷ, θέρμης οὐδ' ὅλως, ὡς ἄν τις δόξαι. Paradoxical as they may sound, the god's remedies eventually work, and this is something that is naturally met by doctors with cautious skepticism. The following is an account of Aelius about one of his personal health issues (*Hieroi Logoi* 1.61–3):

> ὅμοιον δὲ τῷ περὶ τὸ ἦτρον συνέβη καὶ τὸ τοῦ φύματος πολλοῖς ἔτεσι πρότερον. ὁ μὲν γὰρ θεὸς προὔλεγεν ἐκ πολλοῦ δεῖν ὕδερον φυλάττεσθαι, καὶ ἄλλα τε ἔδωκεν ἀλεξιφάρμακα καὶ ὑποδήματα Αἰγύπτια, οἷσπερ οἱ ἱερεῖς χρῆσθαι νομίζουσι. καὶ δὴ καὶ ἔδοξεν αὐτῷ τὸ ῥεῦμα ἀπάγειν κάτω. καὶ γίγνεται φῦμα ἀπ' ἀρχῆς οὐδεμιᾶς φανερᾶς τὸ μὲν πρῶτον οἷον ἄν τῳ καὶ ἄλλῳ γένοιτο, ἔπειτα προῆλθεν εἰς ὄγκον ἐξαίσιον, καὶ ὅ τε βουβὼν μεστὸς ἦν καὶ πάντα ἐξῴδει, καὶ ὀδύναι παρηκολούθουν δειναὶ καὶ πυρετὸς ἔστιν ἃς ἡμέρας. ἐνταῦθα οἱ μὲν ἰατροὶ πάσας φωνὰς ἠφίεσαν, οἱ μὲν τέμνειν, οἱ δὲ ἐπικάειν φαρμάκοις, ἢ πάντως δεῖν ὑπόπυον γενόμενον διαφθαρῆναι. ὁ δὲ θεὸς τὴν ἐναντίαν ἐτίθετο, ἀντέχειν καὶ τρέφειν τὸν ὄγκον· καὶ δηλαδὴ οὐχ αἵρεσις ἦν ἢ τῶν ἰατρῶν ἀκούειν, ἢ τοῦ θεοῦ. ὁ δὲ ὄγκος ἔτι ἐπὶ μᾶλλον ἤρετο καὶ ἦν ἀπορία πολλή. τῶν δὲ φίλων οἱ μὲν ἐθαύμαζον τὴν καρτερίαν, οἱ δὲ ἐνεκάλουν ὡς λίαν ἅπαντα ἐπὶ τοῖς ὀνείρασι ποιουμένῳ, τινὲς δὲ καὶ ὡς ἄτολμον ἐπητιῶντο, ἐπειδὴ οὐ παρεῖχον τέμνειν οὐδ' αὖ φαρμάκων ἠνειχόμην. ὁ δ' αὖ θεὸς διὰ τέλους ἀντεῖχε, κελεύων φέρειν τὸ παρόν.

But as with the abdomen many years before, there was the matter of the tumor. For the god warned for a long time that I should beware of dropsy, and he gave me various drugs and Egyptian slippers, which the priests are accustomed to use. And it seemed best to him to direct the discharge downwards. And a tumor grew from no apparent cause, at first as it might with anyone else, but then increasing to an extraordinary size, and my groin was distended, and everything was swollen and terrible pains ensued, and a fever for some days. At this point, the doctors cried out for all sorts of things, some said surgery, some said cauterisation by drug, or that an infection would arise and I must surely die. But the god gave a contrary opinion and told me to endure and foster the growth. And clearly there was no choice when it came to listening either to the doctors or to the god. But the growth increased even more, and there was much dismay. Some of my friends marvelled at my endurance, others criticized me because I acted too much on account of dreams, and some even blamed me for being cowardly, since I neither permitted surgery nor again suffered any cauterising drugs. But the god remained firm throughout and ordered me to bear with the present circumstances.[121]

On the face of it, Aelius Aristides' passage brings out an antagonistic relationship between temple and secular medicine. Closer inspection of the narrative, however, reveals a more complicated picture. As Manfred Horstmanshoff has illustrated, technical discourse is everywhere present in the text and, more importantly, it is evenly distributed across its various protagonists: Asclepius (e.g. καὶ ἔδοξεν αὐτῷ τὸ ῥεῦμα ἀπάγειν κάτω), Aelius Aristides (φῦμα, βουβὼν etc.),[122] and the doctors (e.g. οἱ μὲν τέμνειν, οἱ δὲ ἐπικάειν φαρμάκοις) all share a medical terminology which is already attested in the Hippocratic Corpus and has numerous parallels in Galen and other medical authors. What is more, instead of acting without intermediaries (which is how the Epidaurian inscriptions typically present him to operate), Aelius' Asclepius performs medicine as a member of a wider therapeutic community of which skilled doctors form part, offering their insight and advice and debating the god's instructions.[123] In turn, Asclepius' 'paradoxical' instructions draw on technical terminology and are informed by medical lore. This is a porous, marvelous world in which doctors and the god *interact* with, rather than exclude each other. As **Georgia Petridou** discusses in her chapter ('Literary Remedies and Rhetorical Prescriptions in Aelius Aristides: Medical Paradoxography or Common Practise?'), even behind some of Asclepius' most 'extraordinary' healing instructions, such as the one according to which (Aelius') breathing problems could be overcome by reading aloud literary texts, one can find solid parallels in secular medicine: as is revealed by medical sources, reading aloud could help someone evacuate excess bodily fluids through perspiration and regulate the body's heat altogether.

The present volume does not aspire to offer an exhaustive discussion of the relationship between medicine and paradoxography in antiquity; the field is new, and there is a lot yet to be done towards illuminating, or even establishing, the dialogue between the two domains. One of the volume's scopes, however, is to provide a first, systematic examination of the 'marvellous' in ancient medical thought in combination with an exegesis of the medical/scientific background that shapes a considerable part of paradoxographical discourse in antiquity. In effect, the present collection of essays hopes to contest the established polarity between the world of marvels and that of 'hard core' science by showing how

121 Translation in Horstmanshoff 2004, 327.

122 On Aelius Aristides as an 'informed patient', see Petridou 2016.

123 Hortmanshoff 2004.

thauma can be present in both, in ways that are often revealing of a complex network of affinities and associations, one which we tend to ignore.

Bibliography

Asper, M. (2017), "Machines on Paper: From Words to Acts in Ancient Mechanics", in: M. Formisano/P.J. van der Eijk (eds.), *Knowledge, Text and Practice in Ancient Technical Writing*, Cambridge, 27–52.

Barton, C.A. (1995), *The Sorrows of the Ancient Romans: The Gladiator and the Monster*, Princeton, NJ.

Beagon, M. (2005), *The Elder Pliny on the Human Animal: Natural History*, Book 7, Oxford.

Beagon, M. (2011), "The Curious Eye of the Elder Pliny", in: R. Gibson/R. Morello (eds.), *Pliny the Elder: Themes and Contexts*, Leiden, 71–88.

Beagon, M. (2014), "Wondrous Animals in Classical Antiquity", in: G.L. Campbell (ed.), *The Oxford Handbook of Animals in Classical Thought and Life*, Oxford, 414–440.

Berrey, M. (2017), *Hellenistic Science at Court*, Berlin/Boston.

Berryman, S. (2009), *The Mechanical Hypothesis in Ancient Greek Natural Philosophy*, Cambridge.

Berthold, H. (2016), "Aristotle's 'Bloody Mirror' and Natural Science in Medieval and Early Modern Europe", in: N.M. Frelick (ed.), *The Mirror in Medieval and Early Modern Culture: Specular Reflections*, Turnhout, 31–71.

Bianchi, O./Thévenaz, O. (eds.) (2004), *Conceptions et représentations de l'extraordinaire dans le monde antique : actes du colloque international*, Lausanne, 20–22 mars 2003, Bern.

Bodnár, I. (2011), "The Pseudo-Aristotelian Mechanics: The Attribution to Strato", in: M.-L. Desclos/W.W. Fortenbaugh (eds.), *Strato of Lampsacus: Text, Translation, and Discussion*, New Brunswick, 443–455.

Bondeson, J. (1997), *A Cabinet of Medical Curiosities*, London.

Bowersock, G.W. (1969), *Greek Sophists in the Roman Empire*, Oxford.

Brisson, L. (2002), *Sexual Ambivalence: Androgyny and Hermaphroditism in Graeco-Roman Antiquity (transl. J. Lloyd)*, Berkeley.

Brock, A.J. (1916), *Galen: On the Natural Faculties* (Loeb Classical Library), Cambridge, MA/London.

Cameron, A. (2004), *Greek Mythography in the Roman World*, Oxford/New York.

Carel, H. (2016), *Phenomenology of Illness*, Oxford.

Chiaradonna, R. (2009), "Galen and Middle Platonism", in: C. Gill/T. Whitmarsh/J. Wilkins (eds.), *Galen and the World of Knowledge*, Cambridge, 243–260.

Cilliers, L./Pieter Retief, F. (2013), "Dream Healing in Asclepieia in the Mediterranean", in: S.M. Oberhelman (ed.), *Dreams, Healing, and Medicine in Greece: From Antiquity to Present*, London/New York, 69–92.

Close, A.J. (1969), "Commonplace Theories of Art and Nature in Classical Antiquity and in the Renaissance", *Journal of the History of Ideas* 30, 467–486.

Cohoon, J.W./Lamar Crosby, H. (1940), *Dio Chrysostom, Discourses 1–36* (Loeb Classical Library), Cambridge, MA/London.

Cole, S.G. (2004), *Landscapes, Gender, and Ritual Space: The Ancient Greek Experience*, Berkeley.
Connell, S. (2015), *Aristotle on Female Animals: A Study of the Generation of Animals*, Cambridge.
Craik, E.M. (2015), *The 'Hippocratic' Corpus: Content and Context*, London/New York.
Dawkins, R. (1998), *Unweaving the Rainbow: Science, Delusion and the Appetite for Wonder*, London.
Dean Jones, L. (1994), *Women's Bodies in Classical Greek Science*, Oxford.
Dean Jones, L. (1995), "Autopsia, Historia and What Women Know: The Authority of Women in Hippocratic Gynecology", in: D. Bates (ed.), *Knowledge and the Scholarly Medical Traditions*, Cambridge, 41–58.
Delattre, C. (2018), "Paradoxographical Discourse on Sources and Fountains: Deconstructing Paradoxes", in: M. Gerolemou (2018), 205–224.
Dickie, M. (2001), *Magic and Magicians in the Greco-Roman World*, London/New York.
Doroszewska, J. (2013), " "...And she became a man": Sexual Metamorphosis in Phlegon of Tralles' *Mirabilia*", *PFLIT* 3, 223–241.
Doroszewska, J. (2016), *The Monstrous World. Corporeal Discourses in Phlegon of Tralles' Mirabilia*, Frankfurt am Main.
Eco, U. (2009), *The Infinity of Lists: An Illustrated Essay*, Rizzoli.
Faraone, C.A. (2011), "Magical and Medical Approaches to the Wandering Womb in the Ancient Greek World", *ClAnt* 30, 1–32.
Felton, D. (2012), "Rejecting and Embracing the Monstrous in Ancient Greece", in: A.S. Mittman/P.J. Dendle (eds.), *The Ashgate Research Companion to Monsters and the Monstrous*, Ashgate, 103–132.
Flashar, H. (1972), *Aristotelis Opuscula II: Mirabilia*, Berlin.
Flemming, R. (2000), *Medicine and the Making of Roman Women*, Oxford.
Flemming, R. (2003), "Empires of Knowledge: Medicine and Health in the Hellenistic World", in: A. Erskine (ed.), *A Companion to the Hellenistic World*, Malden, MA, 449–463.
Flemming, R. (2009), "Demiurge and Emperor in Galen's World of Knowledge", in: C. Gill/T. Whitmarsh/J. Wilkins (eds.), *Galen and the World of Knowledge*, Cambridge, 59–84.
Gaillard-Seux, P. (2010), "Un pseudo-Democrite énigmatique: Bolos de Mendès", in: F. Le Blay (ed.), *Transmettre les savoirs dans les mondes hellénistique et romain*, Rennes, 223–244.
Garland, R. (1995), *The Eye of the Beholder: Deformity and Disability in the Graeco-Roman World*, London.
Gerolemou, M. (2018), (ed.), *Recognizing Miracles in Antiquity and Beyond*, Berlin/Boston.
George, M. (1995), "Wonder as a Source of Philosophy and of Science: A Comparison", *Philosophy in Science* 6, 97–128.
Geus, K./King, C.G. (2018), "Paradoxography", in: P.T. Keyser/J. Scarborough (eds.), *Oxford Handbook of Science and Medicine in the Classical World*, Oxford, 431–444.
Giannini, A. (1963), "Studi sulla paradossografia greca I: Da Omero a Callimaco: Motivi e forme del meraviglioso", *Rendiconti dell'Istituto Lombardo, Academia di Scienze e Lettere* 97, 247–266.
Giannini, A. (1964), "Studi sulla paradossografia greca II", *Acme* 17, 99–140.
Gleason, M. (2009), "Shock and Awe: The Performance Dimension of Galen's Anatomy Demonstrations", in: C. Gill/T. Whitmarsh/J. Wilkins (eds.), *Galen and the World of Knowledge*, Cambridge, 85–114.

Good, B.J. (1994), *Medicine, Rationality and Experience: An Anthropological Perspective*, Cambridge.
Gorrini M. E. (1995), "The Hippocratic Impact on Healing Cults: The Archaeological Evidence in Attica", in: P. van der Eijk *et al.* (eds.), *Hippocrates in Context: Papers Read at the XIth International Hippocrates Colloquium*, Leiden, 135–156.
Gourevitch, D. (1983), "L'aphonie hippocratique", in: F. Lasserre/P. Mudry (eds.), *Formes de pensée dans la Collection Hippocratique*, Geneva, 297–305.
Grant, R.M. (1952), *Miracle and Natural Law in Graeco-Roman and Early Christian Thought*, Amsterdam.
Greenblatt, S. (1991), *Marvelous Possessions: The Wonder of the New World*, Oxford.
Gutzwiller, K. (2007), *A Guide to Hellenistic Literature*, Oxford.
Hankinson, R.J. (1989), "Galen and the Best of All Possible Worlds", *CQ* 39, 206–227.
Hansen, W. (1996), *Phlegon of Tralles' Book of Marvels*, Exeter.
Hanson, A.E. (1990), "The Medical Writer's Woman", in: D.M. Halperin/J.J. Winkler/F.I. Zeitlin (eds.), *Before Sexuality: The Construction of Erotic Experience in the Ancient Greek World*, Princeton, 309–338.
Hanson, A.E. (1991), "Continuity and Change: Three Case Studies in Hippocratic Gynecological Theraphy and Theory", in: S.B. Pomeroy (ed.), *Women's History and Ancient History*, Chapel Hill/London, 73–110.
Hanson, A.E. (1998), "Talking Recipes in the Hippocratic Corpus", in: M. Wyke (ed.), *Parchments of Gender: Deciphering the Body in Antiquity*, Oxford, 71–94.
Harris, W.V./Holmes, B. (eds.), *Aelius Aristides between Greece, Rome, and the Gods*, Leiden/Boston.
Harris, W.V. (2009), *Dreams and Experience in Classical Antiquity*, Cambridge, MA.
Harris, W.V. (2016), "Popular Medicine in the Classical World", in: W.V. Harris (ed.), *Popular Medicine in Graeco-Roman Antiquity: Explorations*, Leiden/Boston, 1–64.
Healy, J.F. (1999), *Pliny the Elder on Science and Technology*, Oxford.
Heidegger, M. (1994), *Basic Questions of Philosophy: Selected "Problems" of "Logic"* (transl. R. Rojcewicz/A. Schuwer), Bloomington.
Helmbold, W.C. (1939), *Plutarch: Moralia, Vol.VI* (Loeb Classical Library), Cambridge, MA/London.
Hett, W.S. (1936), *Aristotle: Minor Works* (Loeb Classical Library), Cambridge, MA/London.
Higbie, C. (2007), "Hellenistic Mythographers", in: R.D. Woodard (ed.), *The Cambridge Companion to Greek Mythology*, Cambridge, 237–254.
Holmes, B. (2008), "Aelius Aristides' Illegible Body", in: W.V. Harris/B. Holmes (eds.), *Aelius Aristides between Greece, Rome, and the Gods,* Leiden/Boston, 81–114
Holmes, B. (2010), *The Symptom and the Subject: The Emergence of the Physical Body in Ancient Greece*, Princeton, NJ.
Holmes, B. (2012), *Gender: Antiquity and its Legacy*, London.
Holmes, B. (2013), "Disturbing Connections: Sympathetic Affections, Mental Disorder, and Galen's Elusive Soul", in: W.V. Harris (ed.), *Mental Disorders in the Classical World,* Leiden, 147–176.
Holmes, B. (2017), "The Generous text: Animal Intuition, Human Knowledge and Written Transmission in Pliny's Books on Medicine", in: M. Formisano/P.J. van der Eijk (eds.), *Knowledge, Text and Practice in Ancient Technical Writing*, Cambridge, 217–230.

Holmes, B. (2013), "In Strange Lands: Disembodied Authority and the Physician Role in the Hippocratic Corpus and Beyond", in: M. Asper (ed.), *Writing Science: Medical and Mathematical Authorship in Ancient Greece*, Berlin, 431–470.
Holmes, B. (2018), "Body", in: P.E. Pormann (ed.) *The Cambridge Companion to Hippocrates*, Cambridge, 63–88.
Horstmanshoff, H.F.J. (2004), "Did the God Learn Medicine? Asclepius and Temple Medicine in Aelius Aristides' *Sacred Tales*", in: H.F.J. Horstmanshoff/M. Stol (eds.), *Magic and Rationality in Ancient Near eastern and Greco-Roman Medicine*, Leiden, 325–341.
Hughes, J. (2017), *Votive Body Parts in Greek and Roman Religion*, Cambridge.
Israelowich, I. (2012), *Society, Medicine and Religion in the Sacred Tales of Aelius Aristides*, Leiden.
Israelowich, I. (2015), *Patients and Healers in the High Roman Empire*, Baltimore.
Jackson, S. (1990), "Myrsilus of Methymna and the Dreadful Smell of the Lemnian Women", *ICS* 15, 77–83.
Jacob, C. (1983), "De l'art de compiler à la fabrication du merveilleux: Sur la paradoxographie grecque", *Lalies* 2, 121–140.
Jacob, C./de Polignac, F. (2000), *Alexandria, Third Century BC: The Knowledge of the World in a Single City*, Alexandria.
Johnson, M.R. (2017), "Aristotelian Mechanistic Explanation", in: J. Rocca (ed.), *Teleology in the Ancient World: Philosophical and Medical Approaches*, Cambridge, 125–150.
Jones, W.H.S. (1923), *Hippocrates. Vol. II* (Loeb Classical Library), Cambridge, MA/London.
Jouanna, J. (1992), "Le statut du thauma chez les médecins de la Collection hippocratique", in: A. Thivel (ed.), *Le miracle grec*, Nice, 223–236.
Kazantzidis, G. (2017), "Empathy and the Limits of Disgust in the Hippocratic Corpus", in: D. Lateiner/D. Spatharas (eds.), *The Ancient Emotion of Disgust*, Oxford, 45–68.
Kazantzidis, G. (2018a), "Haunted Minds, Haunted Places: Topographies of Insanity in Greek and Roman Paradoxography", in: D. Felton (ed.), *Landscapes of Dread in Classical Antiquity: Negative Emotion in Natural and Constructed Spaces*, London, 226–258.
Kazantzidis, G. (2018b), "Medicine and the Paradox in the Hippocratic Corpus and Beyond", in: M. Gerolemou (2018), 31–61.
King, D. (2018), *Experiencing Pain in Imperial Greek Culture*, Oxford.
King, H. (1998), *Hippocrates' Woman: Reading the Female Body in Ancient Greece*, London/New York.
King, H. (2006), "The Origins of Medicine in the Second Century A.D.", in: S. Goldhill /R. Osborne (eds.), *Rethinking Revolutions through Ancient Greece*, Cambridge, 246–263.
King, H. (2013), "Fear of Flute Girls, Fear of Falling", in: W.V. Harris (ed.), *Mental Disorders in the Classical World*, Leiden, 265–282.
Kollesch, J. (1981), "Galen und die Zweite Sophistik", in: V. Nutton (ed.), *Galen: Problems and Prospects*, London, 1–12.
Kovačić, F. (2001), *Der Begriff der Physis bei Galen vor dem Hintergrund seiner Vorgänger*, Stuttgart.
Krevans, N. (2005), "The Editor's Toolbox: Strategies for Selection and Presentation in the Milan Epigram Papyrus", in: K. Gutzwiller (ed.), *The New Posidippus: A Hellenistic Poetry Book*, Cambridge, 81–96.
Laes, C. (2018), *Disabilities and the Disabled in the Roman World: A Social and Cultural History*, Cambridge.
Langholf, V. (1990), *Medical Theories in Hippocrates: Early texts and the 'Epidemics'*, Berlin.

Laqueur, T.W. (1990), *Making Sex: Body and Gender from the Greeks to Freud*, Cambridge, MA.
Laskaris, J. (2002), *The Art is Long: On the Sacred Disease and the Scientific Tradition*, Leiden.
Leigh, M. (2013), *From Polupragmon to Curiosus: Ancient Concepts of Curious and Meddlesome Behaviour*, Oxford.
Llewelyn, J. (1988), "On the Saying That Philosophy Begins in Thaumazein", in: A. Benjamin (ed.), *Post-Structuralist Classics*, London, 173–191.
Llewellyn-Jones, L./Robson, J. (2010), *Ctesias' History of Persia: Tales of the Orient*, London/New York.
Lloyd, G.E.R. (1979), *Magic, Reason and Experience: Studies in the Origin and Development of Greek Science*, Cambridge.
Lloyd, G.E.R. (1983), *Science, Folklore and Ideology*, Cambridge.
Lloyd, G.E.R. (1987), *The Revolutions of Wisdom: Studies in the Claims and Practice of Ancient Greek Science*, Berkeley.
Lloyd, G.E.R. (2003), *In the Grip of Disease: Studies in the Greek Imagination*, Oxford.
Lonie, I.M. (1981), *The Hippocratic Treatises, 'On Generation', 'On the Nature of the Child', 'Diseases IV': A Commentary*, Berlin.
Manuli, P. (1983), "Donne masculine, femminine sterile, vergini perpetue: La ginecologia greca tra Ippocrate e Sorano", in: S. Campese/P. Manuli/G. Sissa (eds.), *Madre Materna: Sociologia e biologia della donna greca*, Turin, 147–192.
Mattern, S.P. (2008), *Galen and the Rhetoric of Healing*, Baltimore.
Mattern, S.P. (2015), "Panic and Culture: *Hysterike Pnix* in the Ancient Greek World", *Journal of the History of Medicine and Allied Sciences* 70, 491–515.
Mayhew, R. (2004), *The Female in Aristotle's Biology: Reason or Rationalization*, Chicago/London.
McKeown, J. (2017), *A Cabinet of Ancient Medical Curiosities: Strange Tales and Surprising Facts from the Healing Arts of Greece and Rome*, Oxford/New York.
Menn, S. (2015), "Democritus, Aristotle, and the *Problemata*", in: R. Mayhew (ed.), *The Aristotelian Problemata Physica. Philosophical and Scientific Investigations*, Leiden/Boston, 1–35.
Montiglio, S. (2000), *Silence in the Land of Logos*, Princeton, NJ.
Murphy, T.M. (2004), *Pliny the Elder's Natural History: The Empire in the Encyclopedia*, Oxford.
Naas, V. (2002), *Le projet encyclopédique de Pline l'ancien*, Rome.
Naas, V. (2011), "Imperialism, *Mirabilia*, and Knowledge: Some Paradoxes in the *Naturalis Historia*", in: R. Gibson/R. Morello (eds.), *Pliny the Elder: Themes and Contexts*, Leiden, 57–70.
Napier, D.A. (1992), *Foreign Bodies: Performance, Art, and Symbolic Anthropology*, Berkeley/Los Angeles.
Neer, R. (2010), *The Emergence of the Classical Style in Greek Sculpture*, Chicago/London.
Nichols, A. (2018), "Ctesias' *Indica* and the Origins of Paradoxography", in: M. Gerolemou (2018), 3–16.
Nielsen, K.M. (2008), "The Private Parts of Animals: Aristotle on the Teleology of Sexual Difference", *Phronesis* 53, 373–405.
Nightingale, A. (2004), *Spectacles of Truth in Classical Greek Philosophy: Theoria in its Cultural Context*, Cambridge.
ní Mheallaigh, K. (2014), *Reading Fiction with Lucian: Fakes, Freaks and Hyperreality*, Cambridge.

Nutton V. (1985), "Murders and Miracles: Lay Attitudes towards Medicine in Classical Antiquity", in: R. Porter (ed.), *Patients and Practitioners. Lay Perceptions of Medicine in Pre-industrial Society*, Cambridge, 23–53.

Nutton, V. (2004) *Ancient Medicine*, London.

Nutton, V. (2009), "Galen's Library", in: C. Gill/T. Whitmarsh/J. Wilkins (eds.), *Galen and the World of Knowledge*, Cambridge, 19–34.

Overduin, F. (2014), "The anti-Bucolic World of Nicander's *Theriaca*", *CQ* 64, 623–641.

Pajón-Leyra, I. (2011), *Entre ciencia y maravilla: el género literario de la paradoxografía griega*, Zaragoza.

Pajón-Leyra (2018), "Turning Science into Miracle in the Voyage of Alexander the Great", in: M. Gerolemou (2018), 275–304.

Parker, R. (1996), *Athenian Religion: A History*, Oxford.

Peck, A.L. (1942), *Aristotle, Vol. XIII: Generation of Animals* (Loeb Classical Library), Cambridge, MA/London.

Pearcy, L. T. (2013), "Writing the Medical Dream in the Hippocratic Corpus and at Epidaurus", in: S.M. Oberhelman (ed.), *Dreams, Healing, and Medicine in Greece: From Antiquity to Present*, London/New York, 93–108.

Peck, A.L./Forster, E.S. (1937), *Aristotle, Vol. XII* (Loeb Classical Library), Cambridge, MA/London.

Petsalis-Diomidis, A. (2010), *Truly Beyond Wonders: Aelius Aristides and the Cult of Asklepios*, Oxford.

Petridou, G. (2015), *Divine Epiphany in Greek Literature and Culture*, Oxford.

Petridou, G. (2016), "Aelius Aristides as Informed Patient and Physician", in: G. Petridou/C. Thumiger (eds.), *Homo Patients: Approaches to the Patient in the Ancient World*, Leiden, 451–470.

Pietrobelli, A. (2017), "Galen's Religious Itineraries", *Religion in the Roman Empire* 3, 221–441.

Porter, J. (2007), "Lucretius and the Sublime", in: S. Gillespie/P. Hardie (eds.), *The Cambridge Companion to Lucretius*, Cambridge, 167–184.

Porter, J. (2016), *The Sublime in Antiquity*, Cambridge.

Potter, P. (2012), *Hippocrates. vol. X.* (Loeb Classical Library), Cambridge, MA/London.

Prier, R. (1989), *Thauma Idesthai: The Phenomenology of Sight and Appearance in Archaic Greek*, Tallahassee.

Rihl, T.E. (2018), "Mechanics and Pneumatics in the Classical World", in: P. Keyser/J. Scarborough (eds.), *The Oxford Handbook of Science and Medicine in the Classical World*, Oxford, 337–358.

Romm, J.S. (1992), *The Edges of the Earth in Ancient Thought: Geography, Exploration, and Fiction*, Princeton.

Rothschild, C.K. (2013), "Hocus Pocus, Galen's *On Prognosis* and the Gospel of Mark", in: T. Nicklas/J.E. Spittler (eds.), *Credible, Incredible: the Miraculous in the Ancient Mediterranean*, Tübingen, 107–142.

Rubenstein, M.-J. (2008), *Strange Wonder: The Closure of Metaphysics and the Opening of Awe*, New York.

Sallis, J. (1995), ". . . A Wonder That One Could Never Aspire to Surpass", in: K. Maly (ed.), *The Path of Archaic Thinking: Unfolding the Work of John Sallis*, Buffalo, 243–274.

Sassi, M. (1993), "Mirabilia", in: G. Cambiano/L. Canfora/D. Lanza (eds.), *Lo spazio letterario della Grecia antica* (vol. 1), Rome, 449–468.

Scarry, E. (1985), *The Body in Pain: The Making and Unmaking of the World*, New York/Oxford.

Schepens, G./Delcroix, K. (1996), "Ancient Paradoxography: Origin, Evolution, Production and Reception", in: O. Pecere/A. Stramaglia (eds.), *La letteratura di consumo nel mondo greco-latino*, Cassino, 375–460.

Schiefsky, M.J. (2007), "Art and Nature in Ancient Mechanics", in: B. Bensaude-Vincent/W.R. Newman (eds.), *The Artificial and the Natural: An Evolving Polarity*, Cambridge, MA, 67–108.

Sharples, R.W. (1988), "Some Aspects of the Secondary Tradition of Theophrastus' *Opuscula*", in: W.W. Fortenbaugh/R.W. Sharples (eds.), *Theophrastean Studies: Fifteen Papers on Natural Science, Physics and Metaphysics, Ethics, Religion and Rhetoric*, New Brunswick/Oxford, 41–64.

Sissa, G. (1990), "Maidenhood Without Maidenhead: The Female Body in Ancient Greece", in: D.M. Halperin/J.J. Winkler/F.I. Zeitlin (eds.), *Before Sexuality: The Construction of Erotic Experience in the Ancient Greek World*, Princeton, 339–364.

Sissa, G. (2013), "The Hymen is a Problem, still. Virginity, Imperforation, and Contraception, from Greece to Rome', *EuGeStA* 3, 67–123.

Smith, W.D. (1994), *Hippocrates: Vol. VII* (Loeb Classical Library), Cambridge, MA/London.

Solmsen, F. (1963), "Nature as Craftsman in Greek Thought", *Journal of the History of Ideas* 24, 473–496.

Sontag, S. (1989), *Aids and its Metaphors*, New York.

Sprague, R. (1985), "Aristotle on Red Mirrors (*On Dreams* 459b24–460a23)", *Phronesis* 30, 323–325.

Stavrianeas, S. (2018), "The Good, the Bad, and the Ugly", in: P. Kontos (ed.), *Evil in Aristotle*, Cambridge, 51–72.

Struck, P. (2016), *Divination and Human Nature: A Cognitive History of Intuition in Classical Antiquity*, Princeton.

Swain, S.C.R. (1996), *Hellenism and Empire: Language, Classicism, and Power in the Greek World, AD 50–250*, Oxford.

Temkin, O. (1956), *Soranus' Gynecology*, Baltimore/London.

Thumiger, C. (2013), "The Early Greek Medical Vocabulary of Insanity", in: W.V. Harris (ed.), *Mental Disorders in the Classical World*, Leiden, 61–95.

Thumiger, C. (2016), "Patient Function and Physician Function in the *Epidemics* Cases", in: G. Petridou/C. Thumiger (eds.), *Homo Patiens: Approaches to the Patient in the Ancient World*, Leiden, 107–137.

Thumiger, C. (2017), *A History of the Mind and Mental Health in Classical Greek Medical Thought*, Cambridge.

Thumiger, C. (2018), "*Stomachikon*, *Hydrophobia* and Other Eating Disturbances: Volition and Taste in Late-Antique Medical Discussions', in: C. Thumiger/P.N. Singer (eds.), *Mental Illness in Ancient Medicine: From Celsus to Paul of Aegina*, Leiden/Boston, 245–268.

Tieleman, T. (2013), "Miracle and Natural Cause in Galen', in: S. Alkier/A. Weissenrieder (eds.), *Miracles Revisited*, Berlin/Boston, 101–114.

Tipton, J.A. (2014), *Philosophical Biology in Aristotle's Parts of Animals*, Heidelberg.

Tredennick, H. (1933), *Aristotle: Metaphysics Books I–IX* (Loeb Classical Library), Cambridge, MA/London.

Tuplin, C. (2004), "Doctoring the Persians: Ctesias of Cnidus, physician and historian", *Klio* 86, 305–347.

Tybjerg, K. (2003), "Wonder-Making and Philosophical Wonder in Hero of Alexandria", *Studies in History and Philosophy of Science* 34, 443–466.

Vanotti, G. (2007), *Aristotele: Racconti Meravigliosi*, Milan.
Van der Eijk, P.J. (2005), *Medicine and Philosophy in Classical Antiquity: Doctors and Philosophers on Nature, Soul, Health and Disease*, Cambridge.
Van der Eijk, P.J. (2009), "'Aristotle! What a Thing for You to Say!' Galen's Engagement with Aristotle and Aristotelians", in: C. Gill/T. Whitmarsh/J. Wilkins (eds.), *Galen and the World of Knowledge*, Cambridge, 261–280.
Vernant, J.-P. (2006), "Some Remarks on the Forms and Limitations of Technological Thought among the Greeks", in: J.-P. Vernant, *Myth and Thought among the Greeks* (transl. J. Lloyd), New York.
Von Staden, H. (1992a), "The Discovery of the Body: Human Dissection and its Cultural Contexts in Ancient Greece", *The Yale Journal of Biology and Medicine* 65, 223–241.
Von Staden, H. (1992b), "Women and Dirt", *Helios* 19, 7–30.
Von Staden, H. (1989), *Herophilus: The Art of Medicine in Early Alexandria*, Cambridge.
Von Staden, H. (1995), "Anatomy as Rhetoric: Galen on Dissection and Persuasion", *JHM* 50, 47–66.
Von Staden, H. (1996), "Body as Machine: Interactions between Medicine, Mechanics, and Philosophy in Early Alexandria", in: *Alexandria and Alexandrianism*, The J. Paul Getty Museum, 85–106.
Von Staden, H. (1997), "Galen and the 'Second Sophistic", in R. Sorabji (ed.), *Aristotle and After*, London, 33–54.
Von Staden, H. (1997), "Teleology and Mechanism: Aristotelian Biology and Early Hellenistic Medicine", in W. Kullmann/S. Föllinger (eds.), *Aristotelische Biologie: Intentionen, Methoden, Ergebnisse*, Stuttgart, 183–208.
Von Staden, H. (1998), "Andréas de Caryste et Philon de Byzance: médecine et mécanique à Alexandrie", in: G. Argoud/J.-Y. Guillaumin (eds.), *Sciences exactes et sciences appliquées à Alexandrie (III siècle av. J.-C. – I siècle ap. J.-C.*, Saint-Étienne, 147–172.
Von Staden, H. (1999), "Rupture and Continuity: Hellenistic Reflections on the History of Medicine", in: P.J. van der Eijk (ed.), *Ancient Histories of Medicine: Essays in Medical Doxography and Historiography in Classical Antiquity*, Leiden, 143–187.
Von Staden, H. (2000), "Body, Soul, and Nerves: Epicurus, Herophilus, Erasistratus, the Stoics, and Galen", in: J.P. Wright/P. Potter (eds.), *Psyche and Soma: Physicians and Metaphysicians on the Mind-Body Problem from Antiquity to Enlightenment*, Oxford, 79–116.
Von Staden, H. (2007), "*Physis* and *Techne* in Greek Medicine", in: B. Bensaude-Vincent/W.R. Newman (eds.), *The Artificial and the Natural: An Evolving Polarity*, Cambridge, MA, 21–49.
Von Staden, H. (2008), "Animals, Women, and Pharmaka in the Hippocratic Corpus", in: V. Boudon Millot/V. Dasen/B. Maire (eds.), *Femmes en médecine*, Paris, 171–204.
Warren, J. (2014), *The Pleasures of Reason in Plato, Aristotle, and the Hellenistic Hedonists*, Cambridge.
Webster, C. (2014), 'Technology and/as Theory: Material Thinking in Ancient Science and Medicine', PhD thesis, Columbia University.
Withington, E.T. (1928), *Hippocrates. Vol.III* (Loeb Classical Library), Cambridge, MA/London.
Witt, C. (2012), "Aristotle on Deformed Animal Kinds", *Oxford Studies in Ancient Philosophy* 43, 83–106.
Witt, M. (2018), "Surgery", in: P.E. Pormann (ed.), *The Cambridge Companion to Hippocrates*, Cambridge, 217–245.

Maria Gerolemou

Technological Wonder in Herodotus' *Histories*

Abstract: Taking as a starting point the assumption that health in antiquity was an acquired good, this chapter aims to examine the concept of the artificially cured or improved human body in Herodotus; this is a product of human *technê*, specifically of health technology. A defining point for the category of this type of body is the concept of the wondrous (θῶμα). As a technological wonder which emphasizes human agency, the cured or improved body threatens to replace the natural body and the *thauma* of nature. In effect, however, there is no substantial difference between the natural and the technological body or, consequently, the natural and the technological wonder; since the latter, the technological, mimics the former, the natural, the only difference that could be observed is the unaccountable behavior of the natural body which opposes the technological predetermined design of the artificial body.

1 Introduction

This chapter examines cases from Herodotus' *Histories* in which the human body, due to its non-physical properties, is regarded as "spectacular", θωμάσιον. Such cases do not concern bodily imperfections or deformities; rather, they concern cases of bodily perfection as the outcome of *technē*. In Herodotus the sick, disabled, or old body is treated as the result of a natural process; on the other hand, healthy bodies are the outcome of an interaction between biological, climatic, economic, and technological forces, and tend to incite feelings of wonder in those who encounter them. Like artistic objects defined through *thauma* in ekphrastic description,[1] these bodies are *made* marvelous, usually by means of bodily cure and, more often, bodily improvement, which I will be calling 'technologies of health'. By the term technology we should understand here the systematized medical knowledge and skills as well as technologies of enhancement such as

1 The description of the shield of Achilles in the *Iliad* is a famous example (18, 478–608). On wonder as a crucial element of *ekphrasis* see, among others, Becker 1995; Hunzinger 2015; Neer 2000, ch. 1.

https://doi.org/10.1515/9783110661774-002

prosthetics and, generally, procedures developed to improve the quality of human body and life. Hence, in speaking of health technologies, I make use of an umbrella term to express the general idea that bodily care and bodily improvement, in a way similar to human societies, depends on non-natural techniques such as education, devices or tools, and training. These technologies mimic, complement, or improve processes of unaccountable agency[2] such as *tychẽ*, chance, which opposes thoughtful design, and automatism,[3] lying behind unconscious natural functions. Body-enhancement technologies in antiquity concentrate on three aspects of life and the body's well-being. Specifically, they are concerned with longevity, greater resistance to various diseases, and improved appearance.

2 Health as prosthetic achievement

Before I examine more closely the connection between wonder, θῶμα, and body, which is perfected through *technẽ*, I will first outline the ways in which health is construed in Herodotus as a non-natural condition. Although, according to Bartoš,[4] an explicit concept of health was absent in the earliest Greek literature, in contrast with the Hesiodic Golden race, where people do not grow old nor do they suffer from illness, and where death is viewed as unnatural (*Op.* 109–120), Herodotus appears to agree on what could be considered a healthy condition with the writer of the Hippocratic text *On Ancient Medicine*. The latter maintains that the body's original state resembles that of disease, since, by its very nature, it undergoes a process of steady degeneration and is in constant need of treatment. On the other hand, health is the outcome of a set of rules related to, e.g., eating and drinking, hygiene, exercise, and so on; more specifically, according to the author of the treatise, health results from following a regimen, or a τετεχνημένα diet, which adjusts itself to various human and environmental conditions (*On Ancient medicine* ch.3. 5–32; *On Regimen in Health* ch.1).[5] For instance, at 14.2 the

2 For this reason, the author of *On the Art* denies that the cause of recovery is spontaneous (*automaton*, 6.10) or due to *tychẽ* (7). See further Holmes 2013. Cf. Schiefsky 2005, 5–13. On the difference between *tychẽ* (confined to 'adult' human world) and *automaton* (confined to nature) according to Aristotle, see Guthrie 1981, vol. 6 on Aristotle, 238–239.

3 However, according to the author of the *De Arte* 6, the automaton is not a cause; it is nothing but a name. On this issue, see Schiefsky 2005, 8.

4 2015, 17.

5 See Miller 1955; Dunn 2005; Schiefsky 2005, 46–55; Holmes 2010, 162–177; Rosen 2016, esp. 252f.; Bartoš 2015, 42.

author of *On Ancient Medicine*, in the context of discussing various types of barley cakes and breads, their materials, and the process of their production, claims "that by each one of these things the human being is affected and altered in one way or another, and a person's whole life depends on them, whether he is healthy, recovering from illness, or sick" (tr. Schiefsky).[6]

A similar idea, generally linking wellbeing to technology, is detected in Aeschylus' *Prometheus Bound*. Prometheus claims credit for teaching humans every kind of craft. More specifically, he stresses that he has "rescued men from shattering destruction" (*PV* 235f., ἐγὼ δ' ὁ τολμῆς ἐξελυσάμην βροτοὺς/ τὸ μὴ διαρραισθέντας εἰς Ἅιδου μολεῖν; see further Sisiphus, TrGF 43 F19).[7] Along the same lines, in fr. DK 68 B 172, Democritus argues that because nature offers many things that can benefit and, at the same time, harm people, humans discovered other solutions, *μηχαναί*, in order to be healthy and safe: for instance, to protect themselves from water, people learned how to swim.[8] Athenaeus, at a later stage, echoes this idea:

> ὃ [sc. βίος] μὲν γὰρ ἀκατάσκευος καὶ καθάπερ ἀνεύρετος ἦν, οὔτ' ἐπιμιξίας οὔσης οὔτε τῶν τεχνῶν διηκριβωμένων, ὃ δὲ πᾶσιν ἐξηρτυμένος πρὸς ῥᾳστώνην καὶ πρὸς ἀπόλαυσιν καὶ πρὸς τὰς ἄλλας διαγωγάς.
>
> [...] Life in heroic times lacked any accoutrements, as it were, and nothing had been invented then, since there had been no contact between people, and no crafts had been refined, whereas life nowadays offers everything a person needs to have an easy existence and enjoy himself and have a good time generally (12.511d, tr. Olson).[9]

The idea that wellbeing, and especially health, is the result of a technical procedure is shared by Herodotus too. In Herodotus, healthy bodies are the outcome of an artful adjustment of the physical human body to remedies, technologies, and to a wide range of environmental factors, including customs and social behavior. Solon, for example, in 1.32.6, implies that the higher the social status of

---

6 See further on that Wöhrle 1990; Wilkins 2015. Bartoš 2015, 15, 93f. (generally on the history of dietetics).

7 On antiprimitivism, see Lovejoy and Boas 1935, 192–221. On progress, see Dodds 1973.

8 ἀφ' ὧν ἡμῖν τἀγαθὰ γίγνεται, ἀπὸ τῶν αὐτῶν τούτων καὶ τὰ κακὰ ἐπαυρισκοί(μεθ' ἄν, τῶν δὲ κακῶν ἐκτὸς εἴημεν. αὐτίκα ὕδωρ βαθὺ εἰς πολλὰ χρήσιμον καὶ δαὖτε κακόν· κίνδυνος γὰρ ἀποπνιγῆναι. μηχανὴ οὖν εὑρέθη, νήχεσθαι διδάσκειν. "From the same things that can benefit us we may also receive evils, and escape from evils. For example, deep water is useful for many things; however, it can also lead to bad situations, specifically, there is a danger of drowning. So a remedy, *mechane*, has been discovered; that is, teaching people how to swim" (tr. Taylor, 1999, p. 19).

9 Tr. C.B. Gulick 1933 (Loeb).

individuals, the better their health; i.e., health is conceived as an attained benefit in the same way that wealth appears to be an accomplished good. This assumption is best illustrated with regard to the proverbial healthy bodies of the Egyptians described by Herodotus (see below), which are directly attributed to the prosperous land they inhabit. The fact that they could work on their fields without spending too much physical effort, since the waters of the Nile rose and watered the earth, must have left them with more free time and income to spend on self-preservation and pleasure. Aristophanes' *Birds* provide an illuminating parallel to the idea that health, like wealth, is considered a 'prosthetic achievement': to the question of the Epops "how will we give humans health which belongs to the gods?", Peisetairos replies that if they have wealth and, therefore, feel happy, health will follow (603–5).

3 Health technologies

The physical body, as I briefly mentioned at the beginning, is determined by natural invisible procedures, such as automatisms, which can be artificially reproduced or improved.[10] This is because natural automatisms, even if they are not intentional and/or governed by an external force or developed according to a prearranged design, still have a discernible pattern and can be imitated easily. On this basis, it is possible for a natural automatic process like motion to be artificially reproduced, on a new developmental logic and based on new laws, by the ability of human *technē* to mimic natural practices.[11] In the Hippocratic Corpus, in order for health to be achieved, the physician manipulates natural automatisms or develops new, artificial ones through prescribed therapies such as diet, exercises, bathing, etc. (*On Regimen* 1.2); this can happen because, according to the author of the *On Regimen* 1.12–24, arts are able to copy the nature of man, along with that nature's invisible forces (1.16, φύσιν τε ἀνθρώπου μιμέονται, 1.17, 1.24). However, *technē* has transformative effects on the body to the point that it can alter or even deform the body's outer form and inner functions; I will briefly return to this point at a later stage in this paper.

The artificially improved body is idealized as the epitome of human *technē*. The belief that the physical body can be transformed by the power of human rea-

10 Cf. Burkert 1972, 44–45 and Bartoš 2014 and 2015, 139–145.
11 See Bartoš 2014 and 2015, 129–163, esp. 141.

son and craft inspires a sense of wonder which replicates and replaces the admiration for the natural body. In fact, given that automatisms cannot be described through a cause-effect chain, they border on the concept of *thauma*, which is similarly identified through the disruption of an obvious relationship between cause and effect. Herodotus often describes natural phenomena as being generated from a process of spontaneous re-iteration. Death and growth, for example, are often defined as automatic processes [2.94, ... τὰ σιλλικύπρια ταῦτα, τὰ ἐν Ἕλλησι αὐτόματα ἄγρια φύεται; 2.66.4, ἐν ὁτέοισι δ' ἂν οἰκίοισι αἰέλουρος ἀποθάνῃ ἀπὸ τοῦ αὐτομάτου (a natural death)]. An artless repetition is also detected in his description of divine miracles: for example, in 1.175, he discusses Pedaseans and explains that when any misfortune befell them or their neighbors, the priestess of Athena would suddenly grow a long beard. This happened three times.[12]

By transferring the unaccountable transformative power of natural or divine forces to the realm of human skill and experience, the marvelous starts to be associated with the latter. In Sophocles' *Antigone*, for instance, the chorus emphasizes how the potential of human technology is beyond imagination (*Ant.* 365, σοφόν τι τὸ μηχανόεν τέχνας ὑπὲρ ἐλπίδ' ἔχων). The technical miracle is miraculous precisely because it is achieved by human activity; as such it substitutes or supplements the natural. Xerxes, in the fifth book of the *Histories*, finds a plane-tree, which he adorns with gold because of its beauty and orders one of his soldiers to preserve it in this state (5.27).[13] What follows, however, supersedes Xerxes' encounter with the tree: this is the technological wonder of the bridge by which Xerxes crosses the Hellespont (7.36) and which is described in terms similar to other wonders of technology in Herodotus, mainly monuments, where what is stressed is the laborious process of the monument's construction and its great size (see, e.g., on the Propylaia of the temple of Athena at Sais, 2.175.1–4).[14]

At this point, a comparison with Thucydides is instructive since he, too, generally takes the poorly constructed nature of the human condition as his starting point, while he considers *technē* to be what improves it, by offering more alterna-

---

12 The association of artificially reproduced automatisms (mostly motion) with miracles goes back to Homer. In the *Iliad*, Hephaestus manufactures twenty tripods which have the ability to move in order to roll automatically to the assembly of the gods and back home (18.373–7), and golden handmaids, looking identical to living girls, who support and help the lame Hephaestus (18.417–20); both products are a *thauma idesthai*, a wonder to see. Cf. the automatically opening doors in *Il.* 5.749–51, 8.393–5; on this issue, see Bielfeldt 2014, 33; see further examples of automatic wonders in Homer in Bur 2016, 28–31.

13 Cf. Aelian *Var. Hist.* 2.14 recounting the same story in a critical manner.

14 See Gerolemou 2018, 141–144.

tives: the most astonishing product of *technē* is, not surprisingly, the city of Athens itself. In 2.37–40, Athens is represented as a *thaumaston* (2.39, 41); its admirable character stems from its self-sufficiency and it is grounded in democracy, an acquired good nurtured further by its own products, i.e. the laws. However, while the body of the Athenian state is something that is artificially created, the Athenian hegemony is represented by the Athenian ambassadors to the Lacedaemonians as *not* acting against nature, especially human nature (1.76); ultimately, Athenian hegemony also becomes naturalized, i.e. becomes a natural necessity.

The attempt to modify the natural, deficient body, i.e. to improve or redesign the body and its automatic functions according to social conditions and cultural expectations, produces a variety of techniques which range from simple imitation of natural automatisms to their manipulation or even abolition through the process of developing completely new bodily skills and habits.[15] In asserting in 2.77, for example, that the Egyptians are the healthiest of all men, Herodotus argues that the natural body's performance can be optimized.[16] The Egyptians' improved bodies, supposedly part of the land's θωμάσια (2.35), are constructed on the basis of a diet which works in accordance with the climate of the country. More specifically, according to Herodotus, it is not merely the absence of major seasonal changes that explains the health of its inhabitants. In addition, "[f]or three following days every month they purge themselves, pursuing after health by means of emetics and drenches; for they think it is from the food which they eat that all sicknesses come to men".[17] Moreover, in order to fight the natural progress of bone decline, the Egyptians had developed a technique to make the bones of the head as strong as possible. At 3.12, Herodotus states that "the Egyptian skulls are so strong that a blow of a stone will hardly break them.[18] And this, the people said (which for my own part I readily believed), is the reason of it: the Egyptians shave their heads from childhood, and the bone thickens by exposure to the sun. This also is the reason why they do not grow bald; for nowhere can one see so few bald heads as in Egypt."[19] This artificial improvement of the natural bone resistance incites wonder (θῶμα δὲ μέγα εἶδον) since it belongs to the realm of craft, i.e. the

15 Noted by Mauss 2006. See also Holmes 2010, 172.
16 On Egyptian health, see Thomas 2000, 45.
17 Tr. A.D. Godley (Loeb); see further Finch 2009.
18 Cf. the Macrocephali, who had the habit of artificially stretching their skulls; on that see Pinna 1988; Jouanna 2003, 7–82; Backhaus 1976, 336; Maas 2015, 335f.
19 Tr. Godley (Loeb).

"humanly possible".[20] In short, while on the face of it several 'marvels' in Herodotus are presented as natural, they turn out in the course of the narrative to be the product of an artificial intervention grounded in *technē*.

In a way similar to the Egyptians, the Libyans also found ways to overcome the natural limits of the body (4.187.2–3). Herodotus discusses the practice of many Libyan nomads to take their children, once they turn four years old, and burn the veins of their scalps or, sometimes, the veins of their temples, in order to protect them from phlegm draining from their heads. According to Herodotus, they claim that this makes their children healthy. In addition to the Hippocratic suggestion in *Acut.* 37, which describes how the Libyans are healthy because they are hot and dry, Herodotus proposes the art of cauterization as a factor that plays a central role in Libyans' health. Eventually, nature, in cooperation with all these non-natural factors, affects the body and, as a result, acquired characteristics become inborn.

The adoption of technologies concerning the body also informs the kind of decisions that are made regarding what is considered an appropriate technique for solving a wide range of bodily matters; these decisions are mostly influenced by cultural differences. Consider, for example, the matter of the aging body. Whereas some nations accept aging as a normal social and biological process, others see it as something distressing or a disease that needs to be treated.[21] Asian Massagetae, for instance, kill the elderly, boil them and feast on them, believing this to be the most blessed way to end one's life (Hdt. 1.214). For the Greeks, a relatively short lifespan is regarded as an essential requirement for human life to be meaningful, while a long life is a cause for worries.[22] Solon, who in Herodotus represents the Greek nation and its customs, implies that prolonging life does not serve any purpose, for, no matter how long we may live, the length of our life would still remain insignificant compared to the end of our life (1.32). Achilles' and Socrates' choice of a short and noble life proves that brevity of life is regarded by the Greeks as an essential feature of humanity (*Il.* 18.8–126; Pl. *Apol.* 28b–d).[23] The Ethiopians, on the other hand, enjoy longevity; they live for 120 years solely on milk and boiled meat which come spontaneously, *automata*, out of the earth; their long lifespan is mostly related to the fact that they wash in the waters of a strangely oily and fragrant spring (Hdt 3.23). The waters of the Ethiopian spring

---

20 Shimron 1989, 37.

21 See Finch 2010; further on the elderly Richardson 1933; Finley 1981; Howell 1986; Falkner and De Luce 1989.

22 See Miller 1955.

23 See Solmsen 1963, 481.

offer the body a 'vital' moisture that does not merely prolong life but also slows aging.[24] While the Ichthiophagoi look amazed at the Ethiopian's tales about their prolonged life (3.23.2, θῶμα δὲ ποιευμένων τῶν κατασκόπων περὶ τῶν ἐτέων), the Ethiopians mock the Persians and their methods for cultivating wellbeing. According to the Ethiopians, the Persians live so few years because they eat dung, i.e. grain; and they would have had an even shorter life if they didn't get the chance to be refreshed by wine, which the Persians do not possess (3.22.4); in conclusion, different cultural habits produce different health technologies.

The copying of the human body and its automatisms in Herodotus is often taken to the extreme. Herodotus tells, for instance, about a Persian seer, Hegesistratus, who was condemned to death but escaped by amputating his own foot and then made a wooden filler to walk 30 miles to the next town (9.37). His wooden foot eventually transforms his disabled body into a symbol of technological awe and medicalized prowess.[25] In this case, technology reconstructs bodily parts and functions, exceeding the limits of the body and extending its capacities by overcoming its natural vulnerability. The transformative capacity of the supportive artificial limbs becomes perhaps more obvious when the artificially reconstructed body-limbs are positioned vis-à-vis the moving limbs of statues. At 2.48, Herodotus points to the fact that during Dionysus' feast in Egypt, astonishingly large mechanical phalluses, parts of the statues of Dionysus, moved automatically, exceeding the natural stillness of the material. However, the ability of the statues' large genitals to move has a sacred explanation, as Herodotus tells us; yet he does not explain why this is so. In the 5th book, he refers further to the statues of the people of Epidaurus, which miraculously knelt and remained in this position, simulating natural motion, when the Athenians were preparing to move them from Aegina (86.3). One could consider these wooden figures as proto-automata; although they are not self-propelled, they possess the option of motion, specifically, of alternate positions.

As I have argued, the belief that technological expertise may be used to improve the body's natural capabilities leads to the development of various body replication and modification techniques that not only repair the body, but move beyond what is typically considered to be a therapeutic medical intervention. On these occasions the restored or improved body becomes an artifact itself and, as

---

24 This appears to be reminiscent of the cold-dry theory of aging discussed in Aristotle, according to which aging is caused by the loss of vital moisture (Arist. *De Juventute et Senectute, De Vita et Morte, De Respiratione* 466a–466b).

25 On prosthesis in antiquity, see Bliquez 1996; Finch 2011; Draycott 2018.

such, is admired. The artificially reconstructed body, being perceived as an artifact, is best exemplified in the story of the Egyptian methods of mummification. Egyptian mummies are described by Herodotus as a sort of a *technosōma* because they represent the maximum technological effort available to transform the body and stop bodily degeneration (2.86–9). There are three types of mummification procedure, depending on the amount of money that a family is willing to spend. The effigies of men, painted and carved in exact imitation of a corpse, two or four feet long and circulated among guests at the symposia, offer another instance of artificially replicated bodies (2.78). The effigies of Spartan kings slain in war are also treated like real bodies and carried out on a bier for all to see (6.58; cf. 3.24).

Nevertheless, to improve or, rather, artificially to replicate the natural body when there is absolutely no need to do so could be considered an act of hubris. For instance, in 6.125 Croesus offers Alcmeon as much gold as he can carry. Alcmeon strews gold dust on his hair and fills all the fold of his tunic, his boots and even his mouth; "when he came out of the treasury, hardly dragging the weight of his boots, he was like anything rather than a human being"[26] (παντὶ δέ τεῳ οἰκὼς μᾶλλον ἢ ἀνθρώπῳ). Bennet, referring to the adamantine chains made by Hephaestus, which bind the Aeschylean Prometheus, associates metal with passivity;[27] in Alcmaeon's case, we could add, gold metal is linked to submissiveness. Croesus bursts into laughter at the sight of this vainly created golden Alcmaeon. The artificial production of the natural body, here through gold, compromises a feature of human agency that contributes to the meaningfulness of wealth, in particular, and of human life, in general.

4 Conclusion

To sum up, natural bodily insufficiency or the non-natural character of health as perceived in Herodotus' *Histories* becomes a point of reference for considering what is necessary or desirable for a properly functioning body. Herodotus concludes that notions of sufficiency change according to various social contexts and that what should be admired is the human ability to develop health technologies

26 Tr. Godley (Loeb).

27 Bennet 2010, 55. Cf. 2.152 where the oracle of Buto says to Psammetichus "that he would have vengeance when he sees men of bronze coming from the sea" (2.152.3). The 'men of bronze' do come indeed. Some Ionians and Carians land on the coast of Egypt, with their armor of bronze; an Egyptian who has never before seen armored men brings news to Psammetichus that men of bronze, χάλκεοι ἄνδρες, have come from the sea (2.152.4).

with the aim of creating alternate body forms and functions to improve bodily capabilities and life quality.

Bibliography

Backhaus, W. (1976), "Der Hellenen-Barbaren-Gegensatz und die Hippokratische Schrift *peri aeron hydaton topon*", *Historia* 25, 170–185.

Barth, H. (1968), "Zur Bewertung und Auswahl des Stoffes durch Herodot (Die Begriffe θῶμα, θωμάζω, θωμάσιος und θωμαστός)", *Klio* 50, 93–110.

Bartoš, H. (2014), "The Concept of Mimesis in the Hippocratic De Victu", *CQ* 64, 542–557.

Bartoš, H. (2015), *Philosophy and Dietetics in the Hippocratic On Regimen: A Delicate Balance of Health*, Leiden.

Becker, A.S. (1995), *The Shield of Achilles and the Poetics of Ekphrasis*, Lanham, MD.

Bennett, J. (2010), *Vibrant Matter: A Political Ecology of Things*, Durham.

Bielfeldt, R. (2014), "Gegenwart und Vergegenwärtigung: dynamische Dinge im Ausgang von Homer", in: R. Bielfeldt (ed.), *Ding und Mensch in der Antike*, Heidelberg, 15–48.

Bliquez, L. (1996), "Prosthetics in Classical Antiquity: Greek, Etruscan, and Roman Prosthetics", *ANRW* II 37.3, 2640–2676

Bur, T. (2016), 'Mechanical Miracles: Automata in Ancient Greek Religion' (Master Thesis), University of Sydney (http://hdl.handle.net/2123/15398).

Burkert, W. (1972), *Lore and Science in Early Pythagoreanism*, Cambridge.

Dodds, E.R. (1973), *The Ancient Concept of Progress and other Essays on Greek Literature and Belief*, Oxford.

Draycott, J. (ed.) (2018), *Prostheses in Antiquity*, London.

Dunn, F. (2005), "On Ancient Medicine and its Intellectual Context", in: P.J. van der Eijk (ed.), *Hippocrates in Context*, Leiden, 49–67.

Falkner, Th.M./de Luce, J. (eds.) (1989), *Old Age in Greek and Latin Literature* (SUNY Series in Classical Studies), Albany, N.Y.

Finch, C.E. (2009), "Herodotus on Diet and Longevity", *Journal of Aging, Humanities, and the Arts* 3, 86–96.

Finch, C.E., (2010), "Evolving Views of Ageing and Longevity from Homer to Hippocrates: Emergence of Natural Factors, Persistence of the Supernatural", *G&R* 57, 355–377.

Finch, J. (2011), "The Ancient Origins of Prosthetic Medicine", *The Lancet* 37.9765, 548–549.

Finley, M.I. (1981), "The Elderly in Classical Antiquity", *G&R* 28, 156–171.

Gerolemou, M. (2018), "Wonder-ful Memories in Herodotus' Histories", in: M. Gerolemou (ed.), *Recognizing Miracles in Antiquity and Beyond*, Berlin, 133–151.

Guthrie, W.K.C. (1981), *A History of Greek Philosophy*. Volume Six. *Aristotle: An Encounter*, Cambridge.

Hartog, Fr. (1988), *The Mirror of Herodotus, The Representation of the Other in the Writing of History* (tr. J. Lloyd), Berkeley/Los Angeles/London.

Holmes, B. (2010), *The Symptom and the Subject: The Emergence of the Physical Body in Ancient Greece*, Princeton.

Holmes, B. (2013), "Causality, Agency, and the Limits of Medicine", *Apeiron* 46, 302–326.

Howell, T.H. (1986), "Celsus on Old Age", *Age and Ageing* 15, 378–379.

Hunzinger, Ch. (2015), "Wonder", in: P. Destrée/P. Murray (eds.), *A Companion to Ancient Aesthetics*, Malden, 422–437.
Jouanna, J. (ed. and trans.) (2003), *Hippocrate, Airs, eaux, lieux*, vol. 2.2 (2nd ed), Paris.
Lloyd, A.B. (1975, 1976), *Herodotus: Book II. Introduction (I) and Commentary (II)*, Leiden.
Lovejoy, A.O./Boas, G. (1935), *Primitivism and Related Ideas in Antiquity* (with supplementary essays by W.F. Albright and P.E. Dumont), Baltimore.
Maas, M. (2015), "The Shaping Hand of the Environment: Three Phases in Classical Antiquity", in: L.L. Brice/D. Slootjes (eds.), *Aspects of Ancient Institutions and Geography. Studies in Honor of Richard J.A. Talbert*, Leiden, 333–346.
Mauss, M. (1973), "The Techniques of the Body", *Economy and Society* 2.1, 70–88.
Miller, H.W. (1949), "On Ancient Medicine and the Origin of Medicine", *TAPA* 80, 187–202.
Miller, H.W. (1955), "Technê and Discovery in On Ancient Medicine", *TAPA* 86, 51–62.
Munson, R.V. (2001), *Telling Wonders: Ethnographic and Political Discourse in the Work of Herodotus*, Ann Arbor.
Neer, R.T. (2010), *The Emergence of the Classical Style in Greek Sculpture*, Chicago.
Pinna, M. (1988), "Ippocrate fondatore della teoria dei climi", *Rivista Geografica Italiana* 95, 3–19.
Richardson, B.E. (1933), *Old age Among the Ancient Greeks*, Oxford.
Rosen, R.M. (2016), "Towards a Hippocratic Anthropology: On Ancient Medicine and the Origins of Humans", in: L. Dean-Jones/R.M. Rosen (eds.), *Ancient Concepts of the Hippocratic*, Leiden, 242–257.
Schiefsky, M. (2005), *Hippocrates On Ancient Medicine: Translated with Introduction and Commentary*, Leiden.
Shimron, B. (1989), *Politics and Belief in Herodotus*, Stuttgart.
Solmsen, F. (1963), "Nature as Craftsman in Greek Thought", *Journal of the History of Ideas* 24, 473–496.
Thomas, R. (2000), *Herodotus in Context: Ethnography, Science, and the Art of Persuasion*. Cambridge.
Wilkins, J. (2015), "Food and Health in Problemata 21–22: Cooking (pepsis) in the Kitchen and "Cooking" (pepsis) in the Body", in: R. Mayhew (ed.), *The Aristotelian Problemata Physica: Philosophical and Scientific Investigations*, Leiden, 255–271.

Katerina Oikonomopoulou

Paradoxography and the pseudo-Aristotelian *Problemata*

Abstract: This chapter discusses in what terms, and on the basis of which epistemic principles, the 'wondrous' is signalled within the pseudo-Aristotelian collection of *Problemata Physica*, and how this concept informs the *Problemata*'s selection and treatment of medical and naturalistic topics. The chapter will argue that if we wish to comprehend the *Problemata*'s notion of the 'wondrous' we need to look beyond aspects of its content that seem to conform to our own concept of the 'paradoxon' – a concept that is partly shaped by the fact that we perceive paradoxography as a distinct form of writing, or genre. As this chapter demonstrates, there is an intimate link between the *Problemata*'s notion of the 'wondrous' and its investigation of causes in nature: far from being collected for their own sake (as in the pseudo-Aristotelian collection *De Mirabilibus Auscultationibus*), wondrous phenomena function within the work as propellers of scientific enquiry, serving to categorise empirical reality and helping to discover the full range and complexity of the mechanisms that govern physical bodies' interior workings and their interactions with the natural environment.

1 Introduction

The 38 books of medical-natural problems that comprise the pseudo-Aristotelian collection of *Problemata*[1] yield rich insights into the common background that informed the relationship between medicine and paradoxography in the ancient Greek and Roman world. This is because, as genres of writing, medical-natural problems and paradoxography share a similar fascination with nature, including

I would like to thank George Kazantzidis for his excellent work on the *Medicine and Paradoxography in the Ancient World* conference, which provided the stimulus for this chapter, and his encouragement. I would also like to thank all the participants in the conference for the many illuminating discussions and comments that helped give shape to this chapter.

1 On the *Probl.*, see detailed introduction, translation and commentary in Flashar 1962; also valuable are the French translation and comments by Louis 1991–1994 (3 vols) and the new Loeb translation by Mayhew 2015 (2 vols); on its medical books, see Marenghi 1965 (Italian translation and commentary); also Ulacco 2007 and Oikonomopoulou 2015.

https://doi.org/10.1515/9783110661774-003

the place of humans in it, and the wondrous inner workings of their bodies.[2] The aim of this chapter is to shed light on key aspects of this shared background, as well as highlight some important differences in approach, by discussing the pseudo-Aristotelian *Problemata*'s concept of the wondrous, and the way it interacts with its scientific outlook. I will be primarily concerned with the ways in which the *Problemata* render wonder instrumental to scientific investigation, and I will discuss the main epistemic notions that inform its notion of the 'wondrous' (a concept that is key to ancient paradoxography but also to ancient science, as we will see). Moreover, I will draw comparisons between the *Problemata* and a Peripatetic collection that falls squarely within the field of ancient paradoxography. This is the pseudo-Aristotelian Περὶ Θαυμασίων Ἀκουσμάτων (*De Mirabilibus Auscultationibus*),[3] a work which, like the *Problemata*, is rich in heterogeneous scientific observation but, as we will come to see, does not yoke its own concept of the wondrous to scientific enquiry as an overarching aim.[4]

2 The *Problemata* and the 'Wondrous'

In a collection of such vast scope as the *Problemata*, one would expect to find ample space reserved for our notion of the 'wondrous'. However, its books make relatively sparse mention of exotic places or animals, or substances of extraordinary properties. Most of the examples are found in books 12–14, 20 and 23–26, and are concerned with the fragrance that is emitted from spices, lands, or animals (12.7, 12.11, 13.4); the curious impact of the environment on human anatomy or ethnic characteristics (14.1–2, 14.4–5); and plants and vegetables with remarkable properties, such as the ability to offer a cure for βασκανία (20.21, 20.34). Other examples discuss unusual meteorological phenomena and their effects on the environment (23.5, 23.6, 23.9, 23.15, 23.32, 23.37, 23.40, 25.2, 25.6, 26.22, 26.37, 26.44, 26.49, with most instances involving discussions of the unique or unusual properties of the sea, e.g. why it burns, or why its colour changes according to the weather or geographic region).[5] Not accidentally, these are also the books in

2 See Kazantzidis in this volume, on the conceptual overlap between medicine and paradoxography in antiquity.
3 On other variants of the title in the MSS (Περὶ παραδόξων ἀκουσμάτων, Θαυμάσια, Συναγωγὴ Ἀκουσμάτων), see Vanotti 2007, 5.
4 See edition, translation and commentary by Flashar 1990 (in German); Vanotti 2007 (in Italian).
5 See Wilson 2015.

which we find references to exotic lands such as Egypt and Ethiopia (14.4), Libya (23.21), Syria and Arabia (14.4), the Pontic region (14.2, 23.6, 25.6), Scythia (20.21) and lands of the north (14.1, 23.9).[6] Only one mention of an exotic animal is made overall, and this is the panther (πάρδαλις), which is discussed as an exceptional case of an animal whose skin is fragrant (13.4).

Wondrous they may be for us, yet there is nothing in the examples listed above to mark them as such for the reader. Put slightly differently, there is nothing in their treatment that serves to distinguish them from problems that do not conform to our notion of the 'wondrous'. In fact, the very terms that one might say serve as markers of the paradoxographical genre in antiquity, namely θαῦμα ('wonder'), θαυμάσιον or θαυμαστόν ('wondrous'),[7] are almost entirely absent from the *Problemata* as a whole. There is only one instance within the entire collection where a phenomenon is described as 'amazing' or 'wondrous', using the term θαυμάσιος:

> Διὰ τί αἱ μὲν βάσεις τῶν πομφολύγων λευκαὶ ἐν τοῖς ὕδασι; καὶ ἐὰν ἐν ἡλίῳ τεθῶσι, σκιὰν οὐ ποιοῦσιν, ἀλλ' ἡ μὲν ἄλλη πομφόλυξ σκιὰν ποιεῖ, ἡ δὲ βάσις οὐ ποιεῖ, ἀλλ' ἡλίωται κύκλῳ. τὸ δὲ ἔτι θαυμασιώτερον, ὅτι οὐδ' ἐάν τι τεθῇ ξύλον εἰς τὸ ὕδωρ ἐν τῷ ἡλίῳ ... τέμνεται ὑπὸ τοῦ ὕδατος ταύτῃ. [...]
>
> Why are the bases of bubbles in water white? And if they are placed in sunlight they do not produce a shadow, but the rest of the bubble produces a shadow, whereas the base does not, but is like sunlight in a circle. But what is still more amazing is that even if a plank is placed into the water in the sunlight there isn't ... [8] it is cut by the water at that point. [...]
>
> (*Problemata* 16.1, 913a18–24, transl. R. Mayhew)

Unfortunately, the missing part of the text only permits an incomplete understanding of the natural phenomenon that is characterised as θαυμασιώτερον ('yet more wondrous') in this problem. Water bubbles must certainly have featured in the discussion somehow, given that they are the main topic of the problem. Nevertheless, the use of the comparative for the adjective θαυμάσιος suggests that the reader is meant to reflect on the problem in its entirety based on the notion that it describes something wondrous (that is, the adjective applies to the opening

6 On such ethnographic information in the *Probl.*, see Leunissen 2015.

7 See *LSJ* s.v., for the adjectives θαυμάσιος and θαυμαστός (both translated as 'wonderful', 'marvellous'). It would be worth noting that θαυμαστός, in view of the fact that it is, grammatically, a verbal adjective, puts the interpreter of θαῦμα to the fore (i.e. it denotes something 'worthy of admiration').

8 Part of the text is missing. See Mayhew 2011, 480 n. 1.

discussion of the bases of bubbles and the fact that they do not produce a shadow as well). Overall, by invoking the concept of θαῦμα, the problem invites its readers to share in its own fascination with nature's workings, involving, besides animate beings, also minute inanimate objects or formations (the subject of book 16 as a whole, entitled 'Problems concerned with inanimate things') such as bubbles.

In striking contrast to what we observe in the *Problemata*, within the pseudo-Aristotelian collection Περὶ Θαυμασίων Ἀκουσμάτων the term θαυμάσιος occurs not only in the title (which can be rendered in English as 'On wondrous things that have been heard'), but also, together with the related term θαυμαστός, at several other places within the work.[9] The frequency of both terms' occurrence is probably tied to the fact that they are used as generic markers, directing the reader towards a response to nature and its extraordinary workings that is emotional as well as intellectual, in that it triggers feelings of awe and amazement.[10] So much can be gleaned if we compare *Problemata* 16.1 with a discussion of lead and its behaviour when it is poured into cold water in the Περὶ Θαυμασίων Ἀκουσμάτων:

> Θαυμαστὸν δέ τί φασιν ἐν Ἰνδοῖς περὶ τὸν ἐκεῖ μόλυβδον συμβαίνειν· ὅταν γὰρ τακεὶς εἰς ὕδωρ καταχυθῇ ψυχρόν, ἐκπηδᾶν ἐκ τοῦ ὕδατος.
>
> Among the Indians an extraordinary occurrence is told of the lead there; for when it is melted and poured into cold water it leaps out of the water.
>
> (*De Mirabilibus Auscultationibus* 61, 835a, transl. W.S. Hett)

The concept of θαυμαστόν is strategically placed at the very beginning of this wondrous ἄκουσμα, which reports that melted lead miraculously leaps out of cold water when it is poured into it. The cause or mechanism is not explained, however. This is typical of the collection as whole: the Περὶ Θαυμασίων Ἀκουσμάτων does not, as a rule, seek to provide explanations for the various θαύματα that it collects, but seeks to entice its audience precisely through the inexplicable or curious nature of the phenomena that it describes. In effect, the

9 See *Mir.* 832b, 833a, 835a, 836a, 836b, 837b, 839a, 844b. See also 838a, 839a, 841b for the use of the verb θαυμάζειν.

10 Cf. Nightingale 2004, 253–268, who argues that the archaic concept of wonder 'is never confined to cognitive experiences: archaic wonder is both cognitive and affective, intellectual and emotional, ranging from the feelings of reverence and awe to admiration and amazement.' (*ibid.*, 256). She contrasts this concept to the Aristotelian notion of wonder, which is tied to the investigation of causes and the search for scientific explanations.

reader of this collection is invited to treat amazement as a key lens through which nature can be experienced (namely, as a collection of miraculous phenomena which exceed, perhaps even preclude, human understanding, and thus effectively render nature an object of admiration).[11] This approach is the reason why the Περὶ Θαυμασίων Ἀκουσμάτων readily conforms to our concept of the 'paradoxographical' and is, hence, quite unproblematically labelled as a work of paradoxography.[12]

The pseudo-Aristotelian problem 16.1 similarly lacks an explanation for the physical attributes and behaviour of bubbles (e.g. why their base has no shadow, when the rest of the bubble does), but in its case it would be reasonable to assume that an attempt to explain the phenomenon might well have featured in the missing part of the text. So much is suggested by the opening question ('Why...?', seeking the causes of a natural phenomenon), which sets the tone for the problem's overall approach; and also by the last segment of the problem (913a24–29, not cited here), which refers the reader to works on optics. The development of an explanation would, moreover, have been in tune with the *Problemata* as a whole, where natural phenomena are not collected for their own sake, but with a view to understanding their causes or so that they can contribute to the investigation of the causes behind other phenomena.[13]

Another important difference is worth noting: Περὶ Θαυμασίων Ἀκουσμάτων 61 locates the wondrous phenomenon that it describes in a far-off place (India),[14] and attributes its knowledge to hearsay (underscored through the use of the verb φασίν, 'they say', cf. the term ἀκουσμάτων in the title). By contrast, in pseudo-Aristotelian problem 16.1, the phenomenon described is presented as something anyone can observe in nature, at every place where there is water. No claim to exclusive or exotic knowledge is made, apart from the fact that the ability adequately to explain the phenomenon requires a scientific manner of thinking (I will discuss this below). This difference in approach reveals the *Problemata*'s placement of wonder squarely within the practice of science instead of locating it predominantly in the remote, unusual, or exotic.

---

11 Cf. Porter 2016, 411–536, discussing wonder's instrumental role in treating nature as a sublime object in a wide range of ancient scientific writings.

12 See detailed discussion of the work's provenance and sources in Flashar 1990, 39–68; and Vanotti 2007, 5–53. See also Kazantzidis 2018 and in this volume.

13 See Menn 2015.

14 See also commentary by Flashar 1990, 97; Vanotti 2007, 159.

Revealing of the *Problemata*'s approach is the fact that, in one instance, namely, the third problem of book 12, it even goes so far as to question the truthfulness of a report concerning a phenomenon that ancient paradoxography would unreservedly characterize as miraculous. The problem enquires:

> <Διὰ τί> λέγεται [γὰρ ὡς] 'εὐώδη γίνεται τὰ δένδρα εἰς ἅπερ ἂν ἡ ἶρις κατασκήψῃ'; πότερον [οὖν] ἀληθές ἐστιν ἢ ψεῦδος; καὶ εἰ ἀληθές, διὰ <τίν'> αἰτίαν ἂν εἴη τὸ συμβαῖνον; ὅτι μὲν οὖν οὔτε πάντα οὔτε ἀεί, δῆλον· πολλάκις γὰρ ἡ ἶρις μὲν γέγονε, τὰ δὲ δένδρα οὐθὲν ἐπίδηλα φαίνεται. ὅταν τε γένηται τοῦτο, οὐκ ἐν πάσῃ γίνεται ὕλῃ, ἐπεὶ συμβαίνει γέ ποτε· διὸ καὶ λέγεται. τὸ δ' αἴτιον κατὰ συμβεβηκὸς τῇ ἴριδι ἀποδοτέον, ἄλλως τε καὶ εἰ μή ἐστί τις φύσις ἡ ἶρις, ἀλλὰ τῆς ὄψεως πάθος ἀνακλωμένης. [...]
>
> <Why> is it said: 'The trees upon which the rainbow has fallen become fragrant'? Now is this true or false? And if it is true, through what cause would there be this occurrence? Now it is clear that this is true neither for all (trees) nor always; for often the rainbow has come, but nothing noticeable appears with respect to the trees. And when this does occur, it does not occur in every wood (since it does happen sometimes, and this is why it is said). But the cause should be assigned to the rainbow only incidentally, especially if the rainbow is not a certain nature, but is an effect of refraction of the organ of sight. [...]
>
> (*Problemata* 12.3, 906a36–b6, transl. R. Mayhew)

The characteristic formulation λέγεται is also common in the Περὶ Θαυμασίων Ἀκουσμάτων, where wondrous tales about places, exotic plants and animals, stones, or substances are as a rule cited as reports or as 'stories that people say', using the verbs φασί (as in the example above) or λέγουσι, as in the following example:

> Λέγεται καὶ τοὺς γῦπας ὑπὸ τῆς τῶν μύρων ὀσμῆς ἀποθνήσκειν, ἐάν τις αὐτοὺς χρίσῃ ἢ δῷ τι μεμυρισμένον φαγεῖν. ὡσαύτως δὲ καὶ τοὺς κανθάρους ὑπὸ τῆς τῶν ῥόδων ὀσμῆς.
>
> Vultures are said to die from the scent of myrrh, if anyone smears it on them, or gives them anything steeped in myrrh to eat. In the same way beetles are said to die from the scent of roses.
>
> (*De Mirabilibus Auscultationibus* 147, 845a35–b3, transl. W.S. Hett)[15]

Questions of truthfulness such as the one problem 12.3 poses (πότερον [οὖν] ἀληθές ἐστιν ἢ ψεῦδος;) do not enter the equation in the Περὶ Θαυμασίων

15 See Flashar 1990, 144; Vanotti 2007, 211. Fragrance emitted from substances is also discussed in *Mir.* 831b, 832a, 841a. Cf. *Probl.* books 12–13 (whose topics are fragrant and malodorous things, respectively).

Ἀκουσμάτων. By contrast, for *Problemata* 12.3 the investigation of causes for the phenomenon would only be meaningful if the phenomenon were true, and the answer, part of which I have quoted, devotes considerable space to clarifying precisely this issue. As it argues, the phenomenon is only partly true: as it explains later on, it happens primarily to trees that have a great quantity of internal heat and which grow in hot and dry places that are renowned for their fragrant plants, such as exotic eastern locations like Syria and Arabia (906b12–20). Notably, the answer employs a logical distinction between accidental cause (κατὰ συμβεβηκὸς) and true cause, which testifies to its commitment to the Aristotelian theory of causality.[16] According to this distinction, the rainbow cannot be considered to be the real cause of the phenomenon, since it is not 'a certain nature' (τις φύσις), but a refraction of the organ of sight. Rather, the true cause is rainwater, which causes the trees to concoct (πέττειν) the water with their internal heat, and thus release fragrance (906b26–34).[17] Far, then, from being excluded from scientific investigation, miraculous phenomena within the *Problemata* appear to be fully 'normalised', in the sense that they are fully integrated into the wide gamut of natural phenomena whose causes the collection's various problem-type enquiries seek to explain by employing scientific observation and scientific reasoning.

The examples just discussed make it clear that, if we wish to comprehend the *Problemata*'s concept of the 'wondrous', we need to look beyond aspects of its material that seem to conform to our own notion of the natural wonder – a concept that is partly shaped by the fact that we perceive paradoxography as a distinct form of writing, or genre. In the remainder of this chapter, I will seek to discuss specifically in what terms, and on the basis of which epistemic notions the wondrous is marked within the *Problemata*, and how this concept informs its selection and treatment of medical and naturalistic topics.

16 On accidental causes in Aristotle, see Freeland 1991; Frede 1992.

17 See also the discussion by Flashar 1962, 552–553.

3 Wonder, Science and Paradoxical Problems

The *Problemata*'s notion of natural wonder must first and foremost be related to Aristotle's own concept of the wondrous and its connection to scientific investigation.[18] At several places within his works Aristotle treats θαῦμα as the main motive and propeller of scientific enquiry.[19] As he remarks in the treatise *On the Parts of Animals*:

> Διὸ δεῖ μὴ δυσχεραίνειν παιδικῶς τὴν περὶ τῶν ἀτιμοτέρων ζῴων ἐπίσκεψιν. Ἐν πᾶσι γὰρ τοῖς φυσικοῖς ἔνεστί τι θαυμαστόν· ... πρὸς τὴν ζήτησιν περὶ ἑκάστου τῶν ζῴων προσιέναι δεῖ μὴ δυσωπούμενον ὡς ἐν ἅπασιν ὄντος τινὸς φυσικοῦ καὶ καλοῦ.
>
> Therefore we must avoid a childish distaste for examining the less valued animals. For in all natural things there is something wonderful ... we should approach the enquiry about each animal without aversion, knowing that in all of them there is something natural and beautiful.
>
> (Aristotle, *De Partibus Animalium* 645a15–24, transl. D.M. Balme)

This is analogous to the notion of θαῦμα that, as Stephen Menn argues, runs through the *Problemata* as well. As he puts it:[20]

> Every problem in our *Physica Problemata* takes up something capable of causing θαῦμα, brings out the θαῦμα that it involves, and then tries to resolve this θαῦμα by offering an explanation ... The process of raising and resolving θαῦμα helps call our attention to the differences we are capable of perceiving in things, and helps lead us to knowledge of their causes. The more the θαῦμα is intensified, the more we will be motivated to seek causes, and the less likely we are to rest content with too vague and general an explanation.

Moreover, according to Hellmut Flashar, the notion of θαῦμα is underscored within the *Problemata* through a characteristic formulation in the enquiries, which he calls 'the paradoxical form'. He describes its typical format as follows:

> 'Why does phenomenon *x* have the effect *xa*, when one would expect it to have the effect *ya*, analogous to phenomenon *y*'?

or:

---

18 See Mansfeld 1992 on physical problems as a genre of scientific writing.

19 See detailed discussion in Llewelyn 2001; Nightingale 2004, 253–268; Menn 2015. See also Kazantzidis in this volume.

20 Menn 2015, 28.

'Why does phenomenon *x* have the effect *y*, when one would expect the opposite?'[21]

This formulation is indeed very common throughout the *Problemata*. The paradoxical nature of certain phenomena is additionally highlighted through the use of key phrases, namely, ἄτοπον ('curious') and [οὐκ] εἰκός/[οὐκ] εὐλόγως ('[not] reasonable/ [not] with good reason'), and sometimes even with the simple contrast μὲν... δὲ...[22] All such phrases underscore the fact that certain phenomena contravene or violate certain logical expectations in terms of the physical processes that seem to underpin them or the physiological responses that they elicit. Their use, instead of the terms θαῦμα/θαυμάσιος/θαυμαστός, foregrounds the cognitive rather than the affective aspect of θαῦμα within the *Problemata*. At the same time, the terms pose broader questions about the deeper epistemic beliefs which underpin the *Problemata*'s perception of the natural world, in terms of its mechanisms. To put it slightly differently, they urge us to consider on what conceptual grounds, and based on what sort of pre-existing categories or preconceptions about how the natural world ought to behave, the Peripatetic scientists who contributed to the *Problemata* considered certain phenomena to be more 'curious' or strange than others.

The three examples that I quote below can help us detect the first principle that underpins the notion of the 'wondrous' within the *Problemata*: namely, that a sort of intuitive physics informs our perception of the world. Processes or phenomena that are counterintuitive are those that generate ἀπορία and call for investigation. Notably, all three underscore the counterintuitive nature of the phenomena that they describe, by using the key terms ἄτοπον, εἰκός, and εὔλογον (all underlined below):

Διὰ τί φρίττουσι καὶ τῷ θερμῷ καὶ τῷ ψυχρῷ προσχεόμενοι; ἄτοπον γὰρ τὰ ἐναντία τοῦ αὐτοῦ εἶναι αἴτια. ἢ διότι ὑπὸ μὲν τοῦ ψυχροῦ προσχεόμενοι τὸ ἐντὸς θερμὸν σβεννύμενον ποιεῖ τὴν φρίκην, ὑπὸ δὲ τοῦ θερμοῦ τὸ ἐκτὸς ψυχρὸν ἀντιπεριιστάμενον εἰς ἓν καὶ ἀθροιζόμενον τῇ φυγῇ ἔσω; ὥστε ὑπὸ τοῦ αὐτοῦ ἄμφω γίνεται, ἀλλ' ὁτὲ μὲν ὑπὸ τοῦ ἔσω, ὁτὲ δὲ ὑπὸ τοῦ ἔξωθεν.

---

21 Flashar 1962, 299: '... Ganz fest ist dabei die Form: "Warum hat das Phänomen *x* die Wirkung *y*, nicht aber entsprechend das Phänomen *xa* die Wirkung *ya*?" Oder: "Warum hat das Phänomen *x* die Wirkung *y*, obwohl doch eigentlich das Gegenteil zu erwarten wäre?" Oft verbindet sich in den *Problemata* gerade mit dieser Form inhaltlich der Charakter des Mirakulösen (θαυμάσιον)'; and *ibid*., 342, when discussing the relationship between question-format and explanations within the *Probl.*: 'Am häufigsten is die paradoxe Form gewählt: "Warum liegt das Phänomen P vor, obwohl das Gegenteil zu erwarten wäre?"'

22 On these phrases, see Flashar 1962, 342–345. On μὲν... δὲ..., see, e.g. *Probl.* 10.6, 891b4–13; Flashar 1962, 343.

Why do people shiver when they are soaked in either hot or cold water? For it is strange that contrary things should be the causes of the same result. Is it because, in being soaked by cold water, the extinguishing of the internal heat produces shivering, but (in being soaked) by hot water, the external cold is enclosed in one place and gathered together by its flight inward? So both are brought about by the same thing, but in one case the cause is internal, in the other external.

(*Problemata* 8.11, 888a31–38, transl. R. Mayhew)

Διὰ τί ἀλγεινοτέρα ἡ πληγὴ τοῦ νάρθηκος ἢ ἐνίων σκληροτέρων, ἐάν τις κατὰ λόγον σκοπῇ τύπτων; εὐλογώτερον γὰρ τὴν τοῦ σκληροτέρου εἶναι ἀλγεινοτέραν· μᾶλλον γὰρ τύπτει. ἢ ὅτι ἡ σὰρξ ἀλγεῖ οὐ μόνον τυπτομένη ἀλλὰ καὶ τύπτουσα; ὑπὸ μὲν οὖν τῶν σκληρῶν τύπτεται μόνον (ὑπείκει γὰρ διὰ τὴν σκληρότητα αὐτῶν), ὑπὸ δὲ τοῦ νάρθηκος ἄμφω αὐτῇ συμβαίνει, τύπτεσθαί τε καὶ διὰ κουφότητα τοῦ βάρους τύπτειν μὴ εἴκουσαν, ὥστε διπλασία γίνεται ἡ πληγή.

Why is the blow from a fennel stalk more painful than from some harder things, if one considers it in proportion in delivering the strike? For it is more reasonable (to expect) that the blow of the harder thing would be more painful, for it delivers more of a strike. Is it because the flesh feels pain not only when being struck, but also when delivering the strike? Therefore, by the hard things it is only struck (for it yields owing to their hardness), but by the fennel stalk both effects are produced in it – it is struck, and owing to the lightness of the weight it also delivers the strike without yielding, so that the blow is double.

(*Problemata* 9.8, 890a36–b7, transl. R. Mayhew).

Διὰ τί τῶν γλυκέων ὄντων ὁμοιοτέρων ἡμῖν ἢ τῶν δριμέων, θᾶττον πληρούμεθα ὑπὸ τῶν γλυκέων; εἰκὸς δὲ ἦν ἧττον· ὑπὸ γὰρ τῶν ὁμοίων ἧττον ἦν εἰκὸς πληροῦσθαι. ἢ ὅτι οὐχ ὁμοίως τό τε ἀγγεῖον πληροῦται ταχύ, ἐξ οὗ πληρούμεθα, καὶ τὸ τρεφόμενον, ἀλλ' ἐνίοτε ἡ μὲν κοιλία πλήρης ἐστίν, οἷον τῶν διψώντων, τὸ δὲ δίψος οὐδὲν ἧττόν ἐστιν. οὐ γὰρ τῷ ταύτην εἶναι πλήρη παυόμεθα διψῶντες, ἀλλὰ τῷ ἕκαστον τῶν τοῦ σώματος τὸ αὑτῷ οἰκεῖον ἐσπακέναι, καὶ ὅταν ἐκεῖνα ἀπολάβῃ ἱκανῶς, τότε παυόμεθα διψῶντες. καὶ πεινῶντες δὲ ὡσαύτως.

Why, although what is sweet is more akin to us than what is acrid, are we filled more quickly by what is sweet? It seems natural that we should be less so, since it seems natural to be filled less by what is akin to us. Is it because the vessel from which we are filled and the body that is nourished are not filled equally quickly, but sometimes the stomach is full, for example in those who are thirsty, but the thirst is no less? For we do not cease being thirsty through the stomach being full, but through each part of the body having drawn in its own proper liquid, and when they have received this sufficiently, then we cease being thirsty. And it's the same way with being hungry.

(*Problemata* 22.2, 930a14–23, transl. R. Mayhew)

Starting with the first problem (8.11), what is at issue is the fact that two opposing processes (hot and cold baths) bring about the same result in the body, namely, shivering. The second problem (9.8) next puts into question the presumption that heavy bodies produce greater pain in the body when they strike it than light bodies. The third problem (22.2) finally wonders how we can feel more quickly sated by nourishment that is sweet, when in fact we should seek more of it, since it is more akin/similar to us (if 'akin/similar' is understood here in the sense of more compatible with/acceptable by the body, by virtue of being more pleasant). In all three cases, we are dealing with bodily responses to the external environment that confound intuitive expectations about how nature should work: shivering is normally associated with cold, not with heat; light objects are not expected to cause more pain to bodies when they strike them than are heavy objects; one should like sweet things and want more of them.

The explanations provided in each case demonstrate that these are phenomena to which causes can be attributed, provided that one goes beyond common intuition and seeks to understand their actual mechanism: thus, the first problem (8.11) employs scientific concepts, such as internal heat (τὸ ἐντὸς θερμὸν),[23] and the notion that substances collect in one place when pressured by opposite forces (ἀντιπεριιστάμενον), so as to call attention to the precise mechanisms that regulate the body's interaction with or reaction to changes in the external environment. The explanation resolves the apparent contradiction by stating that the cause is the same (ὑπὸ τοῦ αὐτοῦ) – meaning that the body becomes cold either when its internal heat is extinguished (because of the cold water) or when the external cold that surrounds it resists (through the mechanism of ἀντιπερίστασις), so to speak, the influence of external heat by 'fleeing' inside the body and thus cooling it.[24] The approach is similar in the second problem (9.8), which emphasises the counterintuitive nature of the physical mechanism according to which the flesh reacts to blows: when hit by harder things, the flesh simply yields (and therefore hurts less); when hit by a fennel stalk, which is a light object, it resists, and this feels like a double blow. Last but not least, the third problem (22.2) attempts to answer its question (in a rather unsatisfactory fashion) by formulating a general theory about the nature of thirst and hunger: thus, it argues

23 Cf. the concept of heat in Aristotle's biology, with Freudenthal 1999, esp. 7–73. See also Ulacco 2007, on heat in connection to disease within the *Probl.*

24 See Flashar 1962, 295–383, on the main scientific concepts that appear within the *Probl.* and their provenance (including the Peripatetic concept of ἀντιπερίστασις).

that the body is nourished through the stomach but takes longer than the stomach to feel full. This explains why thirst and hunger may persist even after we seem to have satisfied them through nourishment or drink.

On the basis of these case-studies, one can argue that a key aim of the so-called 'paradoxical form' in medical-natural problems within the *Problemata* is to illustrate how science can explain mechanisms in nature that intuitive thinking cannot – provided that one follows rules of scientific reasoning, is in command of a rich arsenal of scientific knowledge, and can utilise key scientific concepts flexibly and effectively. Further, the three paradoxical problems share a broader goal of placing the body in nature, by discovering the full range and complexity of mechanisms and principles that govern its interaction with the natural environment. Thus, each offers the opportunity to reflect on key points of contact between medicine and naturalist enquiry.[25]

Secondly, the *Problemata*'s notion of the 'wondrous' is predicated on the presence of unique or exceptional features in bodies or substances that belong in certain categories. When an animal or a substance differs in various respects from animals or substances in the same category, these differences trigger an investigation of their causes,[26] as seen in the following examples:

> Διὰ τί ἡ θάλαττα μόνον τῶν ὑδάτων κάεται, τὰ δὲ πότιμα καὶ ποτάμια οὔ; πότερον ὅτι γῆν πολλὴν ἔχει; δηλοῦσι δὲ οἱ ἅλες. ἢ διότι λιπαρά; δηλοῖ δὲ τὸ ἐν τοῖς ἅλασιν ὑφιστάμενον ἔλαιον.
>
> Why does the sea alone of waters burn, whereas fresh water and river water do not? Is it because it contains a lot of earth? The salt proves this. Or is it because it is oily? The oil forming on salt proves this.
>
> (*Problemata* 23.32, 935a5–8,
> transl. R. Mayhew, cf. 23.15)
>
> Διὰ τί ἄνθρωπος μόνον ἴσχει λεύκην; πότερον ὅτι λεπτοδερμότατον τῶν ζῴων ἐστίν, ἅμα δὲ καὶ πνευματωδέστερον; σημεῖον δέ, ὅτι ἡ λεύκη ἐν τοῖς λεπτοδερμοτάτοις μάλιστα καὶ πρῶτον γίνεται μέρεσιν. ἢ διὰ ταῦτά τε, καὶ ὅτι μόνον πολιοῦται τῶν ζῴων; ἐν γὰρ ταῖς λεύκαις πολιαὶ γίνονται αἱ τρίχες, ὥστε ἀδύνατον, ὅσα μὴ πολιοῦται, λεύκην ἴσχειν.
>
> Why does the human alone have the white disease? Is it because he is the thinnest-skinned of animals, and at the same time very full of breath? Now a sign of this is the fact that the white disease occurs most and first on the parts where the skin is thinnest. Or is it for this reason too, i.e. that the human alone of animals turns gray? For in cases of the white disease

---

25 See Menn 2015 and Oikonomopoulou 2015.

26 Cf. the importance of difference in Aristotle's classification of animals. See esp. Balme 1961 and 1987; Lennox 1999.

> the hair becomes gray, so that those animals whose hair does not turn gray cannot have the white disease.
>
> (*Problemata* 10.5, 891a35–b3, transl. R. Mayhew, cf. 10.33)

The first problem (23.32), from book 23 of the *Problemata*, which is concerned with sea water, enquires after a strange property of sea water (the fact that it is flammable) that differentiates it from drinkable water or water from rivers (ἡ θάλαττα μόνον τῶν ὑδάτων κάεται, τὰ δὲ πότιμα καὶ ποτάμια οὔ). The difference is attributed to the sea's unique properties, namely, the presence of earthy matter (as evinced by the presence of salt) and of oiliness.[27] Analogous examples can be found in book 10 of the *Problemata*, entitled 'Epitome of natural things', which heavily draws on Aristotle's zoological works.[28] There, uniqueness is in the overwhelming majority of cases attributed to humans. Thus, the second problem (10.5) asks why humans alone of all animals have the white disease (λεύκην, 10.5, cf. 10.33).[29] The emphasis on the uniqueness of this feature is what triggers the enquiry, as humans appear as an anomaly or a notable exception in the animal world.[30] The explanation explores the cause by referring to other unique features of humans (they have the thinnest skin among all animals; they are the only animal whose hair turns gray) – thus underscoring their distinctness even more. Human uniqueness is highlighted in other enquiries as well, which stress various features, in terms of which humans stand out: they are the only animal whose nostrils can bleed; their offspring do not resemble their parents; they have the smallest distance between their eyes; they sneeze the most; they don't have a mane; they can emit many voices; they stammer; they can be born lame; they have gallstones, large navels, and so on. It is clear from both examples that uniqueness is construed in terms of the possession of unusual or remarkable features, and less in terms of differences in basic physiological functions or attributes shared across animals.

In fact, it is notable that when such basic physiological functions or attributes are mentioned, humans are not found to be unique, but usually to share features with some animals. So much is clear from problem 10.6, in which humans

---

27 On problems pertaining to the properties of the sea within the *Probl.*, see Wilson 2015.

28 Also in the books that are concerned with the human body (31–38). On book 10, see Stoyles 2015.

29 See Flashar 1962, 507 on the likely source of this problem (Arist. *De Gen. Anim.* 784a27 f.).

30 Cf. Kazantzidis 2018 on the relative absence of human oddities in early paradoxography (including the *De Mirabilibus Auscultationibus*).

and cattle are compared to sheep and goats in terms of a specific feature, namely, the production of milk:

> Διὰ τί αἶγες μὲν καὶ πρόβατα ἀμέλγονται πλεῖστον γάλα, οὐ μέγιστον σῶμα ἔχοντα, ἄνθρωπος δὲ καὶ βοῦς ἔλαττον ὡς κατὰ λόγον; πότερον ὅτι εἰς τὸ σῶμα ἀναλίσκεται, τοῖς δὲ ἄλλοις εἰς τὸ περίττωμα, τοῖς δὲ προβάτοις καὶ ταῖς αἰξὶ τὸ περιγινόμενον τοῦ περιττώματος γάλα γίνεται πᾶν; ἢ ὅτι πολυτοκώτερά ἐστι τῶν μεγάλων, ὥστε πλεῖον σπᾷ περίττωμα διὰ τὸ πλείω τρέφειν; ἢ δι' ἀσθένειαν τῶν σωμάτων πλεῖον περίττωμα γίνεται κύουσιν αὐτοῖς; τὸ δὲ γάλα γίνεται ἐκ τοῦ περιττώματος.
>
> Why do goats and sheep provide the most milk, though they do not have the largest bodies, while humans and cattle give proportionally less? Is it because (in humans and cattle) it is used up on the body, and among the other animals it is used up on residues, but in sheep and in goats all of what remains of the residue becomes milk? Or is it because (sheep and goats) have a greater number of offspring than the large animals, so that they draw off more residue because they have more (offspring) to nourish? Or is it that, owing to the weakness of their bodies, more residue is formed during their gestation period? And the milk comes from residue.
>
> (*Problemata* 10.6, 891b4–13, transl. R. Mayhew)

The criterion for grouping animals together in this problem is their relative similarities and differences, all marked through the employment of a series of contrasts, each applying to a different feature (goats and sheep, vs. humans and bovines, small vs. large body, large vs. small production of milk), and highlighted through the use of the μὲν... δὲ... formulation, itself indicative of the so-called 'paradoxical' form of scientific problem, according to Flashar (see above).[31] What groups humans together with cattle, according to the question, is their comparatively low production of milk, as well as the fact that they are relatively large animals. The problem compares them with smaller animals, such as goats and sheep, which produce comparatively more milk, in order to formulate a paradox, at the root of which lies the presumption (itself based on common sense reasoning) that the quantity of milk an animal produces should be proportionate to the size of its body. The explanation offers a sound (scientific) basis for considering these similarities and differences by attributing them to shared underlying physiological processes. According to this understanding, in humans and cattle the leftover residue (περίττωμα) is used up in the body, when in other animals it is converted either into milk (in the case of goats and sheep) or into more residue. Other enquiries in the same book compare humans to pigs, sheep, horses and

---

31 See also Flashar 1962, 507–508 for a detailed discussion of the problem's concepts and argument.

asses, or birds on the basis of similar reasoning, and employing analogous explanations.

It is clear from all the examples that have been discussed in this section that the wonder that is caused by unique or exceptional attributes in animals or substances serves as a tool for categorising reality. Once more, our intuitive classification of the world in terms of fundamental categories such as 'animal', 'liquids', 'plants' forms the basis for issuing further divisions and sub-divisions: thus, the fact that sea water possesses unique attributes such as flammability means that it constitutes a special category of water – and this aspect is in fact reflected in the *Problemata*'s book-divisions, which reserve a special book (23) for the sea and another one for hot water (24) – but no separate book for fresh waters. Similarly, when we look at the case of humans and animals in book 10, the emphasis on the uniqueness of humans forms a special point of focus for the *Problemata*: where Aristotle sought to develop a systematic method of classifying all animals in his zoological works, the *Problemata* appears to foreground the investigation of humans over that of the other animals. This is, once more, reflected in its book-divisions: book 1 treats medical topics, and the last 8 books (31–38) topics dealing with various parts of the human body (the eyes, the ears, the nostril, the mouth, the face as a whole).[32]

4 Paradoxical Problems vs. Non-paradoxical Ones

Is the so-called 'paradoxical form' of problems the only way to conceive of and locate the 'wondrous' in nature and in animal bodies within the *Problemata*? This question is inevitable once a reader has taken in the collection's vast scope, extending over 38 books, and immense variety of subject-matter, devoted to almost all aspects of nature. In fact, most books of the *Problemata* contain a mixture of problems that have the simple form 'why is x so?' and those that have the 'paradoxical form'. The choices of the collection's compilers may become clearer if we examine cases of parallel or reduplicated problems, which occur at several places across the *Problemata*'s books.[33] Such cases are problems 22.2 and 22.3, the first of which we have already discussed above.

---

32 See Oikonomopoulou 2015, on the *Problemata*'s medical books.

33 The presence of parallel problems or replicated problems is a feature that stems mainly from the fact that the collection is a collective work, in which successive Peripatetic scientists provided input, often revisiting enquiries from a fresh perspective. See Jacob 2004 and Oikonomopoulou 2015 for an overview.

As we already saw, problem 22.2 is formulated as a paradox ('Why, although what is sweet is more akin to us than what is acrid, are we filled more quickly by what is sweet? It seems natural that we should be less so, since it seems natural to be filled less by what is akin to us.'). The enquiry is introduced in such a way that the emphasis falls upon the unreasonableness of the fact that we acquire the feeling of fullness more quickly from sweet foods than by acrid foods. The follow-up problem, 22.3, on the other hand, poses the same question in a simpler format, yet in such a way that it puts into sharper focus the fundamental question of difference that lies at the heart of the problem:

> Διὰ τί θᾶττον πληρούμεθα ἀπὸ τῶν γλυκέων ἢ ἀπὸ τῶν δριμέων;
>
> Why are we full more quickly from what is sweet than from what is acrid?
>
> (*Problemata* 22.3, 930a24, transl. R. Mayhew)

This is a question format that invites equal consideration of the properties of sweet and acrid foods and their respective value as nourishment, and indeed the three alternative answers that follow (930a25–38, not cited here) attempt to address precisely these issues. They distinguish between actual fullness and the fulfilment of desire for food (in the second answer); and they discuss acrid and sweet foods in terms of their respective nourishing properties (the third explanation stating that acrid things are not nourishment proper: τὰ μὲν οὖν δριμέα οὐκ ἔστι τρόφιμα, ἀλλὰ τροφὴν μὲν ὀλίγην ἔχει, τὸ δὲ περίττωμα πολύ, 930a31–32). Therefore, it is reasonable that one never feels full by eating them (εἰκότως οὖν πολλὰ ταῦτα ζητοῦμεν ἐσθίειν, 930a32). Moreover, the answer seeks to address issues raised by the first question, for example by affirming the premise of the problem 22.2 that sweet foods are more akin or similar to us (they constitute nourishment proper, as it says: τὰ δὲ γλυκέα ἅπαντά ἐστι τροφή, 930a34). Seen together as a unit, problems 22.2 and 22.3 illustrate how wonder as an initial response to nature's hidden mechanisms can lead to a persistent line of scientific enquiry, its principal goal being to provide as satisfactory an explanation as possible for these mechanisms.

Clearly then, the so-called 'paradoxical form' that Flashar identifies does not fully account for the *Problemata*'s rich and varied ways of conveying its wonder at seemingly inexplicable aspects of nature, nor does it always guarantee the satisfactory treatment of medical or naturalist topics in the explanations afforded by the collection's compilers. It does, however, achieve the goal of drawing the reader into the scientific observer's world of curiosity, as well as drawing attention to the conceptual principles that guide scientific investigation.

5 Conclusion: *Problemata* and Ancient Paradoxography

The association of wonder with scientific enquiry that runs through the *Problemata* was bequeathed to the subsequent tradition of medical-natural *Problemata*-writing represented by imperial authors such as Plutarch (particularly in his Αἴτια Φυσικά)[34] and pseudo-Alexander of Aphrodisias.[35] These authors too include a blend of topics, some of which fall under our own notion of the paradoxographical, while others convey the notion of wonder at the workings of nature through their treatment of topics from everyday life or the sciences. The role writers of *Problemata* played in shaping the paradoxographical genre in the ancient Greek and Roman world remains to be investigated.[36] Similarly, the role the pseudo-Aristotelian collection Περὶ Θαυμασίων Ἀκουσμάτων played in this tradition deserves to be accounted for in more detail. To return to the earlier comparisons I drew between the *Problemata* with the pseudo-Aristotelian Περὶ Θαυμασίων Ἀκουσμάτων, they seem to suggest that the two collections' differing treatments of the miraculous, in the case of the *Problemata* being close to Aristotle's own notion of θαῦμα, and in the case of the Περὶ Θαυμασίων Ἀκουσμάτων collecting θαυμάσια for their own sake, might represent divisions of knowledge that existed within the Peripatetic school. At the moment, and while there is still no systematic investigation of the relationship between the two works, this too remains an open question.

Bibliography

Balme, D.M. (1961), "Aristotle's Use of Differentiae in Zoology", in: S. Mansion (ed.), *Aristote e les problèmes de méthode*, Louvain, 195–212.

Balme, D.M. (1972: 1992), *Aristotle, 'De Partibus Animalium' I and 'De Generatione Animalium' I (with passages from II.1–3)*, Oxford.

Balme, D.M. (1987), "Aristotle's Use of Division and Differentiae", in: A. Gotthelf /J.G. Lennox (eds.), *Philosophical Issues in Aristotle's Biology*, Cambridge, 69–89.

Flashar, H. (1962), *Aristoteles: Problemata Physica*, Berlin.

34 On Plutarch's *Quaest. nat.*, see Meeusen 2015 and the detailed study and commentary of the text by Meeusen 2016.

35 See Meeusen in this volume.

36 See Meeusen in this volume, for an examination of pseudo-Alexander of Aphrodisias' *Medical Puzzles and Natural Problems.*

Flashar, H./Klein, U. (1990), *Aristoteles: Mirabilia, De Audibilibus*, Berlin.
Frede, D. (1992), "Accidental Causes in Aristotle", *Synthese* 92.1, 39–62.
Freeland, C. (1991), "Accidental Causes and Real Explanations", in: L. Judson (ed.), *Aristotle's Physics: A Collection of Essays*, Oxford, 49–72.
Freudenthal, G. (1999), *Aristotle's Theory of Material Substance: Heat and Pneuma, Form and Soul*, Oxford.
Hett, W.S. (1955), *Aristotle: Minor Works* (Loeb Classical Library), Cambridge, Mass.
Jacob, C. (2004), "Questions sur les questions: archéologie d'une pratique intellectuelle et d'une forme discursive", in: A. Volgers/C. Zamagni (eds.), *Erotapokriseis. Early Christian Question-and-Answer Literature in Context. Proceedings of the Utrecht Colloquium, 13–14 October 2003*, Leuven, 25–54.
Kazantzidis, G. (2018), "Medicine and the Paradox in the Hippocratic Corpus and Beyond", in: M. Gerolemou (ed.), *Recognizing Miracles in Antiquity and Beyond*, Berlin/Boston, 31–61.
Lennox, J. (1999), "The Place of Mankind in Aristotle's Zoology", *Philosophical Topics* 27.1, 1–16.
Leunissen, M. (2015), "The Ethnography of *Problemata* 14 in (its mostly Aristotelian) Context", in: R. Mayhew (ed.), *The Aristotelian Problemata Physica. Philosophical and Scientific Investigations*, Leiden/Boston, 190–213.
Llewelyn, J. (2001), "On the Saying that Philosophy begins in *thaumazein*", *Afterall: A Journal of Art, Context and Enquiry* 4, 48–57.
Louis, P. (1991–1994), *Aristote: Problèmes*, 3 vols, Paris.
Mansfeld, J. (1992), "*Physikai Doxai* and *Problêmata Physika* from Aristotle to Aëtius (and Beyond)", in: W.W. Fortenbaugh/D. Gutas (eds.), *Theophrastus: His Psychological, Doxographical, and Scientific Writings*, New Brunswick, NJ, 63–111.
Marenghi, G. (1965), *Aristotele: Problemi di Medicina: Testo Critico, Traduzione e Commento*, Milan.
Mayhew, R. (2011), *Aristotle: Problems*: vol. 1 (*Books 1–19*), vol. 2 (*Books 20–38*, with D. Mirhady, [Arist.] *Rhet. to Alex.*) (Loeb Classical Library), Cambridge, Mass.
Meeusen, M. (2015), "Plutarch Solving Natural Problems: For What Cause? (The Case of *Quaest. nat.* 29, 919AB", in: M. Meeusen/L. Van der Stockt (eds.), *Natural Spectaculars: Aspects of Plutarch's Philosophy of Nature*, Leuven, 129–142.
Meeusen, M. (2016), *Plutarch's Science of Natural Problems: A Study with Commentary on Quaestiones Naturales*, Leuven.
Menn, S. (2015), "Democritus, Aristotle, and the *Problemata*", in: R. Mayhew (ed.), *The Aristotelian Problemata Physica. Philosophical and Scientific Investigations*, Leiden/Boston, 1–35.
Nightingale, A.W. (2004), *Spectacles of Truth in Ancient Greek Philosophy: 'Theoria' in its Cultural Context*, Cambridge.
Oikonomopoulou, K. (2015), "The *Problemata*'s Medical Books: Structural and Methodological Aspects", in: R. Mayhew (ed.), *The Aristotelian Problemata Physica. Philosophical and Scientific Investigations*, Leiden/Boston, 61–78.
Porter, J.I. (2016), *The Sublime in Antiquity*, Cambridge.
Stoyles, B.J. (2015), "Material and Teleological Explanations in *Problemata* 10", in: R. Mayhew (ed.), *The Aristotelian Problemata Physica. Philosophical and Scientific Investigations*, Leiden/Boston, 124–150.

Ulacco, A. (2007), “Malattia e alterazione del calore naturale: medicina ippocratica e fisiologia aristotelica negli *hosa iatrika* e in altri *Problemata* pseudo-Aristotelici”, in: B. Centrone (ed.), *Studi su Problemata Physica Aristotelici, Elenchos* LVIII, Pisa, 59–88.
Vanotti, G. (2007), *Aristotele, Racconti Meravigliosi*, Milan.
Wilson, M. (2015), “On *Problemata* 23: Little Problems on the Vast Sea”, in: R. Mayhew (ed.), *The Aristotelian Problemata Physica. Philosophical and Scientific Investigations*, Leiden/ Boston, 272–293.

Floris Overduin

In the Realm of the Two-Headed Snake

Pragmatics and Aesthetics of *Mirabilia* in Nicander's *Theriaca* and *Alexipharmaca*

Abstract: This paper aims to shed light on the relationship between the poetry of Nicander of Colophon (second century BCE) and the Hellenistic tradition of paradoxography. While the latter has its own origins (to a certain extent parallel to aetiology) and very different aims and characteristics, paradoxography does appear to have been an important influence on Nicander's poetry. Despite the fact that the *mirabilia* in Nicander hardly follow any of paradoxography's conventions (there is no signposting by the author; his poetry lacks the language of marvel; assumed *paradoxa* hardly stand out), the *mirabilia* themselves are important colours on Nicander's palette, with which the poet provides a smooth blend of the real and the fantastic within his poetics of pharmacological agitation.

1 Introduction

What do the two-headed snake, the flying scorpion, and the lethal 'headpecker' have in common? Not only are they all denizens of the poetic world of the late Hellenistic poet Nicander of Colophon, but they also stand out as *mirabilia*, phenomena that seem to belong to the world of wonders, the world paradoxography aimed to capture, rather than the humdrum common world. Paradoxically, of course, the essence of paradoxography is that the real world cannot be separated from the world of wonders – the essence is that ours *is* a world of wonders. Which role does this world of wonders play within Nicander's epic-didactic poetry? Is it something to be marvelled at, to be questioned, or to be explained? In this chapter first I will briefly contextualize the concept of paradoxography by focusing on its relation with aetiology, as well as marking the differences between the efforts of 'proper' paradoxographers and the paradoxographical activities of poets, for which Nicander will be a particular case. Then I will collect some typical instances of *paradoxa* in Nicander's poetry, in order to try to assess how such paradoxographical elements are put to use by the poet.

https://doi.org/10.1515/9783110661774-004

2 Paradoxography and Aetiology: A Parallel Development?

The development of paradoxography, i.e. an interest in collecting isolated instances of unnatural or counternatural oddities, does not seem to be unrelated to the development of aetiology, i.e. an interest in pointing out the origins of cults and other phenomena, particularly with a focus on etymology and on first inventors or first initiators.[1] To be sure, the concepts of paradoxography and aetiology themselves do not evidently share many features, but their historical progress is closely connected to the facilities offered by the newly founded research institutes, the availability of libraries, which started to appear in the third century BCE.[2] Although aetiology is much older than Callimachus, it is Callimachus who is often considered to be the founder of aetiology as a genre in its own right.[3] Scattered aetiologies existed, but the very composition of a work, a poem, called the *Aetia* ('Causes'), drew the attention of many to aetiology as a specific branch of literature, a collection focused not on narrative but on the shared topic of sorting out the roots of certain customs and habits.[4] Thus a development had come to fruition, from the complete absence of emphatically recorded aetiology in Homer, to a full-blown autonomous genre in the Hellenistic period.

This development of aetiology seems quite similar to the development of paradoxography from a complete absence of true *paradoxa* in Homer to the genesis of paradoxograpy in that same Hellenistic age.[5] And just like *aetia* existed in the fifth century BCE without usually being noticed as such, the classical period knew of plenty of *paradoxa* in literature, without paradoxography existing as a coherent genre before the third century BCE.[6] Aetiology and paradoxography

1 For the characteristics of paradoxography, on which this brief chapter merely touches, see e.g. Schepens/Delcroix 1996, 380–382; Pajón Leyra 2011, 29–32. For paradoxography in Nicander, see also Jacques 2002, lxxviii–xc.

2 Cf. Pajón Leyra 2011, 51–56.

3 Ziegler 1949, 1140; Fraser 1972, 775; Schepens/Delcroix 1996, 383–384.

4 Cf. Harder 2012, 24–27.

5 Next to Callimachus (whose paradoxographical collection was in prose), the genre was advocated early by Philostephanus, Callimachus Junior, and Archelaus (the three of them practitioners of metrical paradoxography) and Bolus of Mendes; see Fraser 1972, 778–780. The prose collection of Aristotle is pseudepigraphic, which may also be the case for Antigonus of Carystus; see n.8. For a general overview of sources, see Pajón Leyra 2011, 99–172.

6 One could argue that a possible exception to this development is the *Indica* of the fifth century BCE doctor and writer Ctesias, a work full of natural *paradoxa*. But it is particulary the present

share a development that only comes to full realisation in a world of books, a world in which one can make literature out of existing literature. Through the process of ἐκλογή, collecting, excerpting and sorting out sources, both aetiologists and paradoxographers picked and mixed their nascent genres into existence.[7] Occasionally, however, the two coincided (or rather: sided), as in one of the stories found in pseudo-Antigonus of Carystus, which is the most prominent and best preserved paradoxographical collection to survive:[8]

> Ἀμελησαγόρας δὲ ὁ Ἀθηναῖος, ὁ τὴν Ἀτθίδα συγγεγραφώς, οὔ φησι κορώνην προσίπτασθαι πρὸς τὴν ἀκρόπολιν, οὐδ' ἔχοι ἂν εἰπεῖν ἑωρακὼς οὐδείς. ἀποδίδωσιν δὲ τὴν αἰτίαν μυθικῶς [...]
>
> ([Antig.] *Mir.* fr. 12.1-2 Musso = *FGrHist* 330 F 1)

> Amelesagoras the Athenian, who wrote the *Atthis*, says that crows do not fly up to the Acropolis, and no one can say that he has seen one there; and he gives the reason in a story [...]
>
> (my transl.)

Within Antigonus' collection, this natural (or rather counternatural) oddity is concerned with the observation that the crow never makes its appearance on the Acropolis, which, though not a particularly spectacular story per se, is unnatural to the observer and therefore qualifies for inclusion in pseudo-Antigonus' collection of *mirabilia*.[9] The fragment is, however, also of interest from an aetiological perspective, since it continues with an *aition* accounting for this

---

state of the *Indica* that gives it the appearance of a paradoxographical work, a collection of selected marvels. In its original shape – a full monograph on India – the *paradoxa* must have been simply exciting elements within a bigger picture. As such the *Indica* must have been somewhat closer to e.g. Herodotus' *Histories*, viz. a historical work containing *paradoxa* rather than a work on *paradoxa*, regardless of the fact that Ctesias' work is much more fantastic and much less reliable throughout.

7 Cf. Schepens/Delcroix 1996, 389–394.

8 This collection, *Ἱστοριῶν παραδόξων συναγωγή*, attributed to Antigonus of Carystus (a late third century BCE scholar, sculptor, and art critic active in Pergamon), is essentially made up of extracts from pseudo-Aristotle's *Περὶ θαυμασίων ἀκουσμάτων* (830a) and from Callimachus' *Θαυμάσια* (*Θαυμάτων τῶν εἰς ἅπασαν τὴν γῆν κατὰ τόπους ὄντων συναγωγή*, fr. 407 Pf.). According to Musso (1985, 9: *neque probabilis est neque vera*) the ascription to Antigonus is false, but cf. Fraser 1972, 454 and Schepens/Delcroix 1996, 401. According to the latter, Antigonus aimed to surpass Callimachus in quality and thrustworthiness, showing that Pergamene scholarship was by no means inferior to that of the Alexandrians.

9 This could be considered a 'negative' *paradoxon*. Instead of signalling a remarkable phenomenon, the *paradoxon* exists in the absence of what one would have expected, which still is remarkable and counternatural.

phenomenon. Here Amelesagoras not only provides an aetiology (ἀποδίδωσιν δὲ τὴν αἰτίαν) to mark the object of wonder, but also subsequently explains it through a story (μυθικῶς).[10] This is somewhat exceptional, as the two genres mostly seem to have led separate, though in a sense parallel, lives. Yet the combination is not unique, and some examples will follow.[11]

3 Status of Paradoxography

Aetiology and paradoxography witnessed similar developments. But whereas aetiology, at least initially, remained primarily associated with poets (notably Apollonius of Rhodes and Callimachus), paradoxographers are generally considered an offspring of the historiographers.[12] This may be related to the fact that Herodotus, whose *Histories* harbour quite a few *paradoxa*, was ultimately first and foremost considered a historian, certainly not a mere collector of oddities. It is therefore natural – although also somewhat limited, as poetry has mainly been overlooked – that studies on paradoxography tended to concentrate on the historiographers. This is clearly reflected in one of the very few studies on paradoxography *per se*, published by Flemish scholars Schepens and Delcroix.[13] Their citation from Schmid and Stählin is indicative, the latter calling paradoxography "ein Parasitengewächs am Baum der historischen und naturwissenschaftlichen Litteratur."[14]

Although the study of Schepens and Delcroix is useful and offers a welcome and stuctured overview of the primary source material, it starts out from the problematic relationship between serious historiography and less serious paradoxo-

10 The aetiological story that follows states that the crow was banned from the Acropolis by Athena, because it reported bad news to her. Athena was just carrying the Lycabettus hill to the Acropolis as a bulwark, but when she was told by the crow that Erichthonius had been revealed (the daughters of Cecrops had opened the chest in which Erichthonius was locked) she threw down the mountain in anger and took out her rage on the crow; [Antig.] *Mir.* fr. 12 Musso.

11 One of the main distinctions between paradoxography and aetiology is of course that the latter's focus is on explaining, whereas the paradoxographers focused on the marvel itself, inspiring awe and wonder. To explain a miracle is to undermine its very nature; cf. Schepens/Delcroix 1996, 391.

12 For an overview of the aetiological nature of the *Argonautica* see e.g. Köhnken 2010, 136–150; for Callimachus see e.g. Harder 2003, 290–292; Harder 2012, 24–26 (with references).

13 Schepens/Delcroix 1996.

14 Schmid/Stählin 1920–1924, 237.

graphy. And although it is to their credit that they focus on the virtues of paradoxography as a viable and acceptable genre *sui generis*, the comparison with serious historiography and proper scholarship is never really out of sight. This approach yields many insights into the nature of the paradoxographers, but it gives little attention to e.g. the influence of paradoxography on contemporary literary developments. Hellenistic book literature not only contributed to the birth and dissemination of paradoxography, but in turn paradoxography also seems to have contributed to the composition of book literature, which contained a fair share of *paradoxa*. The monograph of Pajón Leyra, in addition, serves the study of paradoxography well indeed, particularly in its attention to paradoxography as 'popular science', but the focus is understandably on the paradoxographers, not on *paradoxa* elsewhere.[15]

In this paper I will not focus on paradoxography itself, but on the role of *paradoxa* in the pharmacological poetry of Nicander of Colophon (second century BCE), who, as a didactic-epic poet, wrote two substantial poems in hexameters. The *Theriaca* (958 lines) deals with the treatment of wounds inflicted by venomous animals, whereas the *Alexipharmaca* (630 lines) deals with the treatment of poisoning caused by plants and other natural substances.[16] Although the *mirabilia* found in Nicander do not concern medicine directly, the pharmacological nature of Nicander's poetry at least connects him to this volume's topic. The nature of Nicander's material, i.e. plants and animals, is, moreover the very domain that is often associated with paradoxography: marvels of the natural world. Proto-Hellenistic examples of such natural *paradoxa* can of course easily be found in Herodotus' *Histories* and in the remains of Ctesias' *Indika*. But whereas these authors explicitly highlight their own amazement or disbelief at the phenomena encountered, Nicander does not.[17] By using the technical poetry of Nicander as a case study, I hope to show that for at least some poets the use of *paradoxa* may have served a different purpose than the one we find within the paradoxographical collections.

15 Pajón Leyra 2011.

16 For general details regarding the *Theriaca* see Gow/Scholfield 1953; Jacques 2002; Overduin 2015. For the *Alexipharmaca* see Gow/Scholfield 1953; Jacques 2007. A good general introduction to Nicander and his output is Magnelli 2014, 211–223. Also useful in its details is Touwaide 1991.

17 E.g. Hdt. 3.12, *θῶμα δὲ μέγα εἶδον* πυθόμενος παρὰ τῶν ἐπιχωρίων, remarking on the extraordinary thickness of the skulls of the Egyptians; e.g. Ctes. F1b 5, περὶ δὲ τὸν τόπον ὅπου τὸ βρέφος ἐξετέθη πλήθους περιστερῶν ἐννεοττευόντος, *παραδόξως καὶ δαιμονίως* ὑπὸ τούτων τὸ παιδίον διατρέφεσθαι, remarking on the fact that an exposed baby was miraculously nourished by doves who happened to be nesting nearby.

4 Paradoxography versus Nicander's Poetry

Although Nicander is fond of *paradoxa*, and occasionally incorporates them into his poetry, as a formal epic-didactic poet he is not a paradoxographer, neither in the sense of excerpting nor in the sense of collecting *paradoxa*. It is therefore sensible to point out the relation between Nicander and paradoxography. As a generic marker (even though the term, if not the concept, is of course post-classical), paradoxography can be distinguished from *mirabilia*-based poetry, such as Nicander's, in several respects.[18] Of course it is clear that the two have separate origins; nevertheless, their differences of approach will be considered here, apart from the obvious elements of metre, style, and diction.

(i) A first distinction to be made between paradoxography and Nicander's didactic epic is that marvels (θαύματα, παράδοξα, *mirabilia*) are never referred to as such in Nicander, nor are these phenomena signalled or signposted by terms such as ἴδιος, ξένος, τερατώδης, θαυμαστός, or ἄπιστος.[19] The 'rhetoric of the marvellous' is absent, in whatever shape or form.[20] From a semantic point of view, this undermines the very title of this chapter: there are many things to marvel at in Nicander's poetry, but there is virtually nothing which the poet explicitly *tells* us to marvel at. If these off-beat phenomena are *thaumata* to Nicander, he plainly refuses to tell us as much or to point them out to us as such.

(ii) A second distinction to be observed concerns the signposting of externally obtained knowledge, or more particularly, the lack of such signposting in Nicander. Early epic as well as early lyric traditionally signposted the input of knowledge by referring to the Muse. Divine agency assisted in the conveyance of knowledge. The audience was expected to believe that Muse and poet shared a responsibility in transmitting and disseminating wisdom and knowledge.[21] Even in the Hellenistic era, this idea (or rather this fiction) was still traditionally strong.[22] When the unspoken truth – the use of a prose source rather than the

18 As a *terminus technicus* παραδοξογράφοι was first used by Tzetzes, *Chil.* 2.35.151, and introduced in modern scholarship by Westermann in 1839.

19 For the significance of these nouns and adjectives as markers of *mirabilia*, see Schepens/Delcroix 1996, 381–382.

20 Cf. Schepens/Delcroix 1996, 398.

21 The idea was of course already problematized thoroughly in e.g. Plato's *Ion*.

22 E.g. Apollonius' invocation of a divine agent (A.R. 1.1 and 4.2), the more emphatic plea to Erato to stand by the poet's side (A.R. 3.1), or Aratus' suggestion that he is assisted by Zeus, rather than by the technical treatises of Eudoxus etc.

inspiration of the Muse – was voiced for the first time, it presented a major breach of tradition:

> Κεῖε, τεὸν δ' ἡμεῖς ἵμερον ἐκλύομεν
> τόνδε παρ' ἀρχαίου Ξενομήδεος, ὅς ποτε πᾶσαν
> νῆσον ἐνὶ μνήμῃ κάτθετο μυθολόγῳ
>
> (Call. *Aet.* fr. 75.53–5 Harder [= Pf.])

> Cean, and we heard about this love of yours
> from ancient Xenomedes, who once set down
> the whole island in a mythological record
>
> (transl. Harder)

When Callimachus emphatically (and wittily) plays on the fact that he found his material simply by taking recourse to the library, this not only corroborates the idea of a new age in which book culture could finally replace the time-honoured Muse as a source of knowledge, it also shows that there is no need to pretend otherwise, even within poetry itself.[23] Unlike Callimachus, however, Nicander never mentions any sources. Never does he give the impression that the strange phenomena described in his iological poems are attributable to anyone other than himself. Neither god nor Muse is mentioned, let alone any statement of the poet's resorting to written sources. The paradoxographers, by contrast, relied heavily on referring to credible or perhaps 'creditable' sources for their authority.[24] Pseudo-Antigonus, for example, clearly leans on the authority of Callimachus in the compilation of his selection of *paradoxa*:

> Πεποίηται δὲ τινα καὶ ὁ Κυρηναῖος Καλλίμαχος ἐκλογὴν τῶν παραδόξων, ἧς ἀναγράφομεν ὅσα ποτὲ ἡμῖν ἐφαίνετο εἶναι ἀκοῆς ἄξια.
>
> ([Antig.] *Mir.* fr. 129 Musso)

---

23 On this innovative aspect of Callimachus see e.g. Krevans 2004, 179–181. Morrison 2011, 347 argues that Callimachus' reference to a prose source here is not to be read as a rejection of the Muses, but as a mere change of perspective. The breach with earlier poetry is, however, apparent.

24 For the acknowledgement of sources cf. Schepens/Delcroix 1996, 382–386; the aspect of credibility is discussed in Schepens/Delcroix 1996, 386–389. For Callimachus in particular, the famous fragment ἀμάρτυρον οὐδὲν ἀείδω ('I sing nothing unattested', fr. 612 Pf.) is telling in this context.

> Callimachus of Cyrene also made a compilation of miracles, of which we record all those things that to me seemed worthy of hearing.
>
> (my transl.)

Here Callimachus, in turn, is used as a credible source by Antigonus, albeit with slight reservations. Nicander, however, does not seem to need or to want to use such a mode. Markers such as ψεῦδος and ἀπίθανον are therefore absent too. Nicander's authority is achieved by different means, without a need for sources, let alone credible sources.[25] In this respect he operates differently from traditional epic, differently from Callimachus' approach to external knowledge, and differently from the paradoxographers as well.

(iii) A third difference between Nicander's approach and that of the paradoxographers lies in the fact that the *mirabilia* in Nicander are never treated differently than the other, more credible, elements described. The reader may marvel at the outrageous descriptions the poet presents, but *paradoxa* are never a distinct category. Of course, the very nature of paradoxographical works, the *eklogai* of *mirabilia*, focuses on the collection of extracted elements, suppressing the fact that these *paradoxa* were once minor elements in a longer narrative. But even in Herodotus and Ctesias the *paradoxa* must have stood out compared to more believable elements.[26] In Nicander there is no such distinction. This is an interesting element, because if all other descriptions are credible, then why should one not believe the *in*credibles ones? Or, if one argues the other way around, if some descriptions are incredible, how can one take the other ones at face value? These three distinctions (lack of signposting of *mirabilia* as such, lack of mentioning sources, and lack of distinction between the normal and the marvellous) clearly set Nicander apart from the paradoxographers and their conventions.

What the exact relation between Nicander and the paradoxographers was, despite their differences, is not easy to assess. History has shown that some of

25 These means do not include autopsy either, but at least the poet gives the impression of autopsy as an alternative to the acknowledgement of sources.

26 Cf. Hdt. 3.116, πείθομαι δὲ οὐδὲ τοῦτο ὅκως μουνόφθαλμοι ἄνδρες φύονται, which shows Herodotus expressing his disbelief in one-eyed men. In 2.156 he comments with reservations on the allegedly floating island Chemmis with αὐτὸς μὲν ἔγωγε οὔτε πλέουσαν οὔτε κινηθεῖσαν εἶδον. In 2.131 he reacts to a weird story about wooden maiden statues that lost their hands, just like the maidens – in whose image these wooden colossuses were made – whose hands were chopped off, with ταῦτα δὲ λέγουσι φλυηρέοντες, ὡς ἐγὼ δόκεω. For an analysis of the various 'modes' in which Herodotus deals with disbelief (both his own and that of others), see Packman 1991, with references.

Nicander's marvels ended up in Claudius Aelianus' *Historia Animalium.*[27] As such, inclusion in Aelian could be considered an implicit confirmation of someone's paradoxographical status. But Nicander must also have been familiar with paradoxographical collections, which started to appear a century before his time, and he must have actively included *mirabilia* in his work, probably taken from pre-existing 'wonder-books'. This is hard to prove, but it seems likely, as is confirmed by Schepens and Delcroix, that it was not unusual for poets to borrow from collections of *mirabilia*, as Apollonius of Rhodes must have done with the collected paradoxa in Callimachus.[28]

5 Mirabilia in the Theriaca

I will proceed with looking at some striking passages from Nicander's pharmacological works to assess his paradoxographical *modus operandi* and how the use of *mirabilia* can be (and is) put to use in varying ways.[29] The first passage treated here deals with the so-called *amphisbaena* (Nic. *Ther*. 373–5):

> Τὸν δὲ μετ' ἀμφίσβαιναν ὀλίζωνα βραδύθουσαν
> δήεις ἀμφικάρηνον, ἀεὶ γλήνῃσιν ἀμυδρήν·
> ἀμβλὺ γὰρ ἀμφοτέρωθεν ἐπιπρονένευκε γένειον
> νόσφιν ἀπ' ἀλλήλων· [...]

> After him you shall learn of the *amphisbaena*, less in bulk and slow of gait,
> two-headed, ever dull of eye.
> From either end a blunt chin protrudes,
> the one far from the other [...][30]

The *amphisbaena*, as Nicander tells us, is a two-headed snake, with heads at both ends of its body, causing it to be able to move either way, or so its name implies. The most striking feature of this description *would* seem to be the fact that this snake has two heads, a quality by no means common outside of the mythical

27 Nicander's *Theriaca* is mentioned as a particular source in Ael. *NA* 8.8, 9.20, 10.9, 15.18, but quite a few other stories could be added, for which Nicander may well have been Aelian's source (e.g. *HA* 2.36, 2.37, 3.22).

28 Schepens/Delcroix 1996, 404.

29 My selection in this paper is brief and could be augmented with many more examples. For a short summary of other *paradoxa* in the *Theriaca*, which will not be treated here, see Jacques 2002, lxxxviii–xc.

30 English translations of Nicander's poems, here and elsewhere, from Gow/Scholfield 1953.

world of Odysseus or Heracles. It is, however, even more striking that Nicander does not problematize this odd quality of the *amphisbaena* at all. This snake is treated just like any other, within a catalogue of some thirteen snakes, most of which seem te be real.[31] And although Nicander felt the need to tell us that the snake is ἀμφικάρηνος, thus emphatically stating that the snake is not just two-headed by name but also in real life, he does not question its existence. This, of course, is important, for *mirabilia* are supposed to be special, but they also need to be pictured as occurring in the real world. The point concerning its eyes (its gaze being ἀμυδρή, 'dim') is presented as if it is of equal importance. Nicander does not even consider that the tail may simply *look* like a head rather than actually being one.[32] The details suggest that Nicander based his description on autopsy here, but as the *amphisbaena* is elsewhere only known from Aeschylus' *Agamemnon*, where it is sided with the equally mythical monster Scylla, there is good reason to believe this snake only ever lived in name.[33] If Nicander knew the *amphisbaena* did not actually exist, or that it was really a creature with a tail that *looks* like a head, he clearly did not want to share this information. As a consequence, the unbelievable is blended subtly with the real.

Another such improbable description is found in the section dealing with scorpions.[34] This section, consisting of the treatment of scorpions, spiders, and similar creatures (lizards, murrays, stingrays), forms the main complement to snakes as regards the categories of dangerous animals with which the *Theriaca* is concerned. With regard to the flying scorpion, Nicander states (*Ther.* 799–804):

> Ἔχθιστος δ' ὅ γε ῥαιβὰ φέρει φλογὶ εἴκελα γυῖα
> ἀνδράσι, νηπιάχοις δὲ παρασχεδὸν ἤγαγεν αἶσαν·
> οἷς δὴ καὶ νώτοισι περὶ πτερὰ λευκὰ χέονται
> μάστακι σιτοφάγῳ ἐναλίγκια, ταί θ' ὑπὲρ ἄκρων
> ἱπτάμεναι ἀθέρων λεπυρὸν στάχυν ἐκβόσκονται
> Πήδασα καὶ Κισσοῖο κατὰ πτύχας ἐμβατέουσιν.

31 The veracity of snakes in classical literature, connected to the identification of ancient animals in general, is often problematic, yet a distinction should be made between between animals that are plainly impossible in real life, and animals that may well have existed.

32 Which was probably the case. For the identification of this snake as a (one-headed!) Turkish worm lizard or worm snake, see Leitz 1997, 18–21.

33 A. *Ag.* 1232–4, τί νιν καλοῦσα δυσφιλὲς δάκος | τύχοιμ' ἄν; ἀμφίσβαιναν ἢ Σκύλλαν τινὰ | οἰκοῦσαν ἐν πέτραισι, ναυτίλων βλάβην [...] 'What odious beast may I call her? An amphisbaena, or a Scylla, inhabiting the rocks, a pest to sailors [...]?' (my transl.).

34 For the division of the poem in sections concerning different sorts of venomous animals see Gow/Scholfield 1953, 170–171; Jacques 2002, lxxi–lxxii; Overduin 2015, 539–542.

But the worst enemy of man is the [scorpion] whose crooked legs are like fire:
to children it instantly brings death.
Upon its back white wings unfold themselves
like those of the corn-devouring locusts, which
flitting over the tops of the corn feed on husked grain,
and haunt Pedasa and the vales of Cissus.

As far as its veracity goes, Nicander's account of scorpions may not be on a par with modern entomology, but in this case the poet seems to transgress reality: no serious account has ever been given of flying or winged scorpions. Whether we are dealing at this point with a poet indulging in exaggeration, a careless observer who *thinks* he saw one such scorpion, or a writer who does not believe autopsy is required in order to write poetry, one wonders what Nicander is putting forward here. Several scholars have pointed out that it is too easy to qualify Nicander as a mere versifier, lacking any real knowledge of the phenomena he describes.[35] But here we get the impression, again, that Nicander could not have relied on actual autopsy, or that he was particularly interested in it for that matter. Instead Nicander appears to be a poet who does not shun exciting details, even if they can hardly be considered real. The general element of horror, the poet inspiring fear in potential victims of all kinds of animals, real or made-up, is a constant factor in Nicander's poetics.[36] As the saying goes, the devil is never as black as he is painted; likewise, Nicander's monsters are never as real as he composes them in his pseudo-scientific verse.

Of equally dubious nature is the enigmatic creature discussed in *Theriaca* 759–68, an account of some sort of dangerous moth:

Φράζεο δ' Αἰγύπτοιο τά τε τρέφει οὐλοὸς αἶα
κνώδαλα, φαλλαίνῃ ἐναλίγκια, τὴν περὶ λύχνους
ἀκρόνυχος δειπνηστὸς ἐπήλασε παιφάσσουσαν·
στεγνὰ δέ οἱ πτερὰ πάντα καὶ ἔγχνοα, τοῖα κονίης
ἢ καὶ ἀπὸ σπληδοῖο φαείνεται, ὅστις ἐπαύρῃ.
τῷ ἴκελος Περσῆος ὑποτρέφεται πετάλοισι,
τοῦ καὶ σμερδαλέον νεύει κάρη αἰὲν ὑποδράξ
ἐσκληκός, νηδὺς δὲ βαρύνεται· αὐτὰρ ὁ κέντρον
αὐχένι τ' ἀκροτάτῳ κεφαλῇ τ' ἐνεμάξατο φωτός,
ῥεῖα δέ κεν θανάτοιο καὶ αὐτίκα μοῖραν ἐφείη.

35 E.g. Knoefel/Covi 1991. That said, other scholars have stressed Nicander's lack of real knowledge, e.g. Scarborough 1984.
36 This dimension, Nicander as a 'dark' poet dealing in fear and carousing in horror, has been studied most systematically by Sistakou (2012) 193–250. For Nicander's world as a dark place, particularly in opposition to the bucolic world, cf. Overduin 2014.

> Consider now monsters which the grim land of Egypt fosters,
> like the moth which the evening meal-time brings
> in to flutter round the lamps.
> All the wings are dense and are covered with down,
> even as a man appears who may chance to touch dust or ashes.
> Such in appearance, it is reared among the leaves of Perseus's tree.
> Its terrible head nods ever in grim fashion
> and is hard, and its belly is heavy; its sting
> it plants in the top of a man's neck or on his head,
> and it may easily and on the spot bring the doom of death.

Nicander never calls this creature by its presumed proper name, but according to the scholia it is known as the κεφαλοκρούστης or the κρανοκολάπτης, which translates as something like the 'skull-knocker' or 'head-pecker'.[37] It is winged and has the Persea-tree as its main haunt. Despite these 'facts', there is little reason to believe that such a creature did exist. Again, Nicander does not express any doubts about its existence, but here we have an interesting, and somewhat un-Nicandrean detail: this creature does not live just anywhere, but is located in Egypt, called an οὐλοὸς αἶα in 759, a 'grim land'. The adjective οὐλοός may qualify Egypt as a land where many dangerous and venomous creatures actually live, but one gets the impression that Nicander refers here to Egypt rather as the sort of place where such monsters are *rumoured* to be easily found: Egypt as the country associated with *mirabilia* in Herodotus, or, much later, as the haunt of many sort of snakes in Lucian's *Dipsads*. As stated earlier, it is problematic to call the description of this creature a *mirabilium*, because Nicander never invites the reader to wonder at or be amazed by this head-pecker, but the mention of Egypt in particular shares a well-known dimension of paradoxography. Many phenomena only occur in particular locations, as can easily be concluded from the examples in pseudo-Antigonus. From this viewpoint the inclusion of the 'head-pecker' is not merely an occasion to warn, but also an occasion to give statements about the world the poet wishes to portray, a world of wonders, dangerous though they may be.

Closer to home is Nicander's reference to the phenomenon of the so-called βουγονία in *Theriaca* 738–42:

---

37 Σ in *Ther*. 763a Crugnola: [...] τοῦτο οὖν, φησί, τὸ ζῷον τῇ φαλαίνῃ ὅμοιον, ὁ *κεφαλοκρούστης*, ἐν τοῖς φύλλοις τῆς περσείας τρέφεται. ἔχει δὲ ἐν τῇ κεφαλῇ κέντρον καὶ πτερὰ τέσσαρα. Ἄλλως· σποδοῦ χροιὰν ἔχει τὰ πτερά, οἷαν οἱ ἀπὸ κόνεως μεμολυσμένοι ἴσχουσιν. ὁ *κρανοκολάπτης* δὲ ἐν ταῖς περσείαις ὁρᾶται, πτερὰ ἔχων ὅμοια ταῖς ἐν τοῖς κήποις ψυχαῖς. τὸ κέντρον δὲ ἔχει ἐπὶ τῆς κεφαλῆς καὶ τῷ αὐχένι κρύπτει.

Ἄλλο γε μὴν δύσδηρι, τὸ δὴ σφήκειον ἔπουσι,
πυρσὸν ἅλις, σφηκὶ προσαλίγκιον ὠμοβορῆϊ,
ὃς δὴ θαρσαλέην γενεὴν ἐκμάσσεται ἵππου·
ἵπποι γὰρ σφηκῶν γένεσις, ταῦροι δὲ μελισσῶν
σκήνεσι πυθομένοισι λυκοσπάδες ἐξεγένοντο.

But another kind is an aggressive foe, the one men call the wasp-spider,
reddish and like the ravenous wasp,
which resembles the horse in its high-spirit,
for horses are the origin of wasps and bulls of bees,
which are engendered in their rotting carcasses.

In these lines the poet comments on the nature and origin of bees and wasps, followed by a combined reference to *bougonia* and *hippogonia*, intended to explain the character of these animals.[38] This is new: the unsubstantiated idea that bees are born from the carcasses of cows was old, but the connection between the *spirit* of the wasp and its *origin* is not found in earlier sources. Here the *mirabilium*, although it is not singled out as such, serves to point out that the fierce character of the bull (the father) is reflected in the son (the wasp). This yields an interesting connection between paradoxography and aetiology. The combined reference to the *bougonia* and the *hippogonia* makes us wonder whether Nicander was aware of the comparable phenomena of what may have been known as κροκοδειλογονία, and the idea that snakes are born from the marrow of a dead man's body:

εἰς ὑμᾶς κροκόδειλον ἀποφθίμενον διαλύει,
σκορπίοι, ἡ πάντα ζωοθετοῦσα φύσις.

(*SH* 125)

Thus nature, that brings life to all things,
dissolves the dead crocodile into you, scorpions.

(my transl.)

ἀνδρὸς γὰρ κοίλης ἐκ μυελοῦ ῥάχεως
δεινὸς γίνετ' ὄφις νέκυος δειλοῖο σαπέντος.

(*SH* 129.2–3)

38 For the *bougonia*, probably already a well-established topic before Nicander, see Kitchell 1989 and Overduin 2015, 459–461.

Because out of the hollow spine of a man's marrow
a terrible snake is born, when his sorry corpse has started to rot.

(my transl.)

These fragments from the Ἰδιοφυῆ of Archelaus of Chersonesus, who also composed epigrams on the *bougonia* and *hippogonia*, are dated to the third or second century BCE.[39] They clearly represent a wider tradition of *mirabilia* concerning the unlikely origin of certain species. If Nicander knew his *bugonia* from Archelaus, this would show the influence of paradoxography on a medical-biological poet. But the fact that Nicander does not mention the wondrous engendering of snakes from a man's marrow is problematic: would he have let such an opportunity pass by?[40]

Whether or not Nicander was familiar with Archelaus' Ἰδιοφυῆ is hard to tell, but it is easy to assume that there was a common belief in this sort of engendering, considering all the species (snakes, beetles, wasps, bees) implicated in this process. The fact that Nicander does not mention that scorpions are born from crocodiles may, however, have its own explanation, which is found in *Ther.* 791–796. There Nicander gives his own take on the origin of scorpions, not from crocodiles, but from crabs:

τῶν δὴ καὶ γενεὴν ἐξέμμορον εὖτε λίπωσι
πέτρας καὶ βρύα λεπτὰ πολυστίοιο θαλάσσης.
τοὺς ἁλὸς ἐξερύουσι δελαστρέες ἰχθυβολῆες,
αὐτίκα δ' ἀγρευθέντες ἐνὶ γρώνῃσιν ἔδυσαν
μυοδόκοις, ἵνα τέκνα κακοφθόρα τῶνδε θανόντων
σκορπίοι ἐξεγένοντο καθ' ἕρκεα λωβητῆρες.

39 For the particular nature of Archelaus' paradoxographical activities, see Fraser 1972, 779. The *hippogonia* is treated in *SH* 126, ἐκ νέκυος ταύτην ἵππου γράψασθε γενέθλην, | σφῆκας (= [Antig.], *Mir.* 19.4b.1 Musso); *bougonia* in *SH* 127, βοὸς φθιμένης πεπλανημένα τέκνα. *Bugonia* and *hippogonia* are combined in *SH* 128 (= Var. *R.* 3.16.4), ostensibly a single line epigram (ἵππω<v> μὲν σφῆκες γενεά, μόσχων δὲ μέλισσαι). Cf. Ov. *Met.* 15.361–8, Ph. *De specialibus legibus* 1.292, S.E. *P.* 1.42, Ael. *NA* 1.28, Orig. *Cels.* 4.57.26, 4.59.18, [Gal.] *An animal sit quod est in utero* 19.175.7 etc.

40 That the Ἰδιοφυῆ may have become a paradoxographical category of sorts in itself seems to follow from an example in Plutarch. At the very end of the *Life of Cleomenes*, the polymath states: ἄχρι οὗ κατέπαυσαν αὐτοὺς οἱ σοφώτεροι, διδόντες λόγον, ὡς μελίττας μὲν βόες, σφῆκας δ' ἵπποι κατασαπέντες ἐξανθοῦσι, κάνθαροι δ' ὄνων τὸ αὐτὸ παθόντων ζῳογονοῦνται (Plut. *Cleom.* 60.5 [39.3]), "Until the wise men stopped them, giving the explanation that rotten cows put forth bees and horses wasps, and beetles are brought forth when asses suffer the same fate" (my transl.). Plutarch states that the wise men solved the mystery of the corpse of Cleomenes, whose face was protected by a snake from scavengers and predators. The wise men tell about the *bugonia*, adding that snakes are born from marrow. But they also say, according to Plutarch, that beetles are born from asses. This may have been in Archelaus' Ἰδιοφυῆ too, but it could be a later addition, following in the same tradition.

> It is from them [crabs] that they have their allotted being, whenever they quit
> the rocks and the delicate wrack of the pebble-strewn sea.
> The fishermen with their baits draw them from the salt water;
> but directly they are caught they slip into
> mouseholes, and there the scorpions, the deadly offspring of these dead crabs,
> are born, to work ruin from wall and fence.

Many of these *mirabilia* concern the question of how such animals come about, based on faulty observation and careless copying from earlier sources, followed by an insistence of sticking to an unlikely but attractive explanation instead of providing a proper 'Aristotelian' reinvestigation. Another oddity found in the *Theriaca* is the idea that murries (moray eels) come to land, out of the sea, in order to find a viper to mate with:

> Ναὶ μὴν οἶδ' ὅσα πόντος ἁλὸς ῥόχθοισιν ἐλίσσει,
> σμυραίνην δ' ἔκπαγλον· ἐπεὶ μογεροὺς ἁλιῆας
> πολλάκις ἐμπρήσασα κατεπρήνιξεν ἐπάκτρου
> εἰς ἅλα φυζηθέντας ἐχετλίου ἐξαναδῦσα,
> εἰ ἔτυμον κείνην γε σὺν οὐλοβόροις ἐχίεσσι
> θόρνυσθαι, προλιποῦσαν ἁλὸς νομὸν, ἠπείροισι.

> Furthermore I have knowledge of all the creatures that the sea whirls amid its briny surges, and the horror of the murry, since many a time has it sprung up from the fish-box and, striking them with panic, has hurled toiling fishermen from their boat to seek refuge in the sea, if it be true that this creature couples with deadly-biting vipers on the land, forsaking its salt pasturage.

The murry is indeed an eel-like fish that resembles a snake, but it is still a fish. To imagine that it comes out of the sea to mate on land is therefore hard to believe. Surprisingly, here Nicander adds his comments in the form of εἰ ἔτυμον ('if it is true'). This is the only locus where Nicander allows room for doubt that his biological or pharmacological facts may not be so factual after all. The story of the mating of the murry and the viper is found elsewhere, but not before Nicander.[41] Nicander's phrasing, however, implies that he had heard the story elsewhere and was not its inventor.

41 Cf. Ael. *NA* 1.50, 9.66, Opp. *H.* 1.554–573, Plin. *Nat.* 9.76, 27.14. Seemingly incongruous matches became a topos of their own. Oppian discusses the unlikely love of sea breams for goats (*H.* 4.302–44; cf. Ael. *HA* 1.23), but we also learn about the bustards' love of horses (Ael. *HA* 1.28); cf. Ael. *HA* 5.48. This pattern fits parallel cases of topical antipathies (Ael. *HA* 3.7, 5.48), famous examples of which are the enmity between deer and snakes (Nic. *Ther.* 141–44; [Opp.] *C.* 2.238–41, Ael. *HA* 2.9 etc.), between the asp and the mongoose (Nic. *Ther.* 190–208, Ael. *HA* 5.48), and between the dragon and the eagle (*Il.* 12.201–7, Nic. *Ther.* 448–57, Plu. *De invidia* 3 etc.).

Another *mirabilium*, although, again, not presented as such, is found in *Ther.* 128–136. It concerns the way baby vipers are born:

> Μὴ σύ γ' ἐνὶ τριόδοισι τύχοις ὅτε δάχμα πεφυζώς
> περκνὸς ἔχις θυίῃσι τυπῇ ψολόεντος ἐχίδνης,
> ἡνίκα, θορνυμένου ἔχιος, θολερῷ κυνόδοντι
> θουρὰς ἀμὺξ ἐμφῦσα κάρην ἀπέκοψεν ὁμεύνου.
> οἱ δὲ πατρὸς λώβην μετεκίαθον αὐτίκα τυτθοί
> γεινόμενοι ἐχιῆες, ἐπεὶ διὰ μητρὸς ἀραιήν
> γαστέρ' ἀναβρώσαντες ἀμήτορες ἐξεγένοντο·
> οἴη γὰρ βαρύθει ὑπὸ κύματος, οἱ δὲ καθ' ὕλην
> ᾠοτόκοι ὄφιες λεπυρὴν θάλπουσι γενέθλην.

> May you, at the crossroads, never happen upon – when he has fled her bite –
> the dark male viper, as he seethes at the blow of the sooty female,
> because when the male viper mounts her, she, with a furious fang
> passionately scratching, cuts off the head of her mate.
> But immediately they pursue the outrage of their father
> while being born, the little vipers, since by eating through their mother's thin stomach, they are born motherless: for she alone is burdened with a swollen belly, but snakes in the forest that are oviparous warm their offspring in a shell.

In this passage Nicander deals with the birth of the viper, which, unlike most other snakes, does not produce eggs, but gives birth to her young straight out of the womb, which is normally the end of her, as the young are said to eat their way through their mother's womb and skin. Prior to parturition, the female (ἔχιδνα, 129) has usually bitten off the head of her mate (ἔχις, 129) during conception, immediately after he has inseminated her: the young take revenge for their dead father by causing their mother's death in the process of parturition. The story is not confirmed by Aristotle, which makes it a good candidate for the sort of parturition not found in real life.[42] The biological *mirabilium* first concerns the fact that the babies normally eat through their mother's skin in order to see the light of day. This story is already found in Herodotus, and Nicander has done little more than reproducing it in verse.[43] But here again we see an example of aetiological paradoxography, a *paradoxon* not simply as a thing to marvel about, but also a thing to account for. The solution to the implicit question ('why do baby snakes eat through their mother's skin?') is not only an interesting aetion in itself, it also

42 It is found however, not surprisingly, in pseudo-Aristotle (*Mir.* 846b18); cf. Ael. *NA* 1.24.
43 Hdt. 3.109.

helps to characterize the evil animal world, a world in which snakes are even evil among themselves, and not only against man.[44]

My last example from the *Theriaca* concerns the venomous sting of the sting-ray:

Τρυγόνα μὴν ὀλοεργὸν ἁλιρραίστην τε δράκοντα
οἶδ' ἀπαλέξασθαι· φορέει γε μὲν ἄλγεα τρυγών
ἦμος ἐν ὁλκαίοισι λίνοις μεμογηότα κέντρῳ
ἐργοπόνον τύψησιν, ἢ ἐν πρέμνοισι παγείη
δενδρείου τό τε πολλὸν ἀγαυρότατον θαλέθῃσι·
τοῦ μὲν ὑπὸ πληγῇσιν ἅτ' ἠελίοιο δαμέντος
ῥίζαι σὺν δέ τε φυλλὰς ἀποφθίνει, ἀνδρὶ δὲ σάρκες
πυθόμεναι μινύθουσι· λόγος γε μὲν ὥς ποτ' Ὀδυσσεύς
ἔφθιτο λευγαλέοιο τυπεὶς ἁλίου ὑπὸ κέντρου.

Again, from the death-dealing sting-ray and the ravening seasnake
I can protect you. The sting-ray causes trouble
when it strikes with its sting the toiler labouring at his hauled drag-nets;
or if the sting is fixed in the trunk of some tree which is flourishing in full pride, then, as though the tree were stricken by the fierce beams of the sun,
its roots and with them its leafage whither; on a man his flesh
rots and wastes away. Indeed the story tells how Odysseus of yore
perished from the baneful sting of this monster from the sea.

This sting can make a tree die and a man rot away – a story, not surprisingly, repeated in Aelian's *Historia animalium*.[45] Again, this is the sort of *paradoxon* that sounds like it could be the equivalent of an urban myth, yet could very well be real. And just like earlier *mirabilia* in the *Theriaca*, this one is not simply there to be marvelled at. It helps to colour Nicander's dark unpleasant world.[46] Moreover, it occasions a brief, though welcome, mention of an epic myth, the sort of brief mythical elements that are quite frequent in the *Theriaca*, which are part and parcel of Nicander's subtle poetic palette, rooted in the mythic-heroic tradition of early epic.

44 This negative qualification of the innate evil character of snakes was, of course, already prepared in the mythological part of the *Theriaca*'s proem, where it was stated that snakes were created from the blood of the Titans, probably some variation on the myth of Perseus, who accidentally dropped, in flight, a few drops of blood from the Gorgo's dripping head, which fell to the earth (*Ther.* 8–10); see Jacques 2002, 77–78 and Overduin 2015, 182–183.

45 Ael. *HA* 2.36

46 Cf. Sistakou 2012.

6 The Alexipharmaca

Nicander's *Alexipharmaca*, a shorter but similar poem to the *Theriaca*, is not concerned with venomous animals, but with poisoning. Many treatments are discussed, but most are essentially emetics, much like the good old brimstone and treacle formula. In addition, the poet advises the application of enemas to rid the victim of the unwanted poison. Most descriptions seem to be applicable, or at least to be likely to make a person vomit. But in *Alexipharmaca* 207–223, a passage in which arrow-poison is treated, a *paradoxon* is contained, strikingly, in a simile:

> τοῦ καὶ ἔνερθε γλῶσσα παχύνεται, ἀμφὶ δὲ χείλη
> οἰδαλέα βρίθοντα περὶ στομάτεσσι βαρύνει,
> ξηρὰ δ' ἀναπτύει, νεόθεν δ' ἐκρήγνυται οὖλα·
> πολλάκι δ' ἐς κραδίην πτοίην βάλε, πᾶν δὲ νόημα
> ἔμπληκτον μεμόρηκε κακῇ ἐσφαλμένον ἄτῃ·
> αὐτὰρ ὁ μηκάζει μανίης ὕπο μυρία φλύζων,
> δηθάκι δ' ἀχθόμενος βοάᾳ ἅ τις ἐμπελάδην φώς
> ἀμφιβρότην κώδειαν ἀπὸ ξιφέεσσιν ἀμηθείς

> First, his tongue begins to thicken from the root and weighs upon the lips which are heavy and swollen about the mouth; he suffers from a dry expectoration, and his gums break open from the base. Often too his heart is smitten with palpitations, and it is his fate that all his wits are stunned and overthrown by the evil poison; and he makes bleating noises, babling endlessly in his frenzy; often too in his distress he cries aloud even as one whose head, the body's master, has just been cut off with the sword [...]

The symptoms of one suffering from arrow-poison are convincing enough, as for instance the fact that the victim will scream and cry. But then the victim is compared to a victim of decapitation, who, although beheaded, still screams.[47] Although this image is part of a simile, the poet presents it as a fact which he does not seem to doubt. The inclusion of the image in Nicander is harrowing for another reason: as if the symptoms of poisoning described are not horrifying enough, the poet throws in one more detail, which should elucidate the sort of screaming we are to imagine.[48] But the audience can easily imagine serious screaming without stories of beheading. For the poet, however, to present himself as someone whose wide experience even includes observations concerning

---

47 See also Spatafora 2005, 261–262; Magnelli 2014, 222 underlines Nicander's approach between the paradoxographical and the macabre.

48 For the use of horror in Nicander, see Sistakou 2012.

decapitation adds authority to his status as a credible doctor.[49] The lack of doubt with regard to this *paradoxon* makes us believe that this is not just hearsay, or some cock-and-bull story Nicander tries to sell us: facts, even *paradoxa*, even within a simile, are there to uphold the status of the didactic poet.

7 Conclusion

For a long time scholars have debated over the scientific contents of Nicander's poetry, and this has yielded three scenarios: (1) Nicander was an expert doctor, perhaps even a *theriakos*, who made serious contributions to the field, and was certainly not a mere poet engaged in making a poetic metaphrasis of a treatise on poison and venom.[50] (2) Nicander was a poet, but he did his homework, studying his sources thoroughly. He may not have been a doctor, but he must have known what he was talking about at least to a certain extent.[51] (3) Nicander was much more a poet than an expert: he did his elementary homework, but did not speak from experience or autopsy. He saw no reason to refute unbelievable elements; he may even have included them wilfully, to spice up his poetic material at the cost of veracity. He does not cite sources, which would only detract from his mission to *sound* like a true doctor in his literary role as an omniscient teacher within the epic-didactic framework.[52] The division of these three scenarios is strongly informed by the *paradoxa* in the *Theriaca* and, to a lesser extent, in the *Alexipharmaca*. If it were not for the *im*possibilities in the account of the *amphisbaena*, the *cranocolaptes*, and winged scorpions (along with many other problematical obervations in Nicander's poetry) it would be much easier to take his knowledgeability at face value.

49 The image is surely not based on autopsy and a different origin is in fact suggested by Σ *Al.* 216a Geymonat: Nicander misinterpreted *Il.* 10.457 = *Od.* 22.329 (φθεγγομένου δ' ἄρα τοῦ γε κάρη κονίῃσιν ἐμίχθη, 'and while he was still speaking his head was mingled with the dust'; the previous lines show the victim being struck square on the neck with a sword, with the sinews sheared off); cf. Jacques 2007, 124–125. But perhaps this is not so much a case of misinterpretation as the wilful inclusion of a dramatic *thauma*.

50 This view is summed up most clearly by Jacques 2002, xlix–lii; cf. Jacques 1979.

51 Knoefel/Covi 1991.

52 Overduin 2009; 2015 *passim*; 2016. Nicander's credibility was emphatically criticized by Scarborough: "Nicander shows no expertise whatever in the subjects or specifics of poisons and toxicoloy in the *Theriaca* or *Alexipharmaca*" (1984, 27; cf. alib.).

The question then is: why would Nicander, an ostensibly creditable pharmacologist, include these *paradoxa*? Perhaps he does not consider them to be incredible, or perhaps it is a means of larding his account with exciting elements. The *cranocolaptes* plays on the notion that *paradoxa* are mainly based locally (and, at the same time, in far off places on the borders of the known world), the *bugonia* is used to explain (in a semi-aetiological way) the fierce nature of wasps and bees, the stingray occasions a reference to epic Odysseus, the birth of baby vipers corroborates the general view of snakes as malignant animals. Nicander's *mirabilia* are thus, at least partly, functional, for various reasons within his account. My first case, however, concerning the two-headed *amphisbaena*, is not so easy to explain in this way. Nicander's inclusion of *paradoxa* may just be a way to show his awareness of the existence of *mirabilia* themselves, whether he believed them or not, or had ever seen them. Without giving a verdict, they could be put to good use in his world of popular science. This ultimately shows, in my view, how Nicander is not really concerned with medicine, pharmacology, and biology, but with the creation of his own exciting world, a world that does not need to be entirely truthful, as long as it is convincing from the viewpoint of his own presentation.

Bibliography

Crugnola, A. (1971), *Scholia in Nicandri Theriaka cum glossis*, Milan.

Fraser, P.M. (1972), *Ptolemaic Alexandria* (3 vols.), Oxford.

Geymonat, M. (1974), *Scholia in Nicandri Alexipharmaka cum glossis*, Milan.

Gow, A.S.F./Scholfield, A.F. (1953), *Nicander. The Poems and Poetical Fragments*, Cambridge.

Harder, M.A. (2003), "The Invention of Past, Present and Future in Callimachus' 'Aetia'", *Hermes* 131, 290–306.

Harder, M.A. (2012), *Callimachus. Aetia* (2 vols.), Oxford.

Jacques, J.M. (1979), "Nicandre de Colophon: poète et médecin", *Ktema* 4, 133–149.

Jacques, J.M. (2002), *Nicandre. Oeuvres*. Tome II: *Thériaques*, Paris.

Jacques, J.M. (2007), *Nicandre. Oeuvres*. Tome III: *Les Alexipharmaques*, Paris.

Kitchell, K.F. (1989), "The Origins of Vergil's Myth of the *Bugonia*", in: R.F. Sutton (ed.), *Daidalikon. Studies in Memory of Raymond V. Schoder*, Wauconda, IL, 193–206.

Knoefel, P.K./Covi, M.C. (1991), *A Hellenistic Treatise on Poisonous Animals. The 'Theriaca' of Nicander of Colophon. A Contribution to the History of Toxicology*, Lewiston, NY.

Köhnken, A. (2010), "Apollonius' *Argonautica*", in: J. Clauss/M. Cuypers (eds.), *A Companion to Hellenistic Literature*, Malden, MA.

Krevans, N. (2004), "Callimachus and the Pedestrian Muse", in: M.A. Harder/R.F. Regtuit/G.C. Wakker (eds.), *Callimachus II*. Hellenistica Groningana 7, Leuven, Paris, Dudley, MA.

Leitz, Chr. (1997), *Die Schlangennamen in den ägyptischen und griechischen Giftbüchern*, Stuttgart.

Lloyd Jones, H./Parsons, P. (1983), *Supplementum Hellenisticum*, Berlin.

Magnelli, E. (2010), "Nicander", in: J. Clauss/M. Cuypers (eds.), *A Companion to Hellenistic Literature*, Malden, MA.

Morrison, A. (2011), "Callimachus' Muses", in: B. Acosta-Hughes/L. Lehnus/S. Stephens (eds.), *Brill's Companion to Callimachus*, Leiden/Boston.

Musso, O. (1985), *Antigonus Carystius. Rerum mirabilium collectio*, Napoli.

Overduin, F. (2009), "The Fearsome Shrewmouse. Pseudo-science in Nicander's *Theriaca*?" in: M.A. Harder/R.F. Regtuit/G.C. Wakker (eds.), *Nature and Science in Hellenistic poetry*, Leuven, 79–93.

Overduin, F. (2014), "The Anti-bucolic World of Nicander's *Theriaca*", *CQ* 64, 623–641.

Overduin, F. (2015), *Nicander of Colophon's* Theriaca: *A Literary Commentary*, Leiden/Boston.

Overduin, F. (2016), "Beauty in Suffering: Disgust in Didactic Greek poetry", in: D. Lateiner/ D. Spatharas (eds.), *The Ancient Emotion of Disgust*, Oxford, 141–155.

Packman, Z. (1991), "The Incredible and the Incredulous: The Vocabulary of Disbelief in Herodotus, Thucydides and Xenophon", *Hermes* 119, 399–414.

Pajón Leyra, I. (2011), *Entre ciencia y maravilla. El gênero litterario de la paradoxografia griega*, Zaragoza.

Scarborough, J. (1984), *Pharmacy's Ancient Heritage. Theophrastus, Nicander, and Dioscorides*, Lexington, KY.

Schepens, G./Delcroix, K. (1996), "Ancient Paradoxography: Origin, Evolution, Production and Reception', in: O. Pecere/A. Stramaglia (eds.), *La letteratura di consumo nel mondo greco-latino*. Atti del convegno internazionale Cassino, 14–17 settembre 1994. Cassino, 373–460.

Schmid, W./Stählin, O. (1920–1924), *Griechische Literaturgeschichte 2.1–2*, München.

Sistakou, E. (2012), *The Aesthetics of Darkness: A Study of Hellenistic Romanticism in Apollonius, Lycophron and Nicander*, Leuven.

Spatafora, G. (2005), "Riflessioni sull'arte poetica di Nicandro", *GIF* 57, 231–262.

Touwaide, A. (1991), "Nicandre: de la science à la poésie. Contribution à l'exégèse de la poésie medicale grecque", *Aevum* 65, 65–101.

Westermann, A. (ed.) (1839), Παραδοξογράφοι. *Scriptores rerum mirabilium Graeci*, Brunsvigae/Londini.

Ziegler, K. (1949), "Paradoxographoi", *RE* 18.3, 1137–1166.

Lucia Floridi

Wondrous Healings in Greek Epigrams (and Their Parodic Counterparts)

Abstract: In this paper I explore the connections between temple medicine, inscriptions commemorating – or actually "advertising" – wondrous healings, epigrams, and *paradoxa*. I start with a survey of the (often highlighted) connections between Posidippus' *iamatika* and temple *iamata*, and also indicate the points of contact between healing literature and the work of paradoxographers. I then examine a few epigrams on miraculous healings preserved via the *Greek Anthology* in order to show that they belong to the same subgenre of *iamatika*. I end with examples of parodic distortion of the themes of healing literature in scoptic epigrams dealing with murderous doctors.

1 Posidippus' *iamatika* and temple *iamata*

The publication, in 2001, of the "new Posidippus" has drawn scholars' attention to several epigrammatic categories that were previously unknown, or which had only occasionally been attested: among these is the so-called *iamatika*, "epigrams on healings". This section consists of seven epigrams (95–101 A.-B.) concerning sudden and miraculous healings that testify to the power of Asclepius, the healer-god. Various scholars have noted a connection between this set of poems and the surviving private epigraphs about cures, as well as the prose inscriptions on wondrous healings (*iamata*) set up by temple authorities in sanctuaries, such as the ones at Epidaurus.[1] Posidippus' epigrams stress the miraculous and sudden aspect of healing, just as we find it in most of the temple prose inscriptions, where the exceptional character of the healings is highlighted in order to praise the power of the god.[2] Like other early Hellenistic poets, Posidippus, through the reworking of the tradition of inscribed *iamata*, displays in his epigrams an awareness of the genre's inscriptional roots. This is not surprising, since

1 Zanetto 2002, 73–74; Papalexandrou 2004, 255–258; Bing 2004 (= 2009, 217–233); Di Nino 2005; 2006; 2010, 255–274; Männlein-Robert 2015. Epigraphic *iamata* are collected by Girone 1998. For Epidaurus' *Chronicles* see Herzog 1931; LiDonnici 1989; 1992; 1995; on their didactic purposes see Dillon 1994.
2 Dorati-Guidorizzi 1996, 355.

https://doi.org/10.1515/9783110661774-005

he was himself an ἐπιγραμματοποιός, a professional author of epigrams.[3] Scholars have convincingly shown that the *iamatika*, as featured in the papyrus, are designed as an artfully arranged set of poems which encourage a sequential reading and acquire an additional meaning as a group;[4] however, nothing assures us that they were *all* originally conceived as "fictional" literary epigrams, composed for the scroll from the very beginning.[5] At least some of them could have been inscribed and then collected in a book, as has been suggested for other poems in the papyrus.[6] Consider, for instance, the dedication by Soses of Cos (97 A.-B.):

Ἰητήρια σοὶ νούσων, Ἀσκληπιέ, Κῶιος
  δωρεῖται Σωσῆς ἀργυρέην φιάλην,
οὗ σὺ τὸν ἑξαέτη κάματόν θ' ἅμα καὶ νόσον ἱρήν,
  δαῖμον, ἀποξύσας ὤιχεο νυκτὶ μιῆι.

As a thank-offering for curing his disease, Asclepius,
  Soses of Cos gives you this silver bowl.
His six-year suffering, combined with epilepsy,
  you departed, O god, having wiped it off in a single night.[7]

This is an *anathematikon*, not so different in structure from similar dedications found on stone, and most probably echoing the wondrous healings recorded in temple inscriptions, sometimes based on the (embellished) transcriptions of actual dedications.[8] In particular, it is typical of inscribed *iamata* to highlight the contrast between two temporal dimensions: a long-lasting, chronic disease (τὸν ἑξαέτη κάματον, line 3) is cured by the god very quickly (νυκτὶ μιῆι, line 4). Compare, for instance, the tale that opens the collection of *iamata* from Epidaurus (which, given its prominent placement on the stele, probably played a programmatic role): Cleo was pregnant for five years. She then came to the temple, slept

3 As stated by *IG* IX 1² i 17A = T3 A.-B.; on Posidippus' activity as ἐπιγραμματοποιός, see Garulli 2016.
4 E.g. Bing 2004 (= 2009); Di Nino 2010, 187–274; Wickkiser 2013.
5 E.g. Zanetto 2016, 590.
6 Garulli 2005.
7 The text of Posidippus' epigrams is given according to Austin/Bastianini 2002; the translations are by Austin.
8 On the genesis of the corpus of *iamata* in Epidaurus, see LiDonnici 1989; 1995, 40–75. Particularly interesting, for our purposes, is the first *iama* of Epidaurus' stele, A1 Herzog, where the dedication to the god on the part of the healed person is quoted in the narrative: on this point, see Bing 2004, 280–281.

in the *abaton*,[9] and gave birth to a son, who, as soon as he was born, washed himself at the fountain and walked about with his mother (A1 Herzog). A similar story is that of the mute boy who utters his first words as soon as the opening sacrifices to the god are performed (A5 Herzog). Adverbs such as ἐξαπίνας, or the temporal expression ἁμέρας δὲ γενομένας ὑγιὴς ἐξῆλθε, used as a closing formula in several *iamata*,[10] stress the contrast between the swiftness of the healing and the chronic nature of the illness. The same motif appears in Aeschines *AP* 6.330 = *CEG* 776 (first half of the fourth century B.C.), an acrostic dedication transmitted by the *Greek Anthology*:[11]

> Θνητῶν μὲν τέχναις ἀπορούμενος, εἰς δὲ τὸ θεῖον
> ἐλπίδα πᾶσαν ἔχων, προλιπὼν εὔπαιδας Ἀθήνας,
> ἰάθην ἐλθών, Ἀσκληπιέ, πρὸς τὸ σὸν ἄλσος,
> ἕλκος ἔχων κεφαλῆς ἐνιαύσιον, ἐν τρισὶ μησίν.

> Despairing of human art, and placing all my hope in the Divinity, I left Athens, the mother of beautiful children, and was cured in three months, Asclepius, of an ulcer on my head that had continued for a year, by coming to your grove.
>
> (transl. Paton 1916, modified)

Thanks to the intervention of the god, an ulcer that had afflicted the patient for a full year, and which human doctors had been unable to cure, disappeared in just three months.

Another case in point is the epigram for the Cretan Asclas (99 A.-B.) – not a proper dedication this time, but a narrative aimed at celebrating the power of the healing god, like the inscriptions from Epidaurus:

> Ὁ Κρὴς κωφὸς ἐὼν Ἀσκλ[ᾶς, μη]δ' οἷος ἀκούειν
> αἰγιαλῶν †οιοc† μηδ' ἀνέμων πάταγον,

9 As is known, temple literature is mostly concerned with incubation, i.e. ritual sleep in a sanctuary. In the ancient world, dreams were considered capable of ensuring communication with the superhuman dimension, and they were thus credited with healing powers (on this vast topic, see especially Edelstein/Edelstein 1998^2, II, 142–180, and the recent general reassessment by Oberhelman 2013). By contrast, in Posidippus references to incubation are rare: 98.3 A.-B. (ἐπ' ὀνείρωι); a healing dream is also implicit in 97.4 A.-B. (νυκτὶ μιῆι).

10 LiDonnici 1995, 23. Other examples of *iamata* where Asclepius is said to be able to cure long-lasting diseases are A12, B30, C64 Herzog; see also Girone III.12.4-8 (Lebena, first century B.C.).

11 According to Herzog 1931, 39–41, portions of the epigram can be read in a fragmentary inscription found in the Asclepieion at Epidaurus (see also Longo 1969, 77, n. 45; Girone 1998, 42–45, n. II.1). Based on his re-examination of a photograph of the inscription, however, Bajnok 2014 has denied that the fragment contains the epigram in question.

εὐθὺς ἀπ' εὐχωλέων Ἀσκληπιοῦ οἴκαδ' ἀπήιει,
καὶ τὰ διὰ πλίνθων ῥήματ' ἀκουσόμενος.

The Cretan Asclas being deaf and unable to hear
the surge of the shore or the roar of the winds,
all of a sudden, after praying to Asclepius, returned home
able to pick up words even through a brick-wall.

The healing here is not only miraculously swift (εὐθὺς ἀπ' εὐχωλέων, line 3), but it is also wondrous for the consequences it produces. The man, once deaf, can now hear words through a brick-wall. This apparent hyperbole, in which scholars have sometimes detected some irony on the part of the poet, is a technique borrowed from inscribed *iamata*:[12] the god is not only able to cure those who trust him, but can also endow them with "superpowers". Hagestratus, who suffered from insomnia, caused by headaches, was cured by the god and "not long afterwards won in the *pancratium* at the Nemean games" (B29 Herzog). In other words, not only was he healed of an impairing illness, but he became strong and healthy enough to win an important athletic competition. Hermodicus of Lampsacus, paralysed in the body, was healed and, in a dream, was ordered by the god to bring into the sanctuary the biggest stone that he could carry. He did so, and the big boulder lying in front of the *abaton* was there to confirm this incredible event (A15 Herzog).[13] 98 A.-B. is another interesting example of the connections between Posidippus' *iamatika* and Epidaurus' *iamata*: Architas, having kept a piece of bronze in his thigh *for six years*, escaped his suffering thanks to a dream. A similar case is the one recorded at A12 Herzog: Euhippus bore a spearhead in his jaw *for six years* and was cured by the god in a dream.

As these examples show, the records of Asclepius' healings contain several paradoxical elements: they describe phenomena that occur against *doxa*, human expectations. Paradoxographical writings usually call attention to the anomalous and wondrous nature of an occurrence, using key words, such as θαῦμα or

12 Zanetto 2016, 591.
13 The stone has been found and its weight has been estimated at 240 or 334 kg: Girone 1998, 53. The dedication of a stone by Hermodicus of Lampsacus is also recorded in *IG* IV^2 1.125, found at Epidaurus (Herzog 1931, 100–101; Longo 1969, 79–80, n. 48; Girone 1998, 53–57, n. II.3). The epigraph can be dated to around 200 B.C. (or even earlier), so it is probably a false inscription set up by temple authorities in order to offer confirmation of the miracle.

τέρας (especially with reference to stories where gods intervene, directly or indirectly).[14] No such key words appear in Posidippus' *iamatika* – although elsewhere the poet stresses the wondrous character of what he describes, be it a human artefact or a prodigious event, using this very terminology.[15] In Epidaurus' *iamata* the expression θαυμαστέον ... τὸ θεῖον is used once, at the beginning of the collection, in order to stress Asclepius' power (A1 Herzog).[16]

It is usually assumed that miraculous healings were the object of "aretalogies" – narratives of the deeds of a god which testified to his/her power – and that they constituted an autonomous branch of literature, different from paradoxography.[17] However, no ancient evidence is to be found of this (presumed) distinction between paradoxography and "aretalogy". It is crucial to bear in mind that the very term "aretalogy" was introduced by modern scholars to label a phenomenon for which the ancient sources did not have any specific word.[18] In spite of such a (modern) distinction, the similarities between healing literature and paradoxography are actually quite striking; I list below the most important ones.

1. Both paradoxography and aretalogies give no rational explanation for the *thauma* described. As remarked by Schepens and Delcroix 1996, 391, "the sense of the marvellous cannot survive on a rational basis. It is imperative for the paradoxographer to concentrate on *historia*, the establishing and the recording of facts without explaining them". This is also the rule in accounts of wondrous healings: in order to instil a sense of wonder, *thauma*, what sounds

14 Stories where gods intervene are the realm of the "divine-wonderful", according to Giannini's classification of the deeds narrated by paradoxographers: Giannini 1963. On paradoxography, see also Giannini 1964; 1966 (a critical edition of the texts); Sassi 1992–1993; Schepens/Delcroix 1996; for a book-length study, Pajón Leyra 2011.

15 Just a couple of examples: "marvellous" stones are described by words such as τέρας (8.7 A.-B.) or θαῦμα (15.7 A.-B.); in 31.5 A.-B. τέρας describes the "portent" of a statue of Athena that, in front of her temple, stirred her right foot from the basement, as a good omen for Alexander the Great, who was about to fight against the Persians. On Posidippus and paradoxography, see Krevans 2005, 89–92; Guichard 2006.

16 For the terminology of "wonder" in connection to Epidaurus' *iamata*, see Herzog 1931, 50–51. The language of paradoxography in relation to Asclepius' healing powers is regularly used in later sources, e.g., by Aelius Aristides (e.g. *Or.* 42.8 καὶ μὴν τό γε παράδοξον πλεῖστον ἐν τοῖς ἰάμασι τοῦ θεοῦ...; *Or.* 50.17 ἔργον τοῦ θεοῦ θαυμαστόν). It also appears in many inscriptions recording the wonders of a healing deity: e.g. *SEG* IV 1 (1929), 467.1 = *IDid* 159.1 (third century A.D.) τὸ θαῦμα τοῦτο, on a "miracle" by Apollo; *SEG* VIII 2 (1937), 551.35 = Egypt, *Inscr. Métriques* 175.IV.35 (first century B.C.) θαῦμα δὲ καὶ παράδοξον, on Isis' powers (both texts are discussed by Longo 1969 at, respectively, 133–136 and 177–178).

17 E.g. Longo 1969, 22; Schepens/Delcroix 1996, 382, n. 25.

18 Longo 1969, 11–34 (and 34–56 for a definition of the concept of "aretalogy").

odd, is never explained, it is only narrated. Worshippers are asked to trust in the power of the god and their healing depends on an act of faith; this is best exemplified by the stories, typical of incubatory literature, about incredulous people (ἄπιστοι) who are healed only after changing their mind regarding the god's power.[19]

2. In paradoxographical literature, as many details as possible are added, in order to increase the credibility of the story and the sense of wonder. This can also result in an interest in numbers and measurements, shared by both inscribed *iamata* and Posidippus' *iamatika* (some examples have been mentioned above: the duration of the illness, for instance, is usually indicated, so as to provide both a reliable account of the fact narrated and to build a contrast with the rapidity of the divine intervention).[20]
3. The programmatic search for documentation also entails a tendency to provide evidence for what is narrated: just as paradoxographers tend to specify their sources in order to enhance the reliability of their accounts,[21] in the same way the religious authorities responsible for collections of divine deeds provide as many signs of authenticity as they can. Not only do they tend to indicate their sources, but they also try to establish a connection between the stories and the votive materials visible in the shrine, mostly mentioning thank-offerings that the worshipper can still see.[22]
4. In paradoxography, the phenomenon described tends to be "geographically" isolated, and so "singularised". The same happens in incubatory literature: the exceptionality of the healing provided by the god is enhanced by linking the healing phenomenon to a specific geographic setting (namely, the space consecrated to the healing deity).[23]
5. Finally, the very process of assembling a collection of healing wonders resembles the work of paradoxographers. Both Posidippus and the anonymous temple authorities responsible for the inscriptions mirror the key process put forward by paradoxographers in constructing their collections of "miracles":

19 Dorati/Guidorizzi 1996, 357–358.

20 According to Herzog 1931, 82, numbers in tales imitate medical writing. Although this is possible, the paradoxographical interest in numbers is, to my mind, equally significant. Compare, for instance, Lucian's interest in recording numbers and measurements in his *True History*, a text profoundly indebted to paradoxography (Scarcella 1985 aptly described this attitude toward numbers in Lucian's *True History* as *furor mathematicus*).

21 Schepens/Delcroix 1996, 382–389.

22 Dorati/Guidorizzi 1996, 351.

23 This is particularly evident when the superiority of the sanctuary of Epidaurus over rival shrines is stressed: B21 and B23 Herzog; LiDonnici 1989, 186; Dorati/Guidorizzi 1996, 350–351.

they select, excerpt, and ultimately classify a series of events that belong to the realm of *thaumata*. The facts listed in a paradoxographical work are cut off from their original contexts (usually written sources, such as historiographical/geographical works); nevertheless, they retain a substantial degree of self-sufficiency, even when they form part of a thematic sequence.[24] Similarly, both *iamata* and *iamatika*, "lifted", as they are, from a (supposedly) original context (inscriptions, oral traditions etc.), retain their individuality, while forming at the same time a compact unit.

A telling example of the similarities between paradoxography and the accounts of Asclepius' miracles is provided by Aelianus *NA* 9.33. Acting as a typical paradoxographer, who describes an incredible event while citing his source in order to make the story more believable, Aelianus recounts the story of a woman cured at Epidaurus, derived – as he declares – from a work by the historian Hippys of Rhegium. The story, in which the woman undergoes a dangerous surgical procedure, finds a parallel in Epidaurus' *iamata* (B23 Herzog, on Aristagoras of Troizen).[25] The boundaries between aretalogy and paradoxography appear to be quite blurred, and suggest that the two branches of literature should not be regarded as rigidly distinct.

With this in mind, I now turn to a small group of epigrams of the *Greek Anthology* that deal with healings. Scholars have usually dismissed their importance as testimonies to the fortunes of the subgenre of *iamatika*, probably because here the divine healing power is not that of Asclepius, but that of other deities; even scholars who have recorded their existence have not paid much attention to them, but have only noted in passing their presence in the *Anthology*.[26]

In the next section, I would like to concentrate on the similarities between these epigrams and the tradition of miraculous healings; more specifically, I would like to show how they can be viewed as specimens of an interest in paradoxagraphy on the part of post-Hellenistic epigrammatists. It is worth noting in advance that – with the exception of Aeschines' acrostic dedication, mentioned above – the few *iamata* transmitted via the *Anthology* can all be dated to the Imperial age. This is certainly no surprise, since the Greek epigram of the early Empire shows a strong interest in paradoxography.[27] The few epigrams on healings

---

24 Schepens/Delcroix 1996.

25 Comparative analysis of the two stories in Herzog 1931, 77–84; LiDonnici 1995, 70–74.

26 Among the few exceptions, Conca/Marzi/Zanetto 2005, 483, n. 1 *ad AP* 6.203.

27 Rossi 2002, 164–165; Guichard 2014, 143–146.

that we are about to examine can be considered as yet another manifestation of such an interest.

2 Other *iamata* known via the *Greek Anthology*

AP 6.203 = *GPh* 3134–44 is a poem by Philip of Thessalonica (or by the otherwise unknown Lacon):[28]

Ἡ γρηὺς ἡ χερνῆτις, ἡ γυιὴ πόδας,
πύστιν κατ' ἐσθλὴν ὕδατος παιωνίου
ἦλθέν ποθ' ἑρπύζουσα σὺν δρυὸς ξύλῳ,
τό μιν διεσκήριπτε τὴν τετρωμένην·
οἶκτος δὲ Νύμφας εἷλεν, αἵ τ' †ἐρινόμου†
Αἴτνης παρωρείῃσι Συμαίθου πατρὸς
ἔχουσι δινήεντος ὑγρὸν οἰκίον·
καὶ τῆς μὲν ἀμφίχωλον ἀρτεμὲς σκέλος
θερμὴ διεστήριζεν Αἰτναίη λιβάς,
Νύμφαις δ' ἔλειπε βάκτρον, αἱ δ' ἐπῄνεσαν
πέμπειν μιν ἀστήρικτον ἡσθεῖσαι δόσει.

That old servant-woman, the one lame in the feet, at the good news of healing waters came crawling one day with her oak stick, which propped her maimed body up. Compassion seized the Nymphs who dwell on the foot-hills of < > Etna in the watery home of their whirlpool-sire Symaethus. Etna's hot spring made strong her two lame legs, and she left the Nymphs her stick; so they consented to escort her on her way unsupported, as they rejoiced in her gift.

(transl. Gow/Page 1968)

The epigram is not a proper dedication: it recounts an old woman's offering of a stick to divine dedicatees. It thus bears a structural analogy to Epidaurus' *iamata*, where the (possible) mention of a dedication is subordinated to the narration of a story, attesting to the *arete* of the divinity. The disease from which the old woman suffers is one of those chronic illnesses typically found in miracle inscriptions, where the mention of crutches is also traditional. One could compare it to A16 Herzog, on the lame Nicanor, who was suddenly cured when a boy grabbed his crutch and ran away, or to B35 Herzog, on a man who was carried to the sanctuary in a litter and the next morning was perfectly well. Posidippus 96 A.-B. tells

28 For a discussion of the authorship, see Gow/Page 1968, II, 369.

a similar story:[29] Antichares went to visit Asclepius with a pair of crutches and, after sacrificing to the god, was suddenly able to stand on both legs.[30]

Nevertheless, there are also some differences to be noted. First, the identity of the person healed is not specified, as is usually the case in dedications recording miraculous healings, and in Posidippus' *iamatika*. As far as the Epidaurian *iamata* are concerned, the identity of the person healed is sometimes specified by a proper name and sometimes expressed in generic terms, by words that simply indicate his/her gender, age range, and/or provenance.[31] It has been suggested that tales without names had an oral origin,[32] since oral accounts tend to be vague and indefinite. With an indeterminacy that is typical of fables, the protagonist of our poem is generically defined as an "old servant-woman" (line 1); emphasis is placed on her low social status, which is reminiscent of the tradition of epigrams on poor people, much in fashion since Leonidas of Tarentum. In line with such an indeterminacy, the story is located in a generic past (ποθ', line 3), as is common in popular tales.[33] Both these features – the identification of the human figure through a term that generically designates his/her profession, and the use of the adverb ποτε – are shared by many of the so-called *epideiktika* collected in the first part of book 9 of the *Anthology*;[34] in that section, the influence of school training is particularly evident, which should explain why several poems appear in formats used at school, such as the fable and the *chreia*.[35] Second, the divine healing power here comes not from Asclepius, as in the *iamata* discussed so far, but from the Nymphs. Because of their association with springs, the Nymphs are frequently depicted as healing deities, and they are often represented as Asclepius'

---

29 In the epigram there might also be, as in *AP* 6.203, the *implication* of the offering of an *ex-voto pro sanatione*.

30 That lame people – together with blind people – were typically treated by temple medicine is also testified by A4 Herzog: Ambrosia from Athens, blind in one eye, came as a suppliant to the god. Walking about the sanctuary, she ridiculed some of the healings as being unlikely and impossible, as in the case of *the lame and the blind* becoming well after only having a dream. Then she had a dream herself, was cured, and her scepticism disappeared.

31 E.g. A3 Herzog ἀνήρ; A5 Herzog παῖς ἄφωνος; A13 Herzog Ἀνὴρ Τορωναῖος etc.

32 LiDonnici 1995, 57.

33 In such a context, the very use of the iambic trimeter – related to the tradition of the *ainos* – may be significant, as Luca Mondin has suggested to me (for some general remarks on non-dactylic meters in Greek epigrams, see Floridi/Maltomini 2014, 36–39).

34 On this notoriously problematic definition, see especially Lauxtermann 1998; Rossi 2002.

35 Rossi 2002.

cult partners.[36] The importance of water in healing practices is widely known, and there are frequent allusions to baths in temple literature.[37] However, the epigram, with its celebration of the magical power of a spring, located in a precise geographical setting (i.e. Mount Etna),[38] is also connected to the tradition of paradoxography. Waters with miraculous properties, usually provided with a specific location, are typically present in paradoxographical literature. Already in the early Hellenistic period, Philostephanus of Cyrene, a contemporary of Callimachus, apparently composed a work in elegiac couplets on the waters of a Sicilian λίμνη (*SH* 691 = 34 Capel Badino).[39] Sicily is among the places most frequently mentioned in paradoxographical works: it appears to have been viewed as a "mythical" land, full of wonderful phenomena.[40] The poem can thus be seen as a rhetorical exercise that "translates" into an epigram a paradoxographical interest that was in fashion during the early Imperial period. Although any attempt to identify the poet's sources would be speculative, it cannot be ruled out that he drew directly from a paradoxographical work discussing the wonders of Sicily or the medical properties of various types of water.[41] Be that as it may, miraculous healing, the ethnographic element, and geographical "singularisation" all come together in the poem to produce *thauma*. The distinction between aretalogy and paradoxography becomes particularly blurred here, since the divine agents (the

---

36 Larson 2001, 196–198, 229. At Lebena – where, from the fourth century B.C. onwards, an important cult of Asclepius is attested – the first worship was for the Nymphs and Achelous (Guarducci 1932; 1934, 410; Girone 1998, 112; Larson 2001, 188). Another example of the incorporation of an earlier Nymph cult on the part of Asclepius is provided by Athens: Larson 2001, 129–130.
37 One might think, for instance, of Aelius Aristides' *Hieroi Logoi*, where the theme of the bath plays an important role, or of the panegyric on the water in Pergamum in Aristides *Or.* 53.1–5 (where the Nymphs are mentioned). It might also be worth considering the fourth-century B.C. inscription from the Asclepieion in Cos, intended to safeguard the purity of the water (*LSCG* 152), or Girone III.11, where Asclepius appears in a dream to two different priests – father and son – 47 years apart, to lead them to a source of water near the temple (Girone 1998, 112–115; Longo 1969, 82–83, n. 50; Martínez Fernández 2006, n. 20, 141–150).
38 On thermal waters at the foot of Etna, see Larson 2001, 216–217.
39 The nature of the work cannot be ascertained with confidence: it could have been either a continuous poem or a series of epigrams (Giannini 1964, 110–111; Schepens/Delcroix 1996, 400; Rossi 2002, 165). According to Capel Badino 2010, 38, 192–193, the two couplets on the Sicilian lake could have been part of a larger epigrammatic collection, arranged, like the "new Posidippus", in thematic sections, where a prominent role was played by hydrographic *mirabilia*. The preserved title περὶ τῶν παραδόξων ποταμῶν for a work of Philostephanus (T1 Capel Badino) – to which the verses on the lake obviously cannot be ascribed – would point in this direction.
40 Nymphodorus of Syracuse, for instance, was credited with a paradoxographical work entitled "The Wonders of Sicily"; Polycritus of Mende (*FGrHist* 559 F2) wrote a Σικελικὰ ἐν ἔπεσιν.
41 For such a theme, see Vitruvius 8.3.1-19; 26–27 (Posidonius F123 Jac.).

Nymphs) are basically identified with a natural element (healing water). The celebration of the power of the Nymphs (aretalogy) overlaps with the recounting of the wondrous properties of a spring located in a specific geographical area (paradoxography).

Another example is offered by Antiphilus *AP* 9.298 = *GPh* 1023–8:

Σκίπων με πρὸς νηὸν ἀνήγαγεν ὄντα βέβηλον
οὐ μοῦνον τελετῆς, ἀλλὰ καὶ ἠελίου·
μύστην δ' ἀμφοτέρων με θεαὶ θέσαν· οἶδα δ' ἐκείνῃ
νυκτὶ καὶ ὀφθαλμῶν νύκτα καθηράμενος·
ἀσκίπων δ' εἰς ἄστυ κατέστιχον ὄργια Δηοῦς
κηρύσσων γλώσσης ὄμμασι τρανότερον.

My staff brought me up to the temple, uninitiated not only in the ritual but in the sun's light too. The goddesses made me initiate in both, and I know that on that night I was purged also of the night upon my eyes. Staffless I went down to the city, proclaiming the Mysteries of Demeter more clearly with my eyes than with my tongue.

(transl. Gow/Page 1968)

The inclusion of the epigram in book 9 immediately testifies to the rhetorical nature of the epigram, which was perceived by the Byzantine anthologists (and probably conceived by the author himself) as an "epideictic" recounting of a wondrous event. The poem takes the form of a first-person narrative in which the healing experience clearly aims to elicit *thauma*. Not only is there a miraculous healing provided by certain deities (Demeter and Kore), but – to increase the sense of wonder – the divine act cures two different "disabilities". The lack of sight from which the narrator suffers is both physical (he cannot see the sun's light) and intellectual (he is uninitiated in the mysteries), as lines 1–2 emphatically state. Blindness is one of the diseases most frequently mentioned in the *iamata*,[42] but its association with the cult of Demeter and Kore deserves special attention. The sight bestowed by the goddesses is not limited to the regaining of a physical ability, but extends to the acquisition of a symbolic faculty. The ignorance of the uninitiated is a metaphorical blindness; by contrast, those who have taken part in the rituals are provided with the sight of knowledge. They are called ἐπόπται, "those who see/have seen". Seeing and lack of seeing are central to the initiatory experience of mystery cults. The restored "physical" sight in the epigram symbol-

42 E.g. A4, A9, A18, A20, B22, B32, B40, C65, D69 Herzog; Ar. *Pl.* 400–14 (further examples in Girone 1998, 135 n. 156).

ises the overcoming of an intellectual blindness, the acquisition of the true "vision" granted to the initiates by the goddesses.[43] The miraculous healing, with the sense of the wondrous that it entails, is stressed by the detail of the physical autonomy acquired by the narrator. He arrives with a σκίπων – the typical "companion" of blind people – and leaves ἀσκίπων; the contrast is emphasised by the placement of the two terms in antithesis in a prominent position, i.e. at the beginning of – respectively – lines 1 and 5. The protagonist of the poem is now a μύστης (line 3), both in the sense that he is an initiate in the μυστήρια and that he is admitted to the vision of the sun's light. With a possible allusion to the etymology of the word – μύστης, from μύω, is, according to one interpretation, "the one who closes his lips", i.e. "the one who keeps ritual silence" –[44] the epigram ends with the claim that the Mysteries of Demeter are testified to by the eyes of the speaker more clearly than they would have been by his tongue. Silence about the ceremony in which the initiate has taken part is maintained; nevertheless, the extraordinary experience is communicated to everybody, thanks to the miracle of the recovery of a physical ability that was previously missing.[45]

Recovery from blindness, together with a second "miracle", is also at the core of Antipater of Thessalonica[46] *AP* 9.46 = *GPh* 659–64:

Πηρὸς ἄπαις ἢ φέγγος ἰδεῖν ἢ παῖδα τεκέσθαι
  εὐξαμένη δοιῆς ἔμμορεν εὐτυχίης·
τίκτε γὰρ †εὐθὺς† ἄελπτα μετ' οὐ πολὺ καὶ τριπόθητον
  αὐτῆμαρ γλυκερὸν φέγγος ἐσεῖδε φάους.
Ἄρτεμις ἀμφοτέροισιν ἐπήκοος ἥ τε λοχείης
  μαῖα καὶ ἀργεννῶν φωσφόρος ἡ σελάων.

A blind and barren woman prayed either to see the daylight or to bear a child, and was granted the double blessing. Not long after, against all hope, she gave birth, and on the

43 On the centrality of "vision" in the rites of Eleusis, see Petridou 2013 (319–320 for this epigram). As both literary and material evidence suggest, in certain contexts Demeter may have been credited with the power to heal eye diseases (Petridou 2016). This is probably a consequence of the emphasis on the symbolic sight bestowed on the initiates by the goddess: the blazing light of the revelation at times had the power to cure physical blindness (Clinton 2005, 210).
44 The alternative interpretation for μύστης is "the one who closes his eyes", i.e. "the one who is (ritually) blindfolded": Petridou 2013, 316.
45 A connection between the condition of the μύστης and an ability to walk on one's own feet, highlighted by the very term ἀσκίπων, can already be found in Posidippus' *Seal* (118.24–7 A.-B.).
46 On the poem's authorship, alternatively ascribed to the obscure Callenius or Cyllenius, see Argentieri 2003, 183–184, who notices the affinity of the epigram with Antipater of Thessalonica *AP* 9.268 = *GPh* 209–14 (about a female dog that gave birth while she was killing a deer, thanks to Artemis, patron-goddess of both childbirth and hunting).

same day saw the sweet longed-for radiance of light. Both prayers were heard by Artemis, midwife in child-bed and light-bringer of white-gleaming rays.

(transl. Gow/Page 1968)

A woman addresses a prayer to Artemis – one of the Greek goddesses of childbirth and pregnancy – asking her to restore either her sight or her fertility, and the deity grants her both "miracles". A wish to become pregnant is also one of the most common reasons for visiting healing sanctuaries (e.g. B31, B34, B39, B42 Herzog); the wondrous nature of the facts described is, however, enhanced by the occurrence of a double healing, which does not seem to be typical of healing stories.[47] *Cumulatio* leads to hyperbole, and hyperbole in turn keeps the sense of the wondrous alive. It should be noted, on the other hand, that the geographical location of the story is not specified and a visit to a specific place – be that a temple, as in *AP* 9.298, or a holy spring, as in *AP* 6.203 – is not mentioned. In a similar vein, as in *AP* 9.298, the protagonist of the story is described in generic terms, without any mention of her name. The author focuses on her distinguishing features, i.e. her physical disability (πηρός)[48] and lack of children (ἄπαις), in order to provide a paradigmatic story, a sort of moralising tale on the advantages of piously worshipping the gods. Indeed, the epigram offers an example of rewarded *pietas*, and the narrative serves a moralising purpose, as do many other poems in *AP* 9,[49] according to the rhetorical tradition of didactic fables, anecdotes, and edifying examples that was in fashion in this period. However, the emphasis on the miraculous healing and the stressing of the wondrous elements in the story (namely, the perfect synchronicity of the double healing) are reminiscent of temple literature and reveal an intersection between *iamata* and *paradoxa*.

Imperial epigrams, unlike Posidippus' *iamatika*, betray a stronger influence from rhetorical practices and appear in formats which are in part different from those of the Milan papyrus. The three poems discussed above fit perfectly within the context of the first-century CE "epideictic" epigram, which shows an interest in narrating what is unique and unusual, and which is rhetorically fond of *paradoxa*. Nevertheless, the theme of healing sets them apart from other narrative poems of the same period and connects them to the epigrammatic tradition of *iamatika*, even though, as mentioned above, Posidippus' epigrams are all concerned

47 See Di Nino 2010, 226 n. 253 (with reference to Posidippus 97 A.-B.).

48 This generic term can be applied to different kinds of disability (*LSJ*, s.v. πηρός); it becomes clear from what follows that here it refers to blindness.

49 Rossi 2002, 156–164.

with the powers of Asclepius, while in this case a wider variety of healing deities is celebrated.[50]

The dearth of Imperial epigrams dealing with miraculous healings prevents us from speculating about the overall attitude of their authors towards the subgenre: did these epigrams appear in larger thematic contexts (i.e. did they represent a separate section in an epigrammatic collection, as is the case of Posidippus' *iamatika*)? Did they intend to offer an overall picture of the "miracles" effected by different gods, or did each author select the "wonders" of a single divinity? Were the healing stories perceived to constitute a distinct category, as in the Milan papyrus, or were they just considered "wonders" not so different from the accounts of – for instance – curious manners of death? These questions cannot be answered with any certainty. What can be stated with a certain degree of confidence is that an epigrammatic fondness for *iamata* is not limited to the Hellenistic era and is not characteristic only of Posidippus. Despite the differences, the three poems indicate that an epigrammatic tradition of literary *iamatika* continued after the first Hellenistic age before crossing paths with the rhetorical passion for the recounting of *paradoxa*. Such a clear intersection between *paradoxa* and *iamata* in epigrams should probably warn scholars against classifications that might appear too schematic and should lead us to reconsider the traditional distinction between aretalogy and paradoxography.

3 Parody

A recurring feature of the epigrams discussed above – and of healing literature in general – is the tendency to enhance the wondrous character of the facts narrated by means of hyperbole. The achievements of the healing deity are super-human. Healing gods can do what "normal" doctors cannot: they cure chronic illnesses and they can restore the healed person not only to *good*, but to *extraordinary*

50 The lack of Imperial literary epigrams on Asclepius' healings is most probably the result of mere chance: his cult played an important part in religious life from the sixth-fifth centuries B.C. onwards, at least up to the time of Diocletian (Edelstein/Edelstein 1998², vol. II, 138). An alternative explanation might be that Imperial epigrammatists, in their search for novelty, favoured the stories of gods less renowned for their healing powers over those of the healing god *par excellence*. For a possible mention of Asclepius, however, see the anonymous *AP* 9.511: Παιήων (= Παιάν, an epithet of both Apollo and Asclepius) asks the worshipper to decorate the head of his cult-statue with gold (after a healing, we can infer).

health. Although – as is widely known – scientific medicine and religious medicine were not mutually exclusive in ancient Greece,[51] it is significant that healing literature typically states that a sick person turns to Asclepius (and the like) after having despaired of human remedies – as in the above-quoted Aeschines' epigram.[52] Asclepius, the father figure of human medicine, is able to achieve things beyond the powers of human doctors. The ability to successfully fight illness in a way that is impossible for "real" doctors is also attributed, in a few epigrams on eminent physicians of the *Greek Anthology*,[53] to some legendary figures of healers, such as Hippocrates (Nicodemus or Bassus *AP* 9.53), Galen (Magnus the Physician *APl.* 270), and Praxagoras (Crinagoras *APl.* 273 = *GPh* 2070–7). However, when celebrating the achievements of these eminent physicians – associated with or likened to the patron deities of medicine – Greek epigrams do not exploit the set of themes apt to elicit *thauma* that we find in the *iamata*. These figures might be credited with the power to avert death – a power that Asclepius himself never displays, as exemplified by the fate of Soses of Cos in Posidippus[54] – but their activity takes place in a distant, mythical past – a Golden Age now irredeemably lost. Hippocrates, in Nicodemus (or Bassus) *AP* 9.53, is described as the one who "was the light of humankind; whole peoples were saved by him, and there was scarcity of dead in Hades". In a similar vein, according to Magnus the Physician *APl.* 270, "there was a time", when Galen was alive, when "the earth received men mortal and reared them in immortality. The halls of tearful Acheron were bereaved by the force of your [that is, Galen's] healing hand". A similar motif had already been explored by Crinagoras *APl.* 273, for whom "if mortals had enough such physicians [i.e. as Praxagoras], the boat [i.e. of Charon] would never have crossed the ferry with its load of corpses" (lines 7–8). The counterfactual conditional here basically clarifies that the naturally occurring human desire for immortality is impossible to fulfil. In other epigrams, the claim that the physician was able to avert other people's death is undermined by the very fact that the poems celebrating his deeds are epitaphs: in "Empedocles" or "Simonides" *AP*

51 E.g. Prêtre/Charlier 2009, 192–197; Pajón Leyra 2015, 64, 73–74.

52 E.g. Dorati/Guidorizzi 1996, 354–355; Girone 1998, 44 n. 19. A peculiar variant of this motif is provided by a second-century A.D. inscription from Phrygia (296 Samama): a woman promises an offer to Asclepius, should her sick son be healed without having to consult any doctors – apparently, she does not trust human medicine. Similarly, in *SEG* 47 (second-third centuries A.D.), a first-person narrator declares that he consulted 36 doctors without obtaining any good, and that he was healed by the intervention of the god.

53 Discussed by Plastira-Valkanou 2004.

54 As often remarked by scholars, although he is mentioned in 97 A.-B. as having been healed by the god, the next section of the Milan papyrus reveals that the man is now dead (103 A.-B.).

7.508 = *FGE* 550–3 Pausanias is described as the one "who turned aside from the chambers of Persephone many men wasted by chilling disease" (lines 3–4). As remarked by Plastira-Valkanou (2004, 453), "it sounds ironic ... that he [i.e. Pausanias], who averted death for so many people, was unable to ward off his own and is now buried".

Inscribed epitaphs[55] reflect a similar pattern: here doctors appear as good men, indifferent to money, meticulous in the exercising of their *techne*, sometimes cultivated and learned. However, they are human, with all the failings and shortcomings which their mortality entails. Epitaphs for doctors often underline the limits of medicine and the irony lying in the fact that those who spent their lives curing other people's illnesses cannot cure their own.[56] A second-century A.D. epitaph found at Stratonicea (266 Samama), for instance, claims: "you had learned to take care of others, but you were not able to save yourself from illness, since the Moira is by her very nature stronger than the doctors" (lines 8–10). Likewise, a first-century A.D. epitaph from Halicarnassus (271 Samama) declares: "you sleep, the best of physicians, but Hades is enemy to the living, Hades who did not even protect he who was fighting maladies for the healing of mortals" (lines 4–6). Epitaphs for doctors do not record any "wonders" that have been performed by the deceased:[57] in this respect, *iamata* and human medicine appear clearly distinct.

On the contrary, hyperbolic descriptions of "wondrous" deeds are found in a set of scoptic epigrams on doctors responsible for unsuccessful healings and even for the death of their patients. In these poems, physicians are notorious figures, able to cause harm in the most unexpected (and thus paradoxical) ways.[58] Dion is able to blind not only his patient, but even a statue of Zeus (Lucillius *AP* 11.112). The restoration of sight granted by healing gods, so often celebrated in healing literature, is replaced by the eternal darkness caused by this human counterpart.[59] The blinding of the statue of a god – a comic hyperbole also exploited by

55 Collected by Samama 2003.

56 On this commonplace motif, see Plastira-Valkanou 2004, 453.

57 Nor, for that matter, are their failures usually mentioned: 309 Samama, a bilingual epitaph for a child (Nicomedia, fourth century A.D.), where the surgical operation that led to the death of the 5-year-old boy is mentioned, is an exception (a couple of references to the faults of doctors also appear in Latin funerary inscriptions: see Schatzmann 2012, 142–143, n. 14).

58 Schatzmann 2012, 129–163; Floridi 2014, 218–236, 459–460, 566–568 (with further bibliography).

59 See also Lucillius *AP* 11.115: Simon is more effective than Isis or Harpocrates in depriving people of sight (on the powers of Serapis and Isis see e.g. Bricault 2008; Serapis' "miracles" have been collected by Longo 1969, 101–122).

Lucillius elsewhere – contributes to the efficacy of the joke. It turns upside down the motif of the statue as a prodigy, common in paradoxography,[60] and of the statue as a personification of the healing deity: in incubatory literature, the god regularly appears in dreams in the shape of his cultic statue, so that the boundaries between the god and his/her image tend to be blurred.[61] With comic reversal, here a divine statue – a statue of Zeus, the king of the gods, among whose attributes was that of Σωτήρ, "Saviour" – not only lacks any "superpowers", but cannot even keep away the incompetent eye doctor. Even more interesting, for our purposes, are the poems that exploit the motif of the "murderous touch". The doctor Hermogenes, with the "touch" of his hand, kills the astrologer Diophantus (Lucillius *AP* 11.114); the physician Marcus just touches a statue of Zeus and kills the god, in spite of the latter's divine nature, and of his being made of stone (Lucillius *AP* 11.113). In a further extension of the hyperbole, some doctors do not even need to touch their patients in order to cause their deaths: their very appearance (Hedylus *AP* 11.123 = *HE* 1887–90), or the simple memory of their names (Nicarchus *AP* 11.118), are sufficient to bring about devastating effects.[62] All these epigrams concerned with the physician's "touch" clearly reverse the laudatory motif of the "healing hand" of the good doctor,[63] and of the very god of medicine, Asclepius. In incubatory literature, Asclepius is often credited with healing his patients by touching their bodies or simply stretching his hand out to them.[64] The doctors satirised by scoptic poets are thus implicitly characterised as "anti-Asclepiuses", and their wondrous killings are the perfect reversal of the god's wondrous healings. This is even more evident in Lucillius *AP* 11.257, a poem that plays on the motif of ritual sleep:

> Ἑρμογένην τὸν ἰατρὸν ἰδὼν Διόφαντος ἐν ὕπνοις
> οὐκέτ' ἀνηγέρθη καὶ περίαμμα φέρων.

Diophantus, seeing in a dream Hermogenes the doctor, did not wake up any more – and he was wearing an amulet.

---

60 E.g. [Arist.] *Mir. ausc.* 175; a sweating statue appears in Posidippus 30 A.-B.; Krevans 2005, 91.

61 Dorati/Guidorizzi 1996, 356–357.

62 For similar jokes in Latin epigrams, see Martial 5.9; Ausonius *epigr.* 77 and 78 Green (free translations of – respectively – Lucillius *AP* 11.114 and *AP* 11.113: see my commentary *ad loc.*, with further bibliography).

63 See the epitaph for Galen quoted above.

64 Plastira-Valkanou 2004, 455–456. On the vocabulary of "touch" in Greek and Latin medical texts, see Boehm 2003.

The idea of dying in sleep after having a dream where the murderous doctor, an ominous counterpart of the healing deity, appears, is clearly a reversal of the rite of incubation, and so it should be viewed as a parodic distortion of "temple" themes. Instead of the instantaneous healings following a dream that are celebrated in the literature on miraculous healings, the epigram records an instantaneous death that does not come about as a consequence of any illness, and which therefore lacks any rational cause. The sense of *thauma* is enhanced by the addition καὶ περίαμμα φέρων: an amulet, usually worn to avert illness,[65] paradoxically proves ineffective against the power of a doctor, who should be the very one counting on such "therapeutic" aid.[66]

4 Conclusion

Healing literature, with its set of themes, and with its interest in stories that defy human expectations, shares several elements with paradoxography. It is no coincidence that in his epigrams Posidippus – the author of a series of poems labelled *iamatika*, indebted to the tradition of temple *iamata* – also discusses other kinds of wonders,[67] and that poems on miraculous healings continue to be composed in the Imperial age, when a special fondness for describing the unique and the unusual is attested. The three *iamatika* of the *Greek Anthology* that we have analysed above preserve the main features of the "subgenre", although they also evidence certain differences that testify to a change in cultural background (in particular, the influence of rhetorical training). Both Hellenistic and Imperial *iamatika* suggest that too rigid a distinction between aretalogy and paradoxography cannot be drawn. Wonders about healings do not appear so different from other categories of *mirabilia*: the case of *AP* 6.203, where the celebration of the healing deities – the Nymphs – overlaps with the recounting of the wondrous properties of a natural element – the waters of a specific spring – is particularly telling.

Laudatory epigrams about doctors stress the human nature of the physicians and are clearly distinguished from healing literature. However, further evidence as to the "fortunes" of *iamatika* seems to come from the scoptic tradition, where satire on doctors was widespread. In portraying the failures of human physicians,

65 Dickie 2001, 24–25.
66 The epigram is "translated" by Martial 6.53: Floridi 2014, 460 (with bibliography).
67 See n. 15 above.

some poems exploit hyperboles which seem to reverse motifs found in the *iamata*, in order to draw a humorous picture of Asclepius' human counterparts, and to offer a disastrously "wondrous" counterbalance to the "miracles" of the deities.[68]

Bibliography

Acosta-Hughes, B./Kosmetatou, E./Baumbach, M. (eds.) (2004), *Labored in Papyrus Leaves: Perspectives on an Epigram Collection Attributed to Posidippus (P.Mil.Vogl. VIII 309)*, Cambridge, MA/London.

Argentieri, L. (2003), *Gli epigrammi degli Antipatri*, Roma/Bari.

Austin, C./Bastianini, G. (2002), *Posidippi Pellaei quae supersunt omnia*, Milan.

Bajnok, D. (2004), "Aeschines's Inscription in Epidaurus? An Old Question Revisited", *Graeco-Latina Brunensia* 19, 15–26.

Bing, P. (2004), "Posidippus' *Iamatika*", in: Acosta-Hughes/Kosmetatou/Baumbach 2004, 276–291.

Bing, P. (2009), *The Scroll and the Marble: Studies in Reading and Reception in Hellenistic Poetry*, Ann Arbor.

Boehm, I. (2003), "Toucher du doigt. Le vocabulaire du toucher dans les textes médicaux grecs et latins", in: F. Gaide/F. Biville (eds.), *Manus medica. Actions et gestes de l'officiant dans les textes médicaux latins. Questions de thérapeutique et de lexique*. Actes du Colloque tenu à l'Université Lumière-Lyon II, les 18 et 19 septembre 2001, Aix-en-Provence, 229–240.

Bricault, L. (2008), "Serapide, dio guaritore", in: E. Dal Covolo/G. Sfameni Gasparro (eds.), *Cristo e Asclepio. Culti terapeutici e taumaturgici nel mondo mediterraneo antico fra cristiani e pagani*. Atti del convegno internazionale. Accademia di studi mediterranei, Agrigento 20–21 novembre 2006, Roma, 55–71.

Capel Badino, R. (2010), *Filostefano di Cirene: Testimonianze e frammenti*, Milano.

Clinton, K. (2005), *Eleusis: The Inscriptions on Stone. Documents of the Sanctuary of the Two Goddesses and Public Documents of the Deme*, vol. I, Athens.

Conca, F./Marzi, M./Zanetto, G. (2005), *Antologia Palatina*, vol. I (libri I–VIII), Torino.

Dickie, M.W. (2001), *Magic and Magicians in the Greco-Roman World*, London/New York.

Dillon, M.P.J. (1994), "The Didactic Nature of the Epidaurian Iamata", *ZPE* 101, 239–260.

68 This paper benefited from discussion with other participants in the workshop "Medicine and Paradoxography in the Ancient World" in Patras, in particular with George Kazantzidis, whom I also wish to thank for his invitation; and with the audience in Venice, where it was presented at "Poesia epigrafica. Seminario di studi sull'epigramma greco", organised by Stefania De Vido and Olga Tribulato (Università Ca' Foscari, 16/2/2017), whom I thank for their feedback and hospitality. Thanks are also due to Francesca Angiò and Giuseppe Zanetto for commenting on earlier drafts of this paper, and to Maria Plastira Valkanou for her help with the bibliography.

Di Marco, M./Palumbo Stracca, B.M./Lelli, E. (eds.), *Posidippo e gli altri. Il poeta, il genere, il contesto culturale e letterario*. Atti dell'incontro di studio, Roma, 14–15 maggio 2004, Pisa/Roma 2005 (= *ARF* 6, 2004).
Di Nino, M.M. (2005), "Posidippo e la letteratura incubatoria", in: Di Marco/Palumbo Stracca/Lelli 2005, 47–76.
Di Nino, M.M. (2006), "Tra aretalogia e gioco letterario: l'ottava sezione del P. Mil. Vogl. VIII 309", *ZPE* 155, 26–36.
Di Nino, M.M. (2010), *I fiori campestri di Posidippo: ricerche sulla lingua e lo stile di Posidippo di Pella*, Göttingen.
Dorati, M./Guidorizzi, G. (1996), "La letteratura incubatoria", in: Pecere/Stramaglia 1996, 343–371.
Edelstein, E.J./Edelstein, L. (1998²), *Asclepius. Collection and Interpretation of the Testimonies*, I–II, Baltimore.
Floridi, L. (2014), *Lucillio. Epigrammi*, Berlin/Boston.
Floridi, L./Maltomini, F. (2014: *re vera* 2016), "Sui contenuti e l'organizzazione interna di P.Vindob. G 40611 (CPR XXXIII)", *Aegyptus* 94, 19–62.
Garulli, V. (2005), "Posidippo e l'epigrafia sepolcrale greca", in: Di Marco/Palumbo Stracca/Lelli 2005, 23–46.
Garulli, V. (2016), "Posidippe, auteur épigraphique ?", in: E. Santin/L. Foschia (eds.), *L'épigramme dans tous ses états: épigraphiques, littéraires, historiques*, Lyon, 60–87.
Giannini, A. (1963), "Studi sulla paradossografia greca (I). Da Omero a Callimaco: motivi e forme del meraviglioso", *RILSL* 97, 247–260.
Giannini, A. (1964), "Studi sulla paradossografia greca (II). Da Callimaco all'età imperiale: la letteratura paradossografica", *Acme* 17, 99–140.
Giannini, A. (1966), *Paradoxographorum Graecorum reliquiae*, Milano.
Girone, M. (1998), *Iamata. Guarigioni miracolose di Asclepio in testi epigrafici*, Bari.
Gow, A.S.F./Page, D.L. (1968), *The Greek Anthology. The Garland of Philip*, I–II, Cambridge.
Guarducci, M. (1932), "I predecessori di Asclepio", *Studi e materiali di storia delle religioni* 8, 215–229.
Guarducci, M. (1934), "I miracoli di Asclepio a Lebena", *Historia* 8, 410–428.
Guichard, L.A. (2006), "Posidipo y los prodigios. Una interpretación de P. Mil. Vogl. VIII 309", *Studi di Egittologia e di Papirologia* 3, 121–133.
Guichard, L.A. (2014), "Paradox and the Marvellous in Greek Poetry of the Imperial Period", in: L.A. Guichard/J.L. García Alonso/M. Paz de Hoz (eds.), *The Alexandrian Tradition: Interactions Between Science, Religion, and Literature*, Bern, 141–156.
Herzog, R. (1931), *Die Wunderheilungen von Epidauros: Ein Beitrag zur Geschichte der Medizin und der Religion*, Leipzig.
Krevans, N. (2005), "The Editor's Toolbox. Strategies for Selection and Presentation in the Milan Epigram Papyrus", in: K. Gutzwiller (ed.), *The New Posidippus: A Hellenistic Poetry Book*, Oxford.
Larson, J. (2001), *Greek Nymphs: Myths, Cult, Lore*, Oxford.
Lauxtermann, M.D. (1998), "What is an Epideictic Epigram?", *Mnemosyne* 51, 525–537.
LiDonnici, L.R. (1989), *Tale and Dream: The Text and Compositional History of the Corpus of Epidaurian Miracle Cures*, Pennsylvania.
LiDonnici, L.R. (1992), "Compositional Background of the Epidaurian Iamata", *AJPh* 113, 25–41.
LiDonnici, L.R. (1995), *Epidaurian Miracle Inscriptions. Text, Translation and Commentary*, Atlanta.

Longo, V. (1969), *Aretalogie nel mondo greco*, Genova.
Männlein-Robert, I. (2015), "Poseidippos, *Iamatika*", in: B. Seidensticker/A. Staehli/A. Wessels (eds.), *Der neue Poseidipp: Text, Übersetzung und Kommentar*, Darmstadt, 370–409.
Martínez Fernández, A. (2006), *Epigramas Helenísticos de Creta*, Madrid.
Oberhelman, S.M. (ed.) (2013), *Dreams, Healing, and Medicine in Greece: From Antiquity to the Present*, Farnham/Burlington.
Pajón Leyra, I. (2011), *Entre ciencia y maravilla. El género literario de la paradoxografía griega*, Zaragoza.
Pajón Leyra, I. (2015), "Los dioses en la salud y en la enfermedad: curaciones milagrosas en el mundo griego", in: O. Martínez/M. Montero (eds.), *Adivinos, magos, brujas, astrólogos*, Madrid, 61–78.
Papalexandrou, N. (2004), "Reading as Seeing: P.Mil.Vogl. VIII 309 and Greek Art", in: Acosta-Hughes/Kosmetatou/Baumbach 2004, 247–258.
Paton, W.R. (1916), *The Greek Anthology*, vol. I, London/Cambridge, MA.
Pecere, O./Stramaglia, A. (eds.) (1996), *La letteratura di consumo nel mondo greco-latino*, Atti del convegno internazionale, Cassino 14–17 settembre 1994, Cassino.
Petridou, G. (2013), "'Blessed Is He, Who Has Seen': The Power of Ritual Viewing and Ritual Framing in Eleusis", in: S. Blundell/D. Cairns/N. Rabinowitz (eds.), *Vision and Viewing in Ancient Greece*, *Helios* 40, 309–341.
Petridou, G. (2016), "Demeter as an Ophthalmologist? Eye Votives and the Cult of Demeter and Kore", in: J. Draycott/E.-J. Graham (eds.), *Bodies of Evidence: Ancient Anatomical Votives Past, Present and Future. Medicine and the body in antiquity*, London/New York, 95–111.
Plastira-Valkanou, M. (2004), "The Praise of Eminent Physicians in the *Greek Anthology*", in: A.P. Vasileiadis/P. Kotzia/A.D. Mavroudis/D.A. Christidis (eds.), Δημητρίῳ στέφανος. Τιμητικός τόμος για τον καθηγητή Δημήτρη Λυπουρλή, Thessaloniki, 441–474.
Prêtre, C./Charlier, Ph. (2009), *Maladies humaines, thérapies divines. Analyse épigraphique et paléopathologique de textes de guérison grecs*, Villeneuve d'Ascq.
Rossi, L. (2002), "Composition and Reception in *AP* 9.1–583: *Aphegheseis*, *epideixeis* and *progymnasmata*", in: M.A. Harder/R.F. Regtuit/G.C. Wakker (eds.), *Hellenistic Epigram*, Leuven, 151–174.
Samama, E. (2003), *Les médecins dans le monde grec*, Genève.
Sassi, M.M. (1992–3), "Mirabilia", in: G. Cambiano/L. Canfora/D. Lanza (eds.), *Lo spazio letterario della Grecia antica*, vol. I.2, *L'Ellenismo*, Roma, 449–468.
Scarcella, A.M. (1985), "Luciano, le *Storie Vere* e il *furor mathematicus*", *GIF* 16, 249–257.
Schatzmann, A. (2012), *Nikarchos II: Epigrammata. Einleitung, Texte, Kommentar*, Göttingen.
Schepens, G./Delcroix, K. (1996), "Ancient Paradoxography: Origin, Evolution, Production and Reception", in: Pecere/Stramaglia 1996, 375–460.
Wickkiser, B.L. (2013), "The *Iamatika* of the Milan Posidippus", *CQ* 63, 623–632.
Zanetto, G. (2002), "Posidippo e i miracoli di Asclepio", in: G. Bastianini *et al.* (eds.), *Un poeta ritrovato: Posidippo di Pella*, 'Giornata di studio, Milano 23 novembre 2001,' Milano, 73–78.
Zanetto, G. (2016), "L'epigramma per Asclas di Creta (Posidippo, 99 A.-B.): problemi di testo e contesto", in: A. Casanova/G. Messeri/R. Pintaudi (eds.), *... e sì d'amici pieno. Omaggio di studiosi italiani a Guido Bastianini per il suo settantesimo compleanno*, Firenze, 587–591.

Julia Doroszewska

Beyond the Limits of the Human Body

Phlegon of Tralles' Medical Curiosities

Abstract: This article examines the collection of extraordinary phenomena composed by the 2nd-century CE Greek paradoxographer Phlegon of Tralles. His work best known under the Latin title of *Mirabilia* comprises 35 chapters which almost exclusively record cases of human oddities. Among them are revenants, hermaphrodites, sex-changers, male mothers, various teratological births, multiple pregnancies, and wondrous fertility. The majority of these records constitute medical curiosities in the sense that they are concerned with issues such as human anatomy, physiology, reproduction or sexuality. These features, therefore, allow us to consider Phlegon's work as one which brings paradoxography and medicine together. The aim of this article is to read the miraculous events described by Phlegon through the lens of contemporary medicine and consider them as case studies subject to scientific (or quasi-scientific) explanation rather than prodigies or wonders intended only to amaze.

1 Introduction

The *Mirabilia* by Phlegon of Tralles is hardly comparable to anything, even within its own genre. This second-century CE collection of extraordinary phenomena, which in its present form contains 35 chapters, records almost exclusively cases of human oddities. This feature significantly distinguishes it from other paradoxographical collections which single out various other peculiarities of either animate or inanimate nature, including unusual properties of stones, plants, rivers, and animals. Phlegon's interest, by contrast, more than in anything else lies in the human body.[1] The majority of cases he records constitute, so to speak, medical marvels, in the sense that they are concerned with issues such as human anatomy, physiology, reproduction, or sexuality. For this reason alone, his work may already be considered to bridge paradoxography and medicine.

1 This thematic discrepancy between Phlegon and earlier paradoxographers has been recently explored by Kazantzidis (2018), who explains the shift towards the human (and especially female) body with reference to the influence of the Hippocratic doctrines and discourse, and in particular Hippocratic gynecology.

https://doi.org/10.1515/9783110661774-006

Phlegon seems to have been a compiler by vocation, as one can infer from both his extant fragmentary works, as well as from the titles of his lost treatises.[2] His literary output perfectly falls in line with what Umberto Eco labels a "*vertigine della lista*", literally, a "dizziness of lists",[3] a passion for cataloguing and collecting, which he considers a phenomenon characteristic of the Western mind from Homer onward. As already noted, Phlegon's predilection for 'collecting' human oddities makes him stand out among other paradoxographers, and that in particular when it comes to the intersection of paradoxography and medicine. Now, a brief overview of the topics explored in the *Mirabilia* will give us a more detailed idea about this overlap.

In the *Mirabilia*, the first three chapters concern revenants. The following seven describe hermaphrodites (this motif is to be found also in ch. 2) and sex-changers. Chapters 11–19 report discoveries of huge bones believed to be the remains of giants. Teratological births, including children with redundant body parts (ch. 20, 21 and 25) and with animal features (ch. 22–24) are the subject matter of the subsequent five chapters. The next two recount cases of male parturition, while chapters 28–31 speak of multiple births and wondrous fertility. Chapters 32–33 detail cases of unnaturally fast human development, and the last two (34–35) describe the capture of live centaurs.

Not all these stories lend themselves to be read through the lens of contemporary medicine. Paradoxography as a genre obviously assumes different objectives and different audiences than do medical treatises. Its goal is to astonish and amaze, whereas the ancient doctors focus principally on description and explanation.[4] This does not necessarily mean that the marvelous cannot be explained rationally. The collector of oddities is simply not interested in providing any such explanation regardless of whether one is possible or not. This is precisely what this chapter will aim to do: to furnish a rational account for Phlegon's oddities –

2 The extant works, apart from the *Mirabilia*, are: *On Longevity* (Περὶ μακροβίων), a compilation listing people of extraordinarily long life-span, and the *Olympiads* (Ὀλυμπιάδες), which was a historical chronicle of the Olympic Games from their founding in 776 BCE until the 229th Olympiad (137–40 CE), when Hadrian died. As for the lost works, according to the Suda (s.v. Φλέγων Τραλλιανός) Phlegon wrote some other books (καὶ ἄλλα) which are: *A Description of Sicily* (Ἔκφρασις Σικελίας); *The Festivals of the Romans* (Περὶ τῶν παρὰ Ῥωμαίοις ἑορτῶν), and *A Topography of Rome* (Περὶ τῶν ἐν Ῥώμῃ τόπων καὶ ὧν ἐπικέκληνται ὀνομάτων); translation of the Greek titles by Hansen 1996, 17.

3 In his book *Vertigine della Lista* (2009); the original Italian title in the English edition (tr. A. McEwen, New York: Rizzoli, 2009) is rendered as *The Infinity of Lists*.

4 Schepens/Delcroix 1996, 390–391; Krevans 2005, 91; Kazantzidis 2018, 32.

where such account is possible in the light of ancient knowledge – and thus explore the points where his *thaumata* may be seen as converging with contemporary medical discourse. In what follows, therefore, I intend to discuss Phlegon's cases of apparent death (in the stories of revenants), problems concerning sex and gender (in the accounts of hermaphrodites, sex-changers, male mothers), and teratological births (in the accounts of fetal malformations and 'animal' children). By contrast, I omit the stories of giant bones, which seem to tap into mythological rather than medical knowledge (e.g. the four or five ages of man), and of hippocentaurs (which seem to be well grounded in contemporary scientific discourse, but are analyzed in detail by Shannon in this volume). I also leave aside some stories which indeed appear to be exaggerated accounts of actual medical conditions (like those of abnormally quick maturation compared to modern data on progeria), but seem to have had no point of contact with ancient medical thought.

2 The *Scheintod* or the Apparent Death

The first three stories in the collection, without a doubt, constitute its most complex and elaborate part. Since they display stylistic similarities in their content and phrasing, and given that they present fiction under the guise of historical reality, earlier scholars thought that they were composed by a single author whose identity remains unknown.[5] Although this hypothesis is nowadays questioned, there is a general agreement that all three stories were composed several centuries before Phlegon, most likely in the late Hellenistic period.[6] Their leitmotif is a revenant, an entity (apparently) come back from the dead. The qualifier 'apparently' is of particular importance for the first of these stories, which for this reason may be considered an intriguing specimen of intersection between medicine and paradoxography.

The first story is that of a woman named Philinnion, who dies young and secretly returns, six months after her death,[7] to her parents' house, where she begins a short-lived liaison with a lodger, a young man by the name of Machates.[8]

5 Rohde 1877, 338–339; Wendland 1911, 9–10, and Mesk 1925, 298.
6 Hansen 1996, 66–67.
7 This detail has been supplied by Rohde (1877) from Proclus' retelling of this story (*In R.* 2.115 Kroll), since the beginning of Phlegon's account is missing.
8 On this story's relationship to ancient medicine, see recently Kazantzidis 2018, 46–47 and n. 70.

Machates does not have the slightest suspicion that he is dealing with a dead person, which of course presupposes that her body displayed no symptoms of decay. That Philinnion is actually dead is revealed when her parents suddenly interrupt the lovers' rendezvous and recognize in her their deceased daughter. In this very moment Philinnion drops dead *again* and does not return to life any more. The plot allows for a twofold interpretation: one may either take it as a typical ghost story, or that of an apparent death. The latter, the so-called *Scheintod*, is a motif well-known from the ancient novel.[9] As the story of Philinnion displays certain similarities to the novel, especially regarding content (as it recounts a sensational and romantic event), one is tempted to choose the latter reading.[10] There is, however, one essential difference: in the novel the protagonist who is apparently dead eventually turns out to be alive, whereas in Phlegon, Philinnion, although seemingly alive, proves to be dead in the end. In a sense therefore, it is a reversed motif of apparent death (or rather of apparent life); this is at least what Phlegon's story seems to suggest. Philinnion is just an animated and good-looking corpse which by the action of an otherwise unspecified "divine will" (θεία βούλησις; 1.2, 1.6., 1.12) returns to a state of 'quasi-life', to use William Hansen's expression.[11]

As such, Philinnion's plight seems to have little in common with medicine and more with religion or even magic. Ironically though, a thoroughly medical explanation was for the first time offered in a work dedicated to magic and its history by the 19th-century French occult author, magician, and freemason, Éliphas Lévi. According to Lévi, Philinnion's "apparent life" followed by a very real death is a case of "hysterical coma, accompanied by lucid somnambulism."[12] The girl, as Lévi's argument runs, first suffered from the coma, whereupon she was thought dead and promptly buried; afterwards she started sleepwalking (and began her amorous adventure with Machates), from which she was "roughly awakened" by her parents, which in turn, as Lévi has it, ultimately led to her real death.

The details of Lévi's rationalization of Phlegon need not concern us here, except for one, which incidentally stems from Greco-Roman antiquity and may have indeed served as a bridge between the sensationalist narratives of "apparent

9 In particular Callirhoe (Charito 1.4.12–1.5.1) and Anthia (X.Eph. 3.5–8), who suffer a death-like state from which they subsequently wake; as instances of *Scheintod* in the ancient novel one could also count events where the heroine is mistaken with another person (who died a 'real' death), such as Charicleia (Heliod. 1.30.4–1.31.1) and Leucippe (Ach.Tat. 3.15; 5.7; 7.1–3); cf. e.g. Bowie 1996, 101; Zimmerman 2000, 23; Chew 2014, 70; Létoublon/Genre 2014, 357–358.

10 Although Phlegon's story precedes the development of the novelistic genre.

11 Hansen 1996, 65.

12 Lévi 2006, 182.

death" (or "apparent life") and contemporary medical and scientific discourse. Hysterical coma, or rather "hysterical suffocation" (ὑστερικὴ πνίξ), as the ancient doctors and others would call it, was a doctrine *apparently* developed by the Hippocratics (see below), subsequently expanded by later medical authors, such as Celsus, Aretaeus, Soranus and Galen,[13] and carried on well into the modern times (Lévi himself is a good example of its resilience).[14] As the name itself suggests, this peculiar condition was thought to have been limited to women only and organically related to the (assumed) movements of the womb (ὑστέρα). As Galen tells us, diseases originating in the womb present the physician with a range of symptoms of varying severity:[15]

> τινὰς μὲν ἀναισθήτους τε ἅμα καὶ ἀκινήτους κειμένας, ἀμυδρότατόν τε καὶ μικρότατον ἐχούσας σφυγμόν, ἢ καὶ παντελῶς ἀσφύκτους φαινομένας, ἐνίας δ' αἰσθανομένας τε καὶ κινουμένας καὶ μηδὲν βεβλαμμένας τοῦ λογισμοῦ, λιποδρανούσας τε καὶ μόγις ἀναπνεούσας, ἑτέρας δὲ συνελκομένας τὰ κῶλα.
>
> Some women become unconscious, lying motionless, with a very weak pulse, or even appearing completely without pulse. Some are conscious, able to move and with their reasoning not affected in any way, but feel weak and breath with difficulty; yet others have their body parts constricted
>
> (*Loc.Aff.* 6.5; 8.414 K; tr. R.E. Siegel, modified).

It is, of course, the first variety that interests us the most. Virtually all authors agree on four primary symptoms: loss of consciousness,[16] loss of breath (ἀπνοία),[17] weak or absent pulse,[18] and coolness of the body.[19] The attack usually

---

13 Celsus: CML 1.180 (4.27); Aretaeus: CMG 2.34–36 (2.11); Soranus: CMG 4.109 (*Gyn.* 3.26); Galen: *Loc.Aff.* 6.5 (8.414–418 K).

14 See King 1993, 7–11, 60–63 and Scull 2009 for the modern fortunes of hysteria and hysterical suffocation.

15 A similar variance in the symptoms of hysterical suffocation is noted by Soranus: 'When an attack occurs, sufferers from the disease collapse, show aphonia, labored breathing, a seizure of the senses, clenching of the teeth, stridor, convulsive contraction of the extremities (but sometimes only weakness), upper abdominal distention, retraction of the uterus, swelling of the thorax, bulging of the network of vessels of the face. The whole body is cool, covered with perspiration, the pulse stops or is very small' (3.26; tr. O. Temkin).

16 καρηβαρίη τε καὶ ἀναισθησία (Aretaeus); κατοχή / κατάληψις αἰσθήσεως (Soranus); *sopor* (Celsus); on Galen – see quotation above.

17 ἄπνοια ξυνεῖναι δοκέει (Aretaeus); ἐποχὴ ἀναπνοῆς (Soranus); *exanimat* (Celsus); on Galen – see below.

18 Σφυγμοὶ διαλείποντες, ἄτακτοι, ἐκλείποντες (Aretaeus); ἀσφυξία παντελὴς ἢ βραχὺς ἄγαν ὁ σφυγμός (Soranus); on Galen – see quotation above.

19 ψύξιες καρτεραί (Aretaeus); περίψυξις (Soranus); on Galen – see below.

does not last long, and those who survive recover quickly. Our sources differ on who exactly is mostly affected by the condition. Galen for instance, taking retention of female 'seed' as the etiology, considers widows to be particularly at risk, as they can no longer discharge it through sexual intercourse. Aretaeus by contrast, who traces the cause in the movements of the womb, argues that hysterical suffocation is primarily the affliction of young women, since "as their age, lifestyle and judgment is less stable (πλανωδεστέρη), so is there womb more prone to wandering (ῥεμβώδης)."[20]

Though traditionally ascribed to the Hippocratic doctrines, "hysterical suffocation" as detailed above seems to belong to later developments in ancient medicine.[21] Its most celebrated case, however – a forerunner, as the idea most likely did not yet take root in the medical discourse of that time – belongs to the domain of philosophy. The Platonist Heraclides of Pontus (4th century BC),[22] as Diogenes Laertius tells us, described a case of a woman who lay without breath or pulse (ἄπνουν καὶ ἄσφυκτον) for a month,[23] during which time she was "looked after" (συντηρεῖν)[24] by Empedocles and eventually "came back to life" (ζῶσαν).[25] Galen adds that many doctors who we were present thought that she was already dead, and the only difference was that she kept a little warmth (βραχεῖαν θερμότητα) around the middle of the body.[26] Though Galen does not commit himself to fixing a precise period of the woman's coma, he provides an admirably insightful explanation for its duration: as in hibernating animals, lower body temperature slows

20 ἧισι γὰρ ἡλικίη τὲ καὶ βιοτὴ καὶ γνώμη πλανωδεστέρη, τῇισι καὶ ἡ ὑστέρη ἐστὶ ῥεμβώδης (2.11.6).

21 King 1993, 15–16; one case, however, in *Mul.* 1.7 seems to present symptoms very similar to those outlined above; described as πνίξ, it involves lack of breath and coolness of the body, its onset is sudden, and it affects older women deprived of sexual intercourse; cf. also King 1993, 18–20 on this and other similar cases in the Hippocratic Corpus.

22 The lost work of Heraclides *On Diseases*, the most famous part of which concerned the woman not breathing and nicknamed already in antiquity Ἄπνους, came down to us only in fragments (82–95 Schutrumpf; 76–87 Wehrli); cf. van der Eijk 2009.

23 Pliny, referring to the same case, narrows it down only to a week: *NH* 7.175; cf. Beagon 2005, 375.

24 On this translation see Eijk 2009, 238, n. 3.

25 For more instances of similar situations in antiquity cf. Grmek 1987.

26 τῶν νεκρῶν ἐνὶ μόνῳ διαλλάττουσα, τῷ βραχεῖαν ἔχειν θερμότητα κατὰ τὰ μέσα μέρη τοῦ σώματος (...) καὶ ζήτησιν ἔφη γεγονέναι τοῖς παροῦσιν ἰατροῖς, εἰ μήπω τέθνηκεν (*Loc.Aff.* 6.5; 8.414 K); translation in King 1993, 34.

down breathing and pulse to an imperceptible minimum, which in turn gives the impression of death.[27]

Compared to thirty days, half a year does not seem to be that big a stretch. Heraclides' *The Woman Not Breathing* could therefore provide an accurate medical parallel for Phlegon's *paradoxon* of the revenant lover, one which aptly reveals not only the actual medical knowledge of the Greek and Roman world, but most importantly the assumptions and presuppositions on which its dogmata were based. There are, however, no doctors in the Philinnion story to provide any clues as to the actual or supposed reasons of her state. No medical authority speaks about the girl's death – either about the "final" one, or the "first" one, which is known to us only through the retrospective reconstruction. Philinnion took this secret to the grave – twice.

3 Gender and Sexual Problems: Hermaphrodites, Sex-changers and Male Mothers

3.1 Hermaphrodites

Phlegon, like other ancient authors did not formally distinguish hermaphrodites (i.e. persons having both feminine and masculine genitals)[28] from sex-changers (i.e. persons who first have one, and then develop another). Both are referred to with the same term (ἀνδρόγυνος), and both are treated without any discrimination in the same part of the *Mirabilia* (chapters 4–10). For the sake of clarity, however, I intend to discuss those two categories separately. There are only two cases

27 *Loc.aff.* 6.5 (8.416 K) and *Diff.Resp.* 1.8 (7.773 K) = Heracleides Ponticus F 89 and 90 Schutrumpf (79 and 80 Wehrli) respectively; cf. Debru 1991; van der Eijk 2009, 245.

28 Modern medicine and science recognizes such a disorder in humans and animals; one of them is called 'true hermaphroditism' and is caused by "genetic defects in the differentiation of the genital system" (Harper 2007, 14); it manifests itself in two complete sets of gonadal tissues (ovarian and testicular – which need not take the shape of developed ovaries or testes) as well as, or at least, one complete set with some features of the other sex; the other type, the so-called 'pseudo-hermaphroditism', is characterized by ambiguity of the external genitals which often assume an intermediate form between developed female and male; the gonadal tissues, however, are limited to one sex only, as is the genetic makeup of a person affected with this condition; pseudo-hermaphroditism happens relatively more frequently than true hermaphroditism; see Harper 2007; cf. Androutsos 2006.

of actual hermaphroditism discussed in Phlegon. One of them – for different reasons – is presented in another part of his work (chapter 2). It is a story of an androgynous birth which sets in motion an entire chain of uncanny events, which do not concern us here. The newborn baby has two sets of genitals (αἰδοῖα δύο), male and female (ἀνδρεῖόν τε καὶ γυναικεῖον), and its physical appearance is "amazingly altered" (τὴν φύσιν θαυμαστῶς διηλλαγμένον). As the text vaguely explains, "the upper part, above the genitals, was perfect and male, whereas that around the thighs was female and softer" (τὰ μὲν ἄνω τοῦ αἰδοίου ὁλόκληρά τε καὶ ἀνδρώδη ἦν, τὰ δὲ περὶ τοὺς μηροὺς γυναικεῖα καὶ ἁπαλώτερα). Since the antithesis informing this obscure description is clearly unbalanced – the male body-parts being "complete"/"perfect" (ὁλόκληρά) as opposed to the female ones which are "softer" (ἁπαλώτερα) – a widely accepted emendation seeks to remedy this asymmetry. Instead of the former, Nauck suggested the reading ὅλω⟨ς σ⟩κληρά, that is, "wholly hard,"[29] which indeed elegantly complements the epithet describing the feminine parts. On closer inspection, however, the emendation seems hardly necessary. According to Stramaglia,[30] the antithesis ὁλόκληρα – ἁπαλώτερα is perfectly intelligible, if only the former is taken in the sense "of full health" or "force" (one closely related to the meaning "integral"), which is well documented already in the Hellenistic age. As for the other epithet – "soft", "delicate" (ἁπαλός) – Stramaglia suggests understanding it as a defining feature of femininity. Already in the Hippocratic Corpus (*Mul.*1.37, Littré 8.12.11) we find a woman described as ἁπαλόσαρκος in order to distinguish her from a man, and from Sappho onwards the adjective ἁπαλός typically connotes feminine delicacy or effeminacy. Thus, Phlegon's image of the hermaphrodite seems to underscore the polarization of the male (that is 'in full force') and the female (that is 'soft' and 'delicate'), and that despite the fact that such antithesis makes little sense when it comes to a newborn. The latter's description therefore seems to operate on a symbolic rather than realistic level, as it tells us less about the actual morphology of a hermaphrodite baby and more about the ideological underpinning of the oppositions it is assumed to bridge – or rather undermine. To the ancient Greeks and Romans, in the words of Brisson, these were the basic oppositions on which 'the whole of reality was organized',[31] and therefore the hermaphrodite was as a rule considered an ominous portent whose appearance required swift action on the part of the entire community (hence the collective motion to have

29 Nauck, in: Keller 1877, 63.

30 Stramaglia 1995, 213–214.

31 Brisson 2002, 5.

the child – along with the mother – thrown outside the borders and burnt).[32] Its dangerous potential is stressed even further in the second of Phlegon's two cases of hermaphroditism (chapter 10); though the fate of the androgynous baby is unknown here, the entire state is alerted (the story takes place in Rome in 125 BCE),[33] and the senate orders a reading of the dreaded Sibylline oracles.[34] Other authors who record cases of hermaphroditism are all in agreement as to their ominous significance.[35] In fact, they are not mentioned otherwise than as a prodigy. And the one detail – apart from the dutifully provided date and place – reemerging with dreary consistency in all these accounts is the fate of the hermaphrodites, either slain or (more frequently) drowned.[36]

The grim fate of (actual or alleged) hermaphrodites may seem all the more surprising if we consider the fact that the condition was not unknown to ancient scientific and medical writers. Already in Aristotle we find descriptions of animals with two sets of genitals, though the philosopher is keen on stressing that only one of them is properly developed (κύριον), while the other is always (ἀεί) imperfect and "inoperative" (ἄκυρον).[37] Aristotle's observations correspond well with Leonides' (1st century CE) morphological classification of hermaphrodites, of which he distinguishes three "male" varieties and one "female." His lost work, of uncertain title, is quoted by the Byzantine doctor, Paul of Aegina (7th century CE):[38]

> τεσσάρων γὰρ οὐσῶν κατὰ Λεωνίδην τῶν διαφορῶν αὐτοῦ αἱ μὲν τρεῖς ἐπὶ τῶν ἀνδρῶν συνίστανται, ἡ δὲ μία ἐπὶ τῶν γυναικῶν. ἐπὶ μὲν γὰρ τῶν ἀνδρῶν ποτὲ μὲν κατὰ τὸν περίναιον, ποτὲ δὲ κατὰ μέσον τὸν ὄσχεον θέσις αἰδοίου γυναικείου τετριχωμένου φαίνεται, τρίτη δὲ πρὸς ταύταις, καθ' ἣν ἐπί τινων διὰ τοῦ κατὰ τὸν ὄσχεον οἷοιν αἰδοίου τὰ οὖρα προχεῖται. ἐπὶ δὲ τῶν γυναικῶν ἀνωτέρω τοῦ αἰδοίου κατὰ τὸ ἐφήβαιον ἀνδρείου πολλάκις αἰδοίου θέσις εὑρίσκεται τριῶν τινῶν ἐξεχόντων σωμάτων, ἑνὸς μὲν ὥσπερ καυλοῦ, δυοῖν δὲ καθάπερ διδύμων.

---

32 Bloch 1963, 70, 73; Brisson 2002, 14–15; Allély 2003, 138.

33 During the consulate of Marcus Plautius Hypsaeus and Marcus Fulvius Flaccus.

34 The entire case is discussed at length by Den Boer 1979, 103–108.

35 These are: Livy (27.11.4; 27.37.6; 31.12.6; 31.12.8; 39.22.5), Obsequens (3, 22, 27a, 32, 34, 36, 47, 48, 50, 53) and Tacitus (*Ann.* 12.64); for a useful list of cases of hermaphroditism mentioned in ancient authors, see Grauman 2013, 185; cf. Brisson 2002, 26–27.

36 Drowned: Livy 27.37.5–7; 31.12.6 and 8; Obsequens 22, 27a, 32, 34, 36, 47, 48, 50; slain: Livy 39.22.5 (*necari... iusserunt*); Obsequens 3 (*necatus*); no detail concerning the hermaphrodite's fate: Livy 27.11.4–5; Tac. *Ann.* 12.64; Obs. 53.

37 Aristotle, *GA* 772b; see also Grauman 2013, 191–192; cf. van der Gracht 2012; 'inoperative' is A.L. Peck's translation (Loeb).

38 Paul.Aeg. 6.69.1.

> There are four varieties of it [i.e. hermaphroditism], according to Leonides; three of them occur in men and one in women. In men, sometimes about the perineum and sometimes about the middle of the scrotum, there appear female private parts (αἰδοίου) with hair; and in addition to these there is a third variety, in which the discharge of urine takes place at the scrotum, as if from [female] private parts. In women, the male private parts are frequently found above the [female] private parts, within the pubic hair; there are three bodies of some kind extruding, one has the appearance of a penis, two other – of testes.
> (Paul.Aeg. 6.69 = CMG 9.2.112; tr. F. Adams, slightly modified)

Leonides' types seem to be grounded in empirical observation instead of fanciful speculation: they correspond quite well with the current state of knowledge about pseudohermaphroditism and hypospadias.[39] Obviously, distinguishing the male from the female presupposes that only one set of genitals is properly developed and is (in Aristotle's words) "operative." The Hippocratic Corpus, by contrast, provides an explanation of the 'pathophysiology' of hermaphroditism through the theory of humors: the fetus is formed by way of combining male (ἄρρην) and female (θῆλυ) secretions (ἀποκριθέντα), which – it should be noted – are produced *both* by each of the sexes.[40] That is, the woman produces both female and male secretions, as does the man. This in turn yields a number of possible combinations in the fetus. If both combined secretions are male, the child is a boy and grows to be strong and brilliant; similarly, if both are female, the baby, obviously a girl, becomes very feminine (θηλυκώκατα) and very fair. When they are different, however, one of them has to 'gain mastery' (κρατεῖν). If it is the corresponding secretion – i.e. the male from the father or the female from the mother – that 'gains mastery,' the child still develops properly (as a boy or a girl respectively), though not as brilliantly as in the previous cases. But when the reverse occurs, the child's development becomes fraught with problems. This happens less so if it is the female secretion from the father that prevails: the offspring, a girl, simply grows up to be 'manlier' (ἀνδρεία). But when the male secretion from the mother overcomes the female secretion of the father, the child becomes a hermaphrodite.

39 Both male and female pseudo-hermaphroditism are umbrella terms; the former "manifests variously, but individuals are always genetically male; poor virilization results in variable degrees of feminization, with genitals ranging from those appearing male to those appearing female and with a range of ambiguities in between; female pseudo-hermaphroditism describes individuals who are genetic females, with almost completely female internal genitals; their external genitals usually appear as male because of clitoral enlargement"; see Harper 2007, 14.
40 Hp. *Vict.*1.28.

Other medical writers were apparently uninterested in this condition: Galen seems not to have thought much of it, as he even gives the impression of distancing himself from any speculations on this matter.[41] To him these are only cases of 'so called' (ὀνομαζομένων, καλουμένους) ḥermaphrodites, of which the only actual instances are artifacts.[42] Perhaps he and many of his colleagues considered them to belong to a different register of knowledge, that of myths, marvels, portents, and monstrosities rather than the science (or pseudo-science) of the human body and of its diseases.

3.2 Sex-changers

Sex-changers were considered by Phlegon and other ancient authors to be "successive" hermaphrodites, as they are termed *androgynoi* as well. The *Mirabilia* presents us with six such stories (chapters 4–9), two of which belong to the mythical world – that of the famous seer Teiresias and of the warrior Kaineus – whereas the other four are drawn from the historical period and presented as "genuine." Of the mythical sex changers, Tiresias' is the most complex one, as he undergoes such metamorphosis twice: first he becomes a woman, and then returns to his masculine form. Kaineus' story is much simpler: originally born a girl, by the name Kainis, he was changed by Poseidon into a man at his own request. Scholars agree that the mythical examples are fundamentally different from the historical ones, as they belong to a different register of knowledge. As Delcourt argues:

> in this kind of successive androgyny we must not see a transposition of genuine cases where an adolescent turns out not to be of the sex supposed at his birth. The stories of Kaineus and Teiresias do not spring from concrete experience. They are indeed myths, born of customs or beliefs – and, moreover, each one requires a separate explanation.[43]

Such explanation is sought, for instance, in ritual transvestitism, accompanying an adolescent's rite of passage, alluded to in both stories.[44]

By contrast, the credibility of Phlegon's quasi-historical accounts is established by the addition of precise details of both place and time (in the latter case,

---

41 *Sem.* 4.619 K (= CMG 5.3.1.170); *Hipp. Aph.* 18a.148–149 K; cf. King 2016, 82.
42 "Such as the *so-called* hermaphrodites that artists fashion" (οἵους οἱ πλάσται πλάττουσι τοὺς καλουμένους ἑρμαφροδίτους; tr. Ph. De Lacy); cf. "about the *so-called* hermaphrodites" (περὶ τῶν ἑρμαφροδίτων ὀνομαζομένων); my emphasis.
43 Delcourt 1961, 34.
44 Delcourt 1961, 36; 41–42.

down to the exact year, determined by the names of Roman consuls and Athenian eponymous archon). The most exhaustive account is given in chapter 6: the story took place in Antioch on the Meander in 45 BCE. A 13-year-old maiden of a prominent family, outstanding in beauty (εὐπρεπής) and therefore desired by many, was eventually betrothed to a man chosen by her parents. On the day of their wedding the girl suddenly experienced a great pain in the lower abdomen (κοιλία) which continued on through the three subsequent days and nights. No doctor in the city was able to cure her illness. On the fourth day, around daybreak, the pain became stronger and male genitals burst out from her, turning her into a man. Chapter 7 recounts, although much more briefly, a similar event which happened in the city of Mevania in Italy in 53 CE. A certain Philotis, a maiden whose family came from Smyrna, was betrothed to a man by her parents when suddenly male genitals appeared on her and she became a man. Chapter 8, in an equally concise way, reports that in Epidauros a certain Sympherousa, a child of a poor family, also became a man: as Sympheron, he spent the rest of his life as a gardener. Chapter 9 mentions a woman by the name of Aetete who lived with her husband in Syrian Laodicaea. All of a sudden she became a man and changed her name to Aetetus. Interestingly and quite exceptionally, in this incident the compiler himself marks his presence claiming to have seen this person with his own eyes. Since the event can be dated to 116 CE due to the information provided by Phlegon, it seems plausible that he acquired the story from Aetetus himself or from another local informant, as Hansen suggests.[45]

The two other authors[46] reporting several cases of spontaneous sex-change are Diodorus and Pliny.[47] The former recounts at length two such incidents, embellishing them as well with historical detail: in the times of Alexander Balas (mid II century BCE), one of his companion cavalrymen, a certain Diophantus of Abae (in Arabia) was previously a girl by the name of Herais – at least as far as appearances were concerned. He was even given in marriage to another man, and only after an entire year of conjugal cohabitation suffered from an already familiar illness which brought about his sex-change (or rather revealed his true gender): a swelling in his lower abdomen, accompanied by fever, spontaneously burst, re-

45 Hansen 1996, 120.

46 Brief remarks are also found in Livy (*ex muliere Spoleti virum factum*; 24.10.10), and Ausonius (see below, n. 62).

47 Pliny's account is quoted by Gellius (9.4.15–16), while Diodorus' account is quoted by Photius (*Bibl.* 377a–379a); the latter's quotation is our only source for this lost part of Diodorus' work; for a useful list of sex-changers in ancient literary sources, see Grauman 2013, 185–186.

leasing male genitals from within. A similar fate befell a certain Kallon of Epidaurus, previously known by the feminine counterpart of his name as Kallo. This Kallo was afflicted by the same malady already two years after marriage: this time the tumor was cut open by a doctor,[48] only to reveal, again, male genitals hidden within. Two other such cases, one from Athens and one from the vicinities of Rome, are mentioned briefly by Diodorus who deplores their outcome: both 'sex-changers' were burned alive as monstrosities (*terata*) by their superstitious compatriots, incapable of understanding the true nature of their condition.

Pliny's account,[49] though not as firmly rooted in historical circumstances, provides by contrast the details of its sources, among them also a lost book of *Mirabilia* compiled by a many-time consul, Licinius Mucianus.[50] On the ex-consul's authority, Pliny mentions two cases, one from Argos, of a certain Arescusa/Arescon, who after being given in marriage grew a beard, developed masculine attributes, and eventually himself took a wife; and a similar one (this time without any details) from Smyrna. Pliny also draws on earlier annals for another case (an unnamed girl changing into a boy), and himself testifies to have seen yet another, a person by the name Lucius Constitius, who became a man on the day of his/her marriage. In his account, Pliny seems to be describing what he believes to be instances of actual sex-change, which to him is 'nothing incredible' (*non est fabulosum*). Diodorus by contrast exercises more critical judgement. His report, though sensational and seasoned with intriguing detail, is discursively grounded in contemporary medicine, as he repeatedly speaks of fever swelling, tumors, and even surgical interventions[51] (by contrast, the only intervention mentioned by Pliny is that of an augur, who exiles one of the unfortunate sex-changers). Even more revealingly, Diodorus' professed objective is to dispel superstition (δεισιδαιμονία) among his readers: true change from female to male is not possible (ἀδύνατον), and therefore what seems to be a monstrous marvel (τέρας),[52] is

48 Strictly speaking, by a pharmacist (φαρμακοπώλης), contrasted with the multitude of doctors (ἰατροί) who were not up to the task (32.11.2).

49 Plin. *Nat.* 7.36; cf. Healey 1999, 51; Brisson 2002, 38–40; Beagon 2005, 173–176.

50 Mucianus was a follower and collaborator of Vespasian; apart from the lost *Mirabilia* he also compiled and edited collections of speeches and letters (also lost); he died probably shortly after 75 CE; cf. Beagon 2005, 13–14, 17–18.

51 φλεγμονὴν γὰρ ἰσχυρὰν γενέσθαι περὶ τὸ ἦτρον αὐτῆς. ἐπὶ πλέον δὲ οἰδήσαντος τοῦ τόπου, ἔπειτα πυρετῶν μεγάλων συνεπιγινομένων (32.10.3); μετὰ δὲ ταῦτα φλεγμονῆς αὐτῆι συμβάσης περὶ τὸν κτένα καὶ δεινῶν ἀλγηδόνων ἐπιγενομένων (...) φαρμακοπώλης τις (...) ἔτεμε τὸν ἐπηρμένον τόπον (32.11.2).

52 πολλοὶ γὰρ τέρατα τὰ τοιαῦτα νομίζοντες εἶναι δεισιδαιμονοῦσιν (32.12.1).

only a trick played by nature which hides the true (masculine) nature of an apparent sex-changer behind the superficial arrangement of his body.[53] What Diodorus endeavors therefore is a quasi-scientific, quasi-medical explanation of the oddity of sex-change. Both he and Pliny, however, complement one another quite well when compared to Phlegon: the latter's stories are those of an actual (and not apparent) sex-change (and therefore akin to the marvels of the Roman writer), but in their details remain suspiciously similar to the quasi-medical account of Diodorus.

In spite of Diodorus' rationalizing agenda, however, ancient medical writers seem all but silent on the question of true or even apparent sex-changers. Only the Hippocratic Corpus mentions two – probably authentic – cases of women abruptly developing masculine features (such as facial hair, lack of menses), but apparently without undergoing actual sex change; both are said to have died shortly after:[54]

> ἐν Ἀβδήροισι Φαέθουσα ἡ Πυθέου γυνὴ οἰκουρός, ἐπίτοκος ἐοῦσα τοῦ ἔμπροσθεν χρόνου, τοῦ δὲ ἀνδρὸς αὐτῆς φυγόντος, τὰ γυναικεῖα ἀπελήφθη χρόνον πολύν· μετὰ δὲ ἐς ἄρθρα πόνοι καὶ ἐρυθήματα· τούτων δὲ ξυμβάντων τό τε σῶμα ἠνδρώθη καὶ ἐδασύνθη πάντα, καὶ πώγωνα ἔφυσε, καὶ φωνὴ τρηχέη ἐγενήθη, καὶ πάντα πραγματευσαμένων ἡμέων ὅσα ἦν πρὸς τὸ τὰ γυναικεῖα κατασπάσαι οὐκ ἦλθεν, ἀλλ' ἀπέθανεν οὐ πολὺν μετέπειτα χρόνον βιώσασα. ξυνέβη δὲ καὶ Ναννοῖ τῆι Γοργίππου γυναικὶ ἐν Θάσωι τωὐτόν· ἐδόκει δὲ πᾶσι τοῖσιν ἰητροῖσιν οἷσι κἀγὼ ἐνέτυχον μία ἐλπὶς εἶναι τοῦ γυναικωθῆναι, εἰ τὰ κατὰ φύσιν ἔλθοι· ἀλλὰ καὶ ταύτηι οὐκ ἐδυνήθη πάντα ποιούντων γενέσθαι, ἀλλ' ἐτελεύτησεν οὐ βραδέως.
>
> In Abdera, Phaëthusa the wife of Pytheas, a stay-at-home wife, having borne children in the preceding time, when her husband was exiled stopped menstruating for a long time. Afterwards pains and reddening in the joints. When that happened her body was masculinized and grew hairy all over, she grew a beard, her voice became harsh and though we did everything we could to bring forth menses, they did not come, but she died after surviving for not long after. The same thing happened to Nanno, Gorgippos' wife, in Thasos. It seemed to all the physicians I talked to that there was one hope of feminizing her, if normal menstruation occurred. But in her case too it was not possible, though we did everything, but she died, and quickly.
>
> (Hp. *Epid.* 6.8.32; tr. W.D. Smith with H. King's modifications)

These two medical case studies are markedly different from the marvels of Pliny and from Diodorus' quasi-science. There is no question of a hidden (male) sexual

53 τῆς φύσεως διὰ τῶν τοῦ σώματος μερῶν ψευδογραφούσης (32.12.1).
54 *Epid.* 6.8.32; cf. King 1998, 9–10.

identity, as Phaëthusa is explicitly said to have given birth before (ἐπίτοκος ἐοῦσα); nor is there, in fact, any real sex change at all: the author makes it quite clear that we are still dealing with women who merely developed masculine features and lost some feminine ones (menses), and as a result the task of the physician was only to bring back the latter. Yet both these cases, enjoying a considerable *Nachleben* among the early modern writers, eventually came to be assimilated to the wonders of Pliny and Phlegon, as instances of actual sex-change.[55] According to a physiological and medical theory voiced explicitly by Galen (referred to as one-sex theory), it was believed that there is no substantial difference between male and female genitals other than their topography: the latter are merely an inwardly inverted variant of the former. As Galen himself tells us:[56]

> πάντ᾽ οὖν, ὅσα τοῖς ἀνδράσιν ὑπάρχει μόρια, ταῦτα καὶ ταῖς γυναιξὶν [ἰδεῖν ἔστιν] ἐν ἑνὶ μόνωι τῆς διαφορᾶς οὔσης αὐτοῖς, οὗ παρὰ πάντα χρὴ μεμνῆσθαι τὸν λόγον, ὡς ἔνδον μὲν τὰ τῶν γυναικῶν ἐστι μόρια, τὰ δὲ τῶν ἀνδρῶν ἔξω ἀπὸ τοῦ κατὰ τὸν περίνεον ὀνομαζόμενον χωρίου. θάτερα γὰρ αὐτῶν ὁπότερα βούλει νοήσας πρότερα τὰ μὲν τῶν γυναικῶν ἐκτρέψας ἐκτός, τὰ δὲ τῶν ἀνδρῶν οἷον ἐντρέψας τε καὶ ἐνδιπλώσας ἔσω πάντ᾽ ἀλλήλοις εὑρήσεις τὰ αὐτά.
>
> All the parts, then, that men have, women have too, the difference between them lying in only one thing, namely, that in women the parts are within [the body] whereas in men they are outside, in the region called the perineum. Consider first whichever ones you please, turn outward the woman's, turn inward, so to speak, and fold double the man's, and you will find them the same in both in every respect.
>
> (Galen, *UP* 4.158 K; tr. M.T. May)

This close comparison goes on for much longer and into much greater detail and is rounded off with yet another confident conclusion regarding the female anatomy: 'you could not find a single male part left over that had not simply changed its position.'[57] Why did they change their positions? This is where Galen's debt to Aristotle becomes explicit: like the latter, he finds the answer in the excess of body heat which is characteristic of males,[58] and which causes their genitals to migrate outwards and eventually extrude: "the female is less perfect

55 King 2012, 293; 2016, 83.

56 For the complementary parallels between male and female genitals (testes and uterus), cf. Arist. *GA* 715b, 720a.

57 ἓν γὰρ ουδὲν ἔστιν εὑρεῖν μόριον ἐν τοῖς ἀνδράσι περιττεῦον ἀλλ᾽ ἢ τὴν θέσιν μόνην ἐξηλλαγμένην (*Galen* UP 4.159 K).

58 Which, according to Aristotle, is crucial in the process of producing semen from blood: *PA* 650a; *GA* 775a; on Galen's genitals and body heat see Flemming 2000, 306–307.

(ἀτελέστερον) than the male, for one, principal reason – because she is colder (ψυχρότερον)."[59] Thus, in the end, the female genitals are not only an inverted version of the male, but also the less perfect one, just like the eyes of a mole when compared to those of other animals.[60] And the observation that a woman in general is an imperfect version of the male is one of the most notorious statements of Aristotle.[61]

Incidentally, as noted above, Galen himself seems not to have thought much of the accounts of hermaphroditism – and by extension of sex-changers. His theory nonetheless provided the modern authors with an admirable, quasi-scientific explanation for all instances of sex-change known to them, including the ones drawn from the ancient sources, and that regardless of how they were actually understood in these sources. Could it also provide the background to Phlegon's stories of sex-change? His account, not unsurprisingly, gives no hints whatsoever to link it with Galen's one-sex theory. But seeing that with the exception of Tiresias[62] (who, as a mythological example, belongs to a different register of knowledge), all his cases of sex-change involve a metamorphosis from female to male only, which is also true for other authors mentioning incidents of this kind (Diodorus, Pliny), one may detect a common presupposition – or if you will, prejudice – behind all these sensational cases, one which was aptly labeled by Laqueur as the 'purported telos of perfection.'[63] The female gives way to the male, just as the imperfect, when bettered, leads to perfection. This in turn allows us to appreciate the sex-changing marvels of the ancient authors in an entirely different light: not as random tricks of nature, but as cultural phenomena, endowed with a profound (if disturbing to modern sensibilities) teleological sense.

---

59 In the Hippocratic writings heat is not consistently associated with the male; sometimes women are said to be warmer (θερμοτέρη) than men; cf. *Mul.* 1.

60 Galen's own comparison (*UP* 4.159 K), which probably alludes to Aristotle's zoological observations (*HA* 491b).

61 *GA* 728a; cf. *HA* 538a; for Galen's debt to Aristotle on this point, see Flemming 2000, 306; King 2016, 40–41.

62 Yet another possible exception may be found in Ausonius' vague account of a boy from Beneventum turning into a girl (*unus epheborum virgo repente fuit*); Auson. *Epigr.* 76.13–14.

63 Laqueur 1990, 28.

3.3 Male Mothers

In chapters 26 and 27 Phlegon recounts two cases of men who gave birth. It may be significant that these accounts do not belong to the section on the androgynous individuals, but follow the chapters devoted to various monstrous births. This suggests that the compiler seems to find children born from men to be more of an oddity than their male "mothers," even if they themselves do not display any unusual features. This opinion was apparently shared by Phlegon's contemporaries: as he tells us, one such newborn was embalmed and preserved in Egyptian Alexandria. More importantly, this particular case is recounted by Phlegon on the authority of a Greco-Egyptian doctor, Dorotheos of Heliopolis, who lived most likely in the 1st century CE, and who mentioned it in his lost work *Reminiscences* (*Hypomnemata*). The second case has no such authoritative source to back it, but is instead embellished with the standard credentials regarding both place (Germania) and time (56 CE).[64] Both accounts are brief: apart from the details of place, time, or source, they only provide one small piece of information each, regarding the male mother. One of them is described as a "catamite" (κίναιδος), the other as a slave (δοῦλος) to one of the soldiers. Now the term *kinaidos* was traditionally understood as defining the passive partner in a penetrative homosexual act, which in ancient Greece was opposed to the "proper" manner of consummating such relationship through intercrural sex.[65] In more recent scholarship, however, this assumption has been challenged. As indeed the sources themselves seem to suggest,[66] the term denoted in the first place lewdness and effeminacy, with sexual passivity only as a potential corollary.[67] It is primarily in this sense that in the Hellenistic world, to quote Davidson, "the *kinaidos* becomes increasingly popular and increasingly monstrous, until by Roman times he is almost an

---

64 During the consulate of Quintus Volusius Saturninus and Publius Cornelius Scipio, and the archonship of Konon (*Mir.* 26).

65 The bulk of Winkler's seminal study of *kinaidos* and Greek sexual mores is based on this assumption (1990, 45–70); on intercrural sex, see Dover 1989^2, 98–109 (drawing mainly on iconographic evidence); contra: Davidson 2007, 116–121.

66 Most revealing here is the argument from silence: in the speech *Against Timarchus*, where the eponymous adversary is accused of prostituting himself and of passive homosexuality, the term *kinaidos* is never applied to him; but in the very same speech, indeed on the very same breath, it is used to describe Demosthenes, on account of his lewd affair with a younger lover: ταχύ γ' ἂν Τίμαρχον ἢ τὸν κίναιδον Δημοσθένην εἴασε πολιτεύεσθαι (Aesch. 1.181; cf. 1.131; 3.88, 99, 151).

67 "If fondness for taking it up the bottom is a defining characteristic, it is certainly not the first thing that sprang to the lexicographer's mind, nor the second, nor the third, nor the fourth... Perhaps that just got lost in all the lewdness" (Davidson 2007, 55).

obsession, a bogy man."[68] There is no way of telling how much of a bogy man was there in Phlegon's (or indeed Dorotheos') male mother: the context may indeed suggest passive homosexuality (conceiving a baby through intercrural sex would have been even more of a wonder), but it may also hint at a sense of general effeminacy or indeed sexual ambivalence in the subject. Recently, it has even been suggested that Phlegon's "male" mothers were in fact biological women suffering either from pseudo-hermaphroditism (on which see above) or virilism (that is the development of masculine traits usually due to hormonal disorders).[69] In the other story, an equally brief one, the male mother is said to have been a slave of a soldier stationed in Germany. As such, he may have also been kept for the sake of sexual exploitation by his master. And as in the above case, one cannot rule out the possibility that the case concerns a biological woman suffering from a congenital or acquired condition.

The idea of conception and birth without the presence of women is, of course, pure fantasy, and even ancient doctors (Dorotheos left aside) seems to have disavowed such concepts.[70] This, however, was not necessarily the case with popular beliefs, especially those originating in strongly misogynistic *milieux*, such as the majority of ancient Greek poleis, with classical Athens holding pride of place.[71] According to such folk embryology for instance – most famously expressed in Aeschylus' *Eumenides* – it was only the father who contributed to the creation of life, while the woman merely "keeps the offspring safe, like a stranger on behalf of a stranger."[72] This theory, systematized for the first time by Anaxagoras of Clazomenae[73] is seen to surface in various texts of the classical period (usually as a metaphor).[74] Phlegon's stories of male mothers, regardless of whether there is any shred of truth (and real suffering) behind them, seem to be in the first place nothing more than late heirs to this ultimate misogynistic fantasy.

---

68 Davidson 2007, 55; on the *kinaidos*, see also Halperin 2002, 32–38; Azize/Craigie 2002, 56–59; on his Roman counterpart (*cinaedus*) see Williams 2010², 183–213.

69 Pataricza 2009; 131 and n.7.

70 Connel 2016; 94; cf. Hippocr. *Vict*.1.28; see also Lloyd 1983, 86–94; Leitao 2012, 19–20.

71 Cf. Eur. *Or*. 552; *Hipp*. 618–24; *Med*. 573–575; see also Preuss 1977, 67; Rabinowitz 1993, 173–195.

72 ἅπερ ξένωι ξένη | ἔσωσεν ἔρνος (*Eum*. 660–661); tr. A. Sommerstein.

73 DK 59 A107 = Arist. *GA* 763b–764a; cf. Leitao 2012, 24–25.

74 See Leitao 2012, 18–57, 101–145.

3.4 Teratological Births

Three very brief entries give account of children born with abnormal body features:[75] a four-headed infant with a corresponding number of limbs (ch. 20) and two two-headed babies (ch. 21 and 25), one of which had the redundant head growing out of its left shoulder (ἐπὶ τοῦ ἀριστεροῦ ὤμου κεφαλὴν ἐκπεφυκυῖαν ἔχον). The first and last of these events can be dated to 61 CE (ch. 20) and 112 CE (ch. 25) respectively. Although the description is sparing, all three examples clearly suggest a form of congenital disorder, which is most likely that of conjoined twins.[76] Although, like hermaphrodites, they were usually regarded prodigies[77] and were therefore subject to similarly grim treatment, their condition was of interest to scientific reflection in antiquity. According to Aristotle, extra limbs, such as feet or heads, develop due to a fusion of male and female sperms instead of their separating into distinct embryos: as he argues, such redundancies happen often in animals which are multiparous, such as birds (especially chicken), whereas in human beings they are rare.[78]

Three other chapters (22, 23, 24) tell of "animal" children: a monkey, a baby with the head of Anubis, and a pair of snakes curled up into a ball, all born during the 1st century CE. If these accounts are not pure fantasy, then one must assume that they concern severe malformations of the fetus; similar cases are found in other authors, such as Livy, Pliny, Appian, Plutarch, Valerius Maximus, and Obsequens[79] who mention births of elephants, snakes, and even hippocentaurs. Although Phlegon is not concerned with their fate, in other authors such births were habitually considered as prodigies and were treated accordingly.[80] It seems that such babies were commonly regarded as animals rather than humans, contrary

---

75 On teratology and corporeality in ancient Rome, see Gevaert/Laes 2013; on child malformations see Allély 2003 and 2004.

76 Conjoined twins (sharing one body) is a rare phenomenon, presently estimated to occur from 1 in 50,000 births to 1 in 200,000 births; conjoined quadruplets (as the oddity described by Phlegon in ch. 20) or twins asymmetrically conjoined (i.e. 'parasitic twins,' where one of them is smaller, less developed and dependent on the other, as most likely the case in Phlegon ch. 21) are even more rare; cf. Hanson 1975, 2.1257; Spencer 2003, 376 ff.

77 Allély 2003, 140 (who notes that only severe malformations, like the ones mentioned in Phlegon, were considered prodigies); cf. Bloch 1963.

78 *Generat. anim.* 770a 3–4; 770a 7–10; cf. Garland 1995, 155–156.

79 Livy 37.11 (elephant); Pliny, *Nat.* 7.34 (elephant, snake, hippocentaur); Plutarch, *Marcellus* 28.3 (elephant); Valerius Maximus 1.6.5; Obsequens 57 (snake); cf. Allély 2003, 143; Beagon 2005, 168–172.

80 Cicero, *De divinatione* 1.53; cf. Allély 2003, 140.

to Aristoteles' opinion (*Generat. anim.*769b) that they are only similar to animals.[81] An idea current both in popular belief as well as in scientific reflection held that maternal impressions could have a decisive influence on the physical appearance of the child.[82] Soranus, for instance, quotes an example of a woman who saw monkeys during conception and as a result gave birth to a monkey; this is followed by a story of a Cypriot tyrant who forced his wife to gaze at beautiful statues during intercourse in order to distract her from his own deformity, and thus bear him beautiful children.[83]

3.5 Multiple Pregnancies

Two chapters recount extraordinary cases of consecutive multiple pregnancies: a certain woman is said to have given birth to twenty children in the course of four deliveries, and most of them survived and were reared (ch. 28). This information was excerpted from the Hellenistic paradoxographer Antigonos of Carystus (*Mir.* 110.1). Another woman from the same city brought forth five children at once, three of whom were male and two female, and the Emperor Trajan ordered them to be reared at his own expense. In the following year the same woman gave birth to three more children from a single pregnancy (ch. 29). Like hermaphrodites and congenital malformations, multiple pregnancies were sometimes considered prodigies.[84] This, however, may have depended on the number of children: Pliny tells us that this was the case with quadruplets or more, though Obsequens records as a portent the birth of triplets.[85] Perhaps, as with hermaphrodites, multiple pregnancies in the times of the empire became less a cause for alarm, and more for celebration[86] – provided, of course, that the mother and children survived, which, as Pliny tells us, was unusual even in twin pregnancies, more so if the

---

81 Hansen 1996, 152.
82 Garland 1995, 151.
83 Soranus, *Gyn.* 1.39; cf. Galen, *Ther.Pis.* 14.253–254 K; cf. D.H. *De Imitatione* F 3.1.1 (Usener) – who speaks instead of a farmer's wife; on the authority of pseudo-Plutarch ([*Mor.*] 906a = *Placita Philosophorum*) this idea is traced back to Empedocles (A 81 D–K).
84 Multiple pregnancies, such as triplets, quadruplets, and quintuplets, occur very rarely: a traditional approximation of the incidence of twins is 1:80, triplets 1:6400, and quadruplets (etc.) 1:512.000 (Bush/Pernol 2006, 301–310).
85 *Tergeminos nasci certum est* (...); *super inter ostenta ducitur* (Pliny *NH* 7.33); Obsequens 14; cf. Allély 2003, 145; Dasen 2005, 70–71.
86 Beagon 2005, 164.

babies were of different sex.[87] The latter observation – based on the above-discussed question of difference in body heat between men and women – was probably taken up from Aristotle, who also considered all multiple pregnancies an oddity.[88] The Hippocratic treatises establish the ideal number of children at two at a time, referring it to the structure of the female uterus, divided into two "pouches" (κόλποι),[89] and to the two female breasts.[90] Soranus, however, casually mentions twin and even triplet pregnancies (including those with children of different sex) as something rare but perfectly natural.[91]

4 Conclusion

Despite their conspicuous diversity, all the phenomena reported by Phlegon in the *Mirabilia* have one thing in common: they question the limits of the human body. Diligent recording of that which transgresses the norms of human physical existence seems to be an apt summary of this paradoxographer's literary output. Perhaps, it is a display of some anxiety and helplessness in the face of the immeasurability and unpredictability of the world that pushes humans to collect, accumulate and make lists of facts and things, especially those which are difficult to count and understand, as was observed by Umberto Eco. More importantly, however, the cases discussed above share yet another feature which seems to distinguish them from other marvels and oddities: they were all potentially explicable on the grounds of contemporary medicine. In a different discursive register (one perhaps stripped of some exaggerations and embellishments) they might be considered as case studies, subject to scientific (or quasi-scientific) explanation, rather than prodigies or wonders intended only to amaze. Seen from a different perspective, however, the same case studies may just as well be turned into wonders, questioning the boundaries of life, death, sex, and even species. Such is the intersection between paradoxography and ancient medicine, at the core of which lies Phlegon's peculiar interest in the wonders of the human body.

---

87 The beginning of the text is mutilated: editis geminis raram esse aut puerperae aut puerperio praeterquam alter vitam, si vero utriusque sexus editi sint gemini, rariorem utrique salutem (Pliny NH 7.37).

88 Aritotle, *Historia Animalium* 584b; Generat. anim. 770a.

89 [Hipp.] *Acut.* 1.30.1.

90 [Hipp.] *Aph.* 5.37; 5.38.

91 *Gyn.* 1.43, 2.21.

Acknowledgement: I would like to express my greatest thanks to my colleague and friend Janek Kucharski for all his support and suggestions which significantly contributed to the improvement of this article.

Bibliography

Allély, A. (2003), "Les enfants malformés et considerés comme prodigia à Rome et en Italie sous la république", *Revue des Études Anciennes* 105, 127–156.

Allély, A. (2004), "Les enfants malformés et handicapés à Rome sous le principat", *Revue des Études Anciennes* 106, 73–101.

American Psychiatric Association (1994), *Diagnostic and Statistical Manual of Mental Disorders*, 4th Edition: DSM-4, Washington, DC.

Androutsos, G. (2006), "Hermaphroditism in Greek and Roman antiquity", *Hormones* 5, 214–217.

Azize, J./Craigie, I. (2002), "Putative Akkadian Origin for the Greek words *Kinaidos* and *Puge*", *Antichthon* 36, 56–59.

Beagon, M. (trans., ed.) (2005), *The Elder Pliny. On the Human Animal. Natural History Book 7*, Oxford.

Berger, R./Daroff, R.B. (2013), "The Comatose Patient", in: B.A. Green/L.F. Marshall/T.J. Gallagher (eds.), *Intensive Care for Neurological Trauma and Disease*, 31–46.

Berrios, G.E. (1996), *The History of Mental Symptoms: Descriptive Psychopatology since the Nineteenth Century*, Cambridge.

Bloch, R. (1963), *Les Prodiges dans l'Antiquité classique: Grèce, Étrurie et Rome*, Paris.

Bowie, E. (1996), "The Ancient Readers of the Greek Novel", in: G.L. Schmeling (ed.), *The Novel in the Ancient World*, Leiden, 87–106.

Brisson, L. (1997), *Le Sexe incertain : Androgynie et hermaphroditisme dans l'Antiquité romaine*, Paris.

Brisson, L. (2002), *Sexual Ambivalence: Androgyny and Hermaphroditism in Graeco-Roman Antiquity*, Berkeley/Los Angeles/London.

Bush, M./Pernoll, M.L. (2006), "Multiple Pregnancy", in: A.H. DeCherney *et al.* (eds.), *Current Diagnosis and Treatment Obstetrics and Gynecology* (10th ed.), New York, 301–310.

Connel, S.M. (2016), *Aristotle on Female Animals: A Study of the Generation of Animals*, Cambridge.

Cueva, E.P./Byrne, Sh.N. (2014), *A Companiòn to the Ancient Novel*, Oxford/Malden.

Chew, K.S. (2014), "Achilles Tatius, Sophistic Master of Novelistic Conventions", in: Cueva/Byrne 2014, 62–75.

Dasen, V. (2005), "Blessing or Portents? Multiple Births in Ancient Rome", in: K. Mustakallio *et al.* (eds.), *Hoping for Continuity: Childhood, Education and Death in Antiquity and the Middle Ages*, Rome, 61–74.

Davidson, J. (2007), *The Greeks and Greek Love: A Radical Reappraisal of Homosexuality in Ancient Greece*, London.

Debru, A. (1992), "La suffocation hystérique chez Galien et Aetius: Réécriture et emprunt de «je»", in: A. Garzya (ed.), *Tradizione e ecdotica dei testi medici tardoantichi e bizantini*, Napoli, 79–89.

Delcourt, M. (1938), *Stérilités mystérieuses et naissances maléfiques dans l'antiquité classique*, Liège/Paris.
Delcourt, M. (1961), *Hermaphrodite: Myths and Rites of the Bisexual Figure in Classical Antiquity* (tr. J. Nicholson), London.
Den Boer, W. (1979), *Private Morality in Greece and Rome : Some Historical Aspects*, Leiden.
Doroszewska, J. (2016), *The Monstrous World: Corporeal Discourses in Phlegon of Tralles' Mirabilia*, Frankfurt am Main.
Dover, K.J. (1989^2, orig. 1978), *Greek Homosexuality*, Cambridge, Mass.
Erdas, D. (2002), *Cratero il Macedone : Testimonianze e frammenti*, Tivoli.
Flemming, R. (2000), *Medicine and the Making of Roman Women*, Oxford.
Garland, R. (1995), *The Eye of the Beholder: Deformity and Disability in the Graeco-Roman World*, Ithaca/New York.
Grmek, M. (1987), "Les indicia mortis dans la medicine gréco-romaine", in F. Hinard (ed.), *La Mort, les mort et l'au-delà dans le monde romaine*, Caen, 129–144.
Laes, C./Gevaert, B. (2013), "What's in a Monster? Pliny the Elder, Teratology and Bodily Disability", in: Laes/Goodey/Rose 2013, 211–230.
Grauman, L.A. (2013), "Monstrous Births and Retrospective Diagnosis: The Case of Hermaphrodites in Antiquity", in: Laes/Goodey/Rose 2013, 211–230.
Halperin, D.M. (2012), *How to Do the History of Homosexuality*, Chicago.
Hansen, W. (1996), *Phlegon of Tralles' Book of Marvels*, Exeter.
Hanson, J.W. (1975), "Incidence of Conjoined Twinning (Letter)", *The Lancet* 2, 1257.
Harper, C. (2007), *Intersex*, Oxford/New York.
Healey, J.F. (1999), *Pliny the Elder on Science and Technology*, Oxford.
Kazantzidis, G. (2018), "Medicine and the Paradox in the Hippocratic Corpus and Beyond", in: M. Gerolemou (ed.), *Recognizing Miracles in Antiquity and Beyond*, Berlin, 31–61.
Keller, O. (1877), *Rerum naturalium scriptores Graeci 1*, Lipsiae.
King, H. (1998), *Hippocrates' Woman: Reading the Female Body in Ancient Greece*, London.
King, H. (2012), "Knowing the Body: Renaissance Medicine and the Classics", in: P. Olmos (ed.), *Greek Science in the Long Run: Essays on the Greek Scientific Tradition (4th c. BCE–17th c. CE)*, Newcastle-upon-Tyne, 281–300.
King, H. (2016), *The One-Sex Body on Trial: The Classical and Early Modern Evidence*, London.
Krevans, N. (2005), "The Editor's Toolbox: Strategies for Selection and Presentation in the Milan Epigram Papyrus", in: K. Gutzwiller (ed.), *The New Posidippus: A Hellenistic Poetry Book*, Oxford, 81–96.
Laqueur, T.W. (1990), *Making Sex: Body and Gender from the Greeks to Freud*, Cambridge, MA.
Laes, C./Goodey, C.F./Lynn Rose, M. (eds.) (2013), *Disabilities in Roman Antiquity: Disparate Bodies a capite ad calcem*, Leiden/Boston.
Leitao, D.D. (2012), *The Pregnant Male as Myth and Metaphor in Classical Greek Literature*, Cambridge.
Létoublon, F./Genre, M. (2014), "Respect these Breasts and Pity Me", in: E.P. Cueva/S.N. Byrne (eds.), *A Companion to the Ancient Novel*. Malden, MA/Oxford, 352–370.
Lévi, É. (2006), *Magic: A History of its Rites, Rituals, and Mysteries* (translated with a Preface and Notes by A. E. Waite), Mineola/New York.
Lloyd, G.E.R. (1983), *Science, Folklore and Ideology: Studies in the Life Sciences in Ancient Greece*, Cambridge.
Lonie, I.M. (1965), "Medical Theory in Heraclides of Pontus", *Mnemosyne* 18, 126–143.
Mattern, S. (2008), *Galen and the Rhetoric of Healing*, Baltimore.

Mesk, J. (1925), "Über Phlegons Mirabilia I–III", *Philologus* 80, 298–311.
Pataricza, D. (2009), "Father or Mother? Stories of Male Pregnancies in Phlegon's *De Mirabilibus*", *Acta Classica Universitatis Scientiarum Debreceniensis* 45, 129–133.
Preuss, A. (1977), "Galen's Criticism of Aristotle's Conception Theory", *Journal of the History of Biology* 10.1, 65–85.
Rabinowitz, N. (1993), *Anxiety Veiled: Euripides and the Traffic in Women*, Ithaca.
Rohde, E. (1877), "Zu den Mirabilia des Phlegon", *RhM* 32, 329–340.
Schepens, G./Delcroix, K. (1996), "Ancient Paradoxography: Origin, Evolution, Production and Reception", in: O. Pecere/A. Stramaglia (eds.), *La letteratura di consumo nel mondo greco–latino: Atti del convegno internazionale*, Cassino, 14–17 settembre 1994, 373–460.
Scull, A. (2009), *Hysteria: The Biography*, Oxford.
Spencer, R. (2003), *Conjoined Twins: Developmental Malformations and Clinical Implications*, Baltimore/London.
Stramaglia, A. (1995), "Sul περὶ θαυμασίων di Flegonte di Tralle : Problemi di Tradizione, Lingua ed Esegesi", *Studi Classici e Orientali* 45, 191–234.
Stramaglia, A. (2010), *Phlegon Trallianus : Opuscula de Rebus Mirabilibus et de Longaevis*, Berlin/New York.
Van der Eijk, P. (2009), "The Woman not Breathing", in: W.W. Fortenbaugh/E. Pender (eds.), *Heraclides of Pontus: Discussion*, New Brunswick, 237–250.
Van der Gracht, S. (2012), "Setting Aside the Loom: Hermaphroditism in Ancient Medicine", in: L. Peterman/K. Sun/F.W. Stahnisch (eds.), *Proceedings of the 18th Annual «History of Medicine Days» Conference 2009*, Newcastle upon Tyne, 247–262.
Wendland, P. (1911), *De fabellis antiquis earumque ad Christianos propagatione*, Gottingae.
Williams, C.A. (2010^2, orig. 1999), *Roman Homosexuality*, New York/Oxford.
Winkler, J. (1990), *The Constraints of Desire: The Anthropology of Sex and Gender in Ancient Greece*, New York/London.
Zimmerman, M./Panayotakis, S./Keulen, W. (eds.) (2000), *ICAN 2000: The Ancient Novel in Context. Abstracts of the Papers to be Read at the Third International Conference on the Ancient Novel to be held at the University of Groningen*, The Netherlands, 25–30 July 2000, Groningen.

Kelly E. Shannon-Henderson

Phlegon's Paradoxical Physiology

Centaurs in the *Peri Thaumasion*

Abstract: This essay examines how medical-scientific discourses about the nature of hybrid bodies lie in the background of Phlegon's discussion of a centaur (*Mir.* 34–35). Centaurs have a long history as a byword for creatures that cannot possibly exist. Palaephatus, Lucretius, the paradoxographer Heraclitus, Artemidorus, Minucius Felix, Lucian, and Galen all object to the creature on the grounds that its hybrid body would be physically impossible, disadvantageous, and unsustainable by any known diet. A careful examination of Phlegon's description of the centaur shows that, although he cites none of these authors by name, he is aware of, and reacting explicitly to, these pre-existing medical-scientific discussions of centaurs. This reveals Phlegon to be aiming at an educated readership whose recognition of the medical-scientific background to the creature he describes will deepen their appreciation of the θαῦμα it represents.

1 Introduction

Phlegon of Tralles, active during the lifetime of Hadrian,[1] is atypical among paradoxographers in ways that make his Περὶ θαυμασίων ("On Marvels") a good test case for investigating the contact between paradoxography and medicine: his subject matter is derived entirely from human physiology.[2] This is a departure from the material favored by paradoxography in the Callimachean tradition, which dealt mostly with marvels in the natural world (e.g. marvellous springs or unusual properties of stones or plants). These could also bring medical and paradoxographical discourse into contact, since some marvellous properties of

I am very grateful to the audience at the University of Alabama Department of Modern Languages and Classics Work-In-Progress Seminar (especially Jessica Goethals, Alessandra Montalbano, and Tatiana Summers), and to George Kazantzidis, for their observations on this essay.

1 For Phlegon's life and works, see further Shannon 2013, 2–3 and references there cited. The latest event referred to in his text is dated to AD 116 (*Mir.* 9).

2 This has been noted by Giannini 1964, 129–130; Hansen 1996, 11; Schepens/Delcroix 1996, 431; Doroszewska 2016, 10–11.

https://doi.org/10.1515/9783110661774-007

plants or stones have medical applications,[3] yet these medical θαῦματα do not encompass what I will refer to as *physiology*: an interest in unusual manifestations of the human body and its functioning, especially in the area of anatomy. Even paradoxographers who *do* include material on the human body do so in a different way from Phlegon. For example, Apollonius' Ἱστορίαι θαυμασίαι ("Amazing Stories", *FGrHist* 1672), a text of uncertain date and authorship composed in the 2nd century BCE or later, includes some examples that verge on the medical, such as his observation that a person's earwax takes on a sweet taste when he or she is ill (Apollonius 28). Yet such anecdotes, as Spittler argues, do not strain the reader's credibility and "are generally interesting rather than amazing".[4] In other words, many examples of "medical" material found in paradoxographical texts indeed show overlap between those genres, but not in a way that challenges or calls into question the general principles of knowledge about the human body or its treatment that are set out in medical or natural-scientific texts.[5]

Phlegon's human θαῦματα, by contrast, are amazing in a way that occasionally strains credibility. He describes dead people returning to life (*Mir.* 1–3); spontaneous sex changes (4–9) and intersex babies (10); monstrously large bones (11-19); unusual births, including deformed babies (20–21, 25), humans producing animal offspring (22–24), men giving birth (26–27), and astounding multiple births (28–31); and unusually speedy aging processes (32–33). But the example from Phlegon's text on which I will focus here is the final one, arguably even more extreme than the others: a centaur found in Arabia whose preserved body Phlegon claims is still on display in the emperor's storehouse in Rome (*Mir.* 34–35). Although the centaur may seem fantastical, Phlegon's description can be shown to be strongly informed by traditional and contemporary medical and natural-scientific discourse about the impossibility of hybrid creatures. While Phlegon never explicitly acknowledges these common anti-centaur arguments, he refutes them point by point; a medical/scientific counter-explanation that sought to disprove such a creature's existence on physiological grounds thus lurks in the background of Phlegon's description.

---

3 E.g. Apollonius (*FGrHist* 1672) *Mir.* 29 (on a plant called ἀριστολοχία) with commentary of Spittler 2016, *ad loc.*

4 Spittler 2016, introduction. See also Kazantzidis 2018, 32–33, 35 on Phlegon as abnormal among paradoxographers in his focus on human marvels.

5 On this issue in general, see Kazantzidis 2018.

2 The Proverbial and Physiological Impossibility of Centaurs

For a long span of centuries beginning at least with Aristotle and stretching until Galen's medical writings in the later second century CE,[6] the impossibility of centaurs and other hybrid creatures found in myth was a common *topos* in medical, natural-scientific, and other rationalizing texts.[7] By the time Cicero asked, "What difference does it make whether we think of a god or of a hippocentaur?" (*N.D.* 1.105),[8] the centaur had apparently become a commonplace for a creature which did not and could not exist, and this use of centaurs as a rhetorical *topos* for non-existence continued into the Roman era.[9] As a result of these discussions, by Phlegon's time the idea that centaurs were so outlandish that they could function as a rhetorical commonplace of the impossible had been around for centuries, and a common set of objections to their existence had been developed related to the physiological difficulties that such a creature would have to overcome in order to survive. This centuries-long discourse forms the background of medical-scientific "knowledge" about centaurs, a body of commonly-held truths about hybrid creatures that would tacitly inform Phlegon's presentation of his "real-life" centaur.

While Aristotle does not discuss centaurs in his extant biological writings, there is evidence that he may have been among the first to be interested in the physiological problem they presented. He had used the example of "whether a centaur or a god exists" as one of the four main types of questions a philosopher can ask (*APo.* 89b 32), showing clear interest in the question of the creature's existence. Aristotle also composed two works, now lost, entitled "On composite creatures" (Ὑπὲρ τῶν συνθέτων ζῴων) and "On mythical creatures" (Ὑπὲρ τῶν

6 For Galen's dates (b. 129 CE, d. sometime in the 210s), see Hankinson 2008, 1 and references there cited.

7 These texts come from a variety of genres and are not what would normally be considered "medical," but they can be grouped together by their common approach: all refute the existence of centaurs by explaining why their bodies could not possibly exist.

8 All translations are my own unless otherwise stated.

9 Pease 1963, 434 (on a similar reference to centaurs at Cic. *Div.* 2.49): centaurs "came to be regarded by the rationalists as types of the *non-ens*"; see passages cited there and at Pease 1958, 482–84. Salient examples include Pl. *Phdr.* 229d; Theon *Prog.* 95.3; Sen. *Ep.* 58.15 (on which see Inwood 2007, 120–123); Plut. *Mor.* 830d; Lucian *Herm.* 72. Even Galen, who also engaged in more detail with the physiological feasibility of centaurs (see below), sometimes used the creature merely as a shorthand for something impossible (Gal. *MM* 10.144K, 10.153K).

μυθολογουμένων ζῴων, Diog. Laert. 5.25), probably while he was in the process of writing *Historia Animalium*, which contains many legendary or paradoxical anecdotes about animals and their behavior. Probably the lost works were intended, as Moraux hypothesizes, to assemble a representative sample of mythological creatures "and confront these mythological traditions with the results of his observations."[10] Moraux also speculates that another treatise also entitled "On mythical creatures" (Περὶ τῶν μυθολογουμένων ζῴων) attributed to Straton,[11] head of the Academy in Athens in the 280s and 270s BCE, may have been based on these lost works of Aristotle; this would suggest that natural-scientific and philosophical discourse about mythical and hybrid creatures continued to interest Aristotelian thinkers.

Palaephatus, a mythographer active in the era of Aristotle or not long after[12] who sought to rationalize the unbelievable tales found in mythology, shows clearly the influence of this Aristotelian thinking. Palaephatus is perhaps best known for advancing the common theory that stories about centaurs developed out of a misconception generated when humans riding on horseback were seen for the first time by primitive peoples.[13] In general, his refutations of myths revolve around linguistic or metaphorical re-interpretations of old stories, but his chapter on centaurs also voices objections that can be described as physiological, and show the clear stamp of Aristotelian ideas about biology:[14]

> Περὶ Κενταύρων. φασὶν ὡς θηρία ἐγένοντο καὶ ἵππου μὲν εἶχον τὴν ὅλην ἰδέαν πλὴν τῆς κεφαλῆς, ταύτην δὲ ἀνδρός. εἴ τις οὖν πείθεται τοιοῦτον γενέσθαι θηρίον, ἀδύνατον· οὔτε γὰρ ἄλλως αἱ φύσεις σύμφωνοι ἵππου καὶ ἀνδρός, οὔτε ἡ τροφὴ ὁμοία, οὔτε διὰ στόματος

---

10 Moraux 1951, 108–109 ("faire appel aux traditions mythologiques et de les confronter avec les résultats de ses observations").

11 See Diog. Laert. 5.59.

12 Stern 1996, 1–5 argues for an Aristotelian date, but notes that what we have of Palaephatus today is probably a later epitome. Hawes 2014a, 129–132 places him among the Peripatetics and argues for a date of composition in the 340s or 330s.

13 Palaeph. 1; the same argument is made by, e.g., D.S. 4.70.1, Plin. *Nat.* 7.202, Minucius Felix *Octavius* 20.3, Heraclit. *Incred.* 5. For a similar modern argument, see Scobie 1978.

14 Compare Palaephatus' observations on the centaur with Aristotle's biological ideas as summarized by Furth 1987, 27–28, especially Aristotle's beliefs that "biological individuals [are] permanently endowed with a highly definite specific nature" (cf. below on the "fixity of species" argument in Palaephatus), and that "the intricate constitutive nature that typifies such things is very highly species-specific" (cf. Palaephatus on the φύσεις of man and horse that are not "harmonious" [σύμφωνοι]). Schrijvers 1983, 361, 363 and Li Causi 2005, 96–97 also argue for Palaephatus' indebtedness to Aristotle. Osmun 1956, 134 argues for the mainly philological nature of Palaephatus' evidence in the case of the centaurs, without acknowledging the role played by physiology.

> καὶ φάρυγγος ἀνθρωπείου δυνατὸν ἵππου τροφὴν διελθεῖν. εἰ δὲ τοιαύτη ἰδέα τότε ἦν, καὶ νῦν ἂν ὑπῆρχε.
>
> (Palaeph. 1).

> Concerning Centaurs: They say that these are beasts and have the complete appearance of a horse except for the head, which is a man's. So if someone thinks that such a beast exists, it is impossible: for neither are the natures of horse and man harmonious in other respects, nor is their food similar, and a horse's food could not pass through a human mouth and throat. And if such a shape existed at one time, it would also exist nowadays.

Palaephatus' centaurs' only human parts are their heads, rather than the entire torso they are frequently depicted as having in artistic representations.[15] The idea that the "natures" (φύσεις) of man and horse are not "harmonious" (σύμφωνοι) is not elaborated upon, save in the particular case of diet and nourishment as it relates to anatomy: a human body and a horse body require different types of food (τροφή), and the digestive tract of each creature is specifically suited to its diet in such a way that the same mouth and throat could not process the same food. As we shall see, this dietary objection becomes a key feature of later objections to centaurs. Palaephatus' argument that centaurs would still exist today if it were possible for them to exist at all echoes an observation also made in the introduction to the Περὶ ἀπίστων: "As for all the forms and shapes which are said to have once existed which do not exist now – such things never existed. For if something existed at one time, it also exists now and will exist in the future" (Palaeph. pr.: ὅσα δὲ εἴδη καὶ μορφαί εἰσι λεγόμεναι καὶ γενόμεναι τότε, αἳ νῦν οὐκ εἰσί, τὰ τοιαῦτα οὐκ ἐγένοντο. εἰ γάρ <τί> ποτε καὶ ἄλλοτε ἐγένετο, καὶ νῦν τε γίνεται καὶ αὖθις ἔσται).[16] Palaephatus insists upon continued existence as proof that a creature is real and not merely mythological. This idea, as we shall see, would also be carried through in later discourse about centaurs.

Lucretius (5.878–924) picks up some of the arguments presented by Palaephatus, and argues against the existence of centaurs for several physiological reasons. It is likely that Lucretius' dismantling of the myth of centaurs was directly inspired by Palaephatus' criticism, as several scholars have noted, while Epicurus' ideas about the unbreakability of the laws of nature, and a related concept of the fixity of species, are also at play.[17] As Campbell has noted, whereas

15 For centaurs in ancient art, see Baur 1912; Osborne 1994; Morawietz 2000.

16 Palaephatus attributes the idea to Melissus, a fifth-century Presocratic philosopher, and Lamiscus of Samos, a fourth-century Pythagorean; both are very poorly known (Stern 1996, 29).

17 See Schrijvers 1999, 31 (who persuasively argues that Lucretius' discussions of the Chimera [5.901–906] and Cerberus [3.1011–13] as biological impossibilities also derive from Palaeph. 28, 39); and Campbell 2003, 141. For Lucretius' knowledge of and interest in medicine and medical

Lucretius might have been expected to argue that centaurs are impossible using the atomic theories on display in the rest of his poem, in fact his "argument is firmly in the rationalist tradition, which concentrates on criticism at the macroscopic level."[18] Lucretius argues that "centaurs have never existed, nor can beings composed of heterogeneous body-parts, with double nature and twofold body, exist at any time" (5.878–90: *sed neque centauri fuerunt nec tempore in ullo | esse queunt duplici natura et corpore bino | ex alienigenis membris compacta*). Lucretius' case against centaurs is largely based on the idea that equine bodies and human bodies grow, age, and decay at different rates; if a horse is considered mature at three while a human is still a juvenile at that age, how would the process of aging be experienced by a body that had characteristics of both organisms (5.883–92)?[19] But he also repeats some of the same arguments Palaephatus used: the idea that centaurs do not exist now and have never existed in the past (5.878) clearly owe something to Palaephatus' arguments. Lucretius further argues (5.916–922) that the law against hybrid creatures is a fixed law of nature, preventing *semina* of different kinds of organisms from being mixed together both in the primordial past and today, and concludes that "each thing proceeds in its own way, and by a fixed law of nature all preserve their distinctions" (5.923–4 *sed res quaeque suo ritu procedit, et omnes | foedere naturae certo discrimina servant*). Palaephatus' argument of impossibility based on diet also leaves a stamp on Lucretius' argument. His observation (5.884–5) that boys at the age of three occasionally will still obtain nourishment by breastfeeding is perhaps meant to "remind [...] the reader of the traditional criticism that the nourishment of each part of a Centaur would require different foods."[20] The point is made more explicitly a few lines later when Lucretius states that "the same things are not pleasant to the limbs" for all creatures, "for you can often see beard-wearing flocks [of goats] grow fat upon hemlock, which for a human is bitter poison" (5.890–891 *neque sunt eadem iucunda per artus: | quippe videre licet pinguescere saepe cicuta | barbigeras pecudes, homini quae est acre venenum*). Campbell has suggested that Lucretius shifts his dietary argument away from horses to goats in order to provide "an extreme case of the necessity for different foods... rather than stating the

---

disciplines (including physiology) as revealed in his poetry, see Kilpatrick 1996. Lucretius' argument about the fixity of species and the impossibility of hybrid creatures also appears at 2.700–717. On Lucretius and hybrid creatures, see further Campbell 2007, 39–52. For the relevance of Epicurus, see Schrijvers 1983, 360.

18 Campbell 2003, 142; 148–149.

19 Bailey 1947, 1468. Holmes 2013, 165 n. 28 notes that this argument is unparalleled and therefore possibly unique to Lucretius.

20 Campbell 2003, 150.

more obvious, but less dramatic, point that horses and humans cannot survive on one another's food, as is traditional in arguments against Centaurs."[21] Lucretius' argument here is further strengthened by the fact that he has already expressed a similar argument at 2.700–717: hybrid creatures (*semiferas hominum species*) such as the chimera cannot really exist, in part because each creature has a distinct type of food containing the right type of atoms necessary to maintain its particular body and motions.[22]

Lucretius, therefore, in deploying the fixity-of-species argument and the dietary argument to refute the existence of centaurs, represents a further step in the fixing of common physiological objections to centaurs that is strongly indebted to Palaephatus and the Aristotelian biological thinking that probably gave rise to his criticisms. These ideas would continue to be expressed for the next three centuries. Heraclitus, a rationalizing mythographer of the first or second century CE[23] in the spirit of Palaephatus, who also composed a treatise entitled Περὶ ἀπίστων, in his discussion of centaurs reprises not only Palaephatus' horseback-riding hypothesis but also some of his physiological arguments against centaurs. He argues that it is impossible for a creature of two different "natures" (φύσεις) to be born alive and survive (Heracl. *Incred.* 5: δύο γὰρ διηλλαγμένας φύσεις εἰς ἓν συνελθούσας ἀδύνατον ζῳογονηθῆναι καὶ τραφῆναι); use of the verb τρέφω, which can refer to the nourishing activity of food,[24] may also be an implicit reference to the dietary argument against centaurs' existence. Similar arguments are made by Artemidorus, who discusses centaurs in his *Oneirocritica* in the context of offering interpretations of dreams involving the creatures: "It is not possible for a centaur to come into being at all; even if it did, it would be impossible for it to be reared" (Artem. 4.47 οὐδαμῶς γὰρ ἐνδέχεται Ἱπποκένταυρον γενέσθαι, εἰ δὲ καὶ γένοιτο, ἀδύνατον τὸ τραφῆναι).[25] The fixity-of-species argument persists as well. Minucius Felix, a Christian apologist writing in the late second or early third century CE, would deploy it against the existence of "centaurs, horses intermixed with their human [riders]" (*centauros equos suis hominibus inplexos*) by claiming that "if these things had happened, they would [still] happen [today]; and they

21 Campbell 2003, 156.
22 See Lucr. 2.711–12, with Bailey 1947, 914.
23 For the dating, see Hawes 2014b, 94 and references there cited.
24 LSJ s.v. τρέφω III.5.
25 Cf. also Artem. 2.44, with Harris-McCoy 2012, 491.

have not happened for the precise reason that they cannot happen [now]" (*Octavius* 20.3–4 *quae si essent facta, fierent; quia fieri non possunt, ideo nec facta sunt*).[26]

Authors also focus their attention on the most anatomically complex part of a centaur: the midsection, where horse and human parts meet. Heraclitus describes this anatomical dividing point in the mythological beasts with more precision than his predecessors: "They had men's [bodies] above the flanks, but below that point it was all horse" (τὰ μὲν ἐπάνω τῶν λαγόνων ἀνδρῶν ἔχοντας, τὸ δ' ἀπὸ <τούτου> τοῦ μέρους πᾶν ἵππων). Lucian, in describing a famous picture of a family of centaurs by the fifth-century BCE painter Zeuxis, particularly praises the artist's ability to harmoniously join the horse and human anatomy of the mother centaur in a convincing and aesthetically pleasing way:

> καὶ ἡ μίξις δὲ καὶ ἡ ἁρμογὴ τῶν σωμάτων, καθ' ὃ συνάπτεται καὶ συνδεῖται τῷ γυναικείῳ τὸ ἱππικόν, ἠρέμα καὶ οὐκ ἀθρόως μεταβαίνουσα καὶ ἐκ προσαγωγῆς τρεπομένη λανθάνει τὴν ὄψιν ἐκ θατέρου εἰς τὸ ἕτερον ὑπαγομένη.
>
> (Lucian *Zeux*. 6).
>
> The mixing and junction of the bodies, where the horse-section is joined and attached to the woman-section, deceives the sight as it moves between them gently and not all at once, and gradually changes, led on by degrees from one to the other.

Although Lucian is speaking of a fantastical artistic depiction rather than a flesh-and-blood centaur, his praise for Zeuxis' ability to depict the complex anatomy of a centaur's midsection[27] suggests that his attention to this area of the creature's body is part of a larger discourse of skepticism. If the part of the centaur where the human and horse sections join were not the part of its anatomy that proverbially causes disbelief, Lucian would not have singled out Zeuxis' depiction of that particular part for his praise. Thus we see a common physiological discourse about centaurs that emerges in a variety of generic modes, including art criticism: what Palaephatus, Lucretius, Heraclitus, Minucius Felix, Artemidorus, and Lu-

---

26 See Schrijvers 1999, 31 for the connection between Minucius Felix's ideas and those of Lucretius and Palaephatus; cf. Campbell 2003, 141.

27 This section of the body seems to have been a particular challenge for artists attempting to depict centaurs, but was one for which Zeuxis' noted talents of blending color and light and shadow equipped him very well (Schörner 2002, 103–104; Pretzler 2009, 166–167). For another *ekphrasis* of a picture of female centaurs, cf. Philostr. *Im*. 2.3, with Pretzler 2009, 167–168: "Philostratus seems aware of most of the difficulties in painting centaurs… which are emphasized in Lucian's description."

cian all have in common is a shared set of cultural assumptions, relying ultimately on Aristotelian biological ideas, about why centaurs cannot possibly exist in real life.

Where we see these ideas reiterated in the most detail, however, is in a medical writer who can be securely dated to within half a century of Phlegon: Galen.[28] Galen's criticism of centaurs appears in his treatise *On the Uses of the Parts of the Body*, and his objections to the creature's existence based on the superfluity and incompatibility of its body parts adhere to his teleological views on physiology: the principle that "nothing in an animal's body is useless or inactive" (Gal. *UP* 3.268K).[29]

> τί δὴ οὖν οὐ καὶ τέτταρα σκέλη καὶ χεῖρας ἐπ' αὐτοῖς ἔσχεν, ὥσπερ οἱ Κένταυροι; ὅτι πρῶτον μὲν ἀδύνατος τῇ φύσει τῶν τοσοῦτον διαφερόντων σωμάτων ἡ μίξις. οὐ γὰρ δή, ὥσπερ οἱ πλάσται τε καὶ οἱ γραφεῖς, σχήματά τε καὶ χρώματα μόνον αὐτῶν ἔμελλε συνθήσειν, ἀλλὰ καὶ τὰς οὐσίας ὅλας κεράσειν ἀμίκτους τε καὶ ἀκράτους ὑπαρχούσας... ἡμεῖς δ', οἷς ἀληθείας, οὐ μυθολογίας μέλει, σαφῶς ἴσμεν οὐσίαν ἀνθρώπου τε καὶ ἵππου παντάπασιν ἄμικτον ὑπάρχουσαν. εἰ δὲ καὶ συγχωρήσαιμεν ἐν γοῦν τῇ κυήσει καὶ μίγνυσθαι καὶ τελεοῦσθαι τὸ ζῷον τοῦτο τὸ οὕτως ἄτοπόν τε καὶ ἀλλόκοτον, ἀλλὰ τίσι γε τροφαῖς θρέψεται τὸ γεννηθέν, οὐκ ἂν εὕροιμεν. ἢ πόαις μέν τισι καὶ κριθαῖς ὠμαῖς τὰ κάτω τὰ ἵππεια, ταῖς δ' ἑφθαῖς καὶ τοῖς ἀνθρωπείοις ἐδέσμασι τὰ ἄνω; ἄμεινον μέντ' ἂν οὕτως ἦν αὐτῷ καὶ δύο στόματα γεγονέναι, τὸ μὲν ἀνθρώπειον, τὸ δ' ἵππειον. κινδυνεύσει γὰρ οὖν καὶ δύο καρδίας ἔχειν, εἴ τι δεῖ τοῖς στέρνοις τεκμαίρεσθαι.
>
> (Gal. *UP* 3.169K, 3.171K)

> But why, then, do [humans] not have four legs plus hands as well, like the centaur? The reason is that, in the first place, a commingling of such widely different bodies was impossible for Nature. For it was not merely their shapes and colors that she would have had to combine, as sculptors and painters do; she would also have been obliged to blend their very substances, which are absolute and will not mingle... We who are concerned with truth rather than mythology know well that the substance of a man is utterly unable to mingle with that of a horse. And even if we were to grant that this animal, so unnatural and monstrous, could be conceived and brought to term, we would not find any food to feed it once it had been born. Would the lower, horselike parts be nourished with grass and raw barley, and the upper parts on cooked barley and food fit for men? In that case, however, it would be better for the animal to have two mouths, one human and the other that of a horse; and if we must judge from the presence of two breasts, it would probably also have two hearts.[30]

---

28 For Galen's dates, see above, n. 5; for Phlegon, see above, n. 1.

29 On Galen's teleological view of physiology, derived from Hippocratic principles, see Grant 1952, 12–13; Debru 2008, 266–267.

30 Translation adapted from that of Tallmadge May 1968.

One of Galen's arguments against centaurs is that their bodies (σώματα) and indeed their "nature" (οὐσία) are physically too different to be combined; this is clearly a nod to the now-traditional idea of centaurs' "unharmonious natures." In specifying particular foods that would pose a problem, Galen also considers the proverbial problem of the centaur's diet in more detail than his predecessors. Emphasizing the differences between cooked and raw barley also connects Galen's argument about centaurs to his general ideas on diet as expressed in his other treatises, particularly *On the Properties of Foodstuffs* (*Alim.Fac.*): for humans, cooking food is essential to making it more digestible, and barley in particular can case flatulence if not cooked properly.[31] Galen elsewhere also states that wild plants are not nutritious for humans, as they are bad for the stomach and hard to digest.[32] We can presume, then, that the grass Galen mentions as centaur-food would, both according to common sense and in his considered medical opinion, not be an appropriate food for humans. Galen even takes the dietary objection to its logical extreme by claiming that a centaur would need two mouths and two chests containing two digestive tracts in order to be capable of nourishing itself properly. The fact that he extends this even further – two chests means two hearts! – speaks to the anatomical difficulties hinted at in Heraclitus and Lucian; while what bothers Galen about centaurs is not the particular junction of human chest and horse legs, his comment about the two hearts reveals a similar mental difficulty with the practicalities of conjoining two anatomies that are so different into one creature. A similar thought may lie behind Galen's explicit mention of the unlikelihood of any one creature having six limbs. Indeed, it is not merely the creature's body that defies Galen's objections, but also the related problem of its locomotion: as the text continues (Gal. *UP* 3.172K), Galen also connects centaurs' physiology to what he imagines their behavior would be, and objects that centaurs, if they existed, would gain nothing from their extra limbs, as their four legs would not be able to negotiate steep hills as well as a human's two.

Galen represents the culmination of many centuries of thought about centaurs and the physiological problems with their existence. There are no centaurs because it is impossible to combine either the φύσεις or the individual body parts of human and horse; because no single diet could sustain such a composite creature; and because they would be poorly adapted to move around if these fantastical creatures had to inhabit the real world. Galen's objections to centaurs are perhaps the strongest and most detailed, but they do not exist in a vacuum: their

31 Gal. *Alim.Fac.* 6.501K; see Grant 2000, 65. See also Grant 2000, 7–8. Gal. *Ptis.* is devoted exclusively to the proper preparation of a barley soup beneficial to patients.
32 Gal. *Alim.Fac.* 6.622K (grass is not specifically listed); Grant 2000, 137–138.

origins can be traced back to ideas that grew out of the Aristotelian biological tradition.

3 Phlegon Responds

Let us now examine Phlegon's account of a "real-life" centaur. The report is the stuff of paradoxography in many ways: it is located in Arabia (on the fringes of the known world, where the bizarre is often encountered), and in keeping with the generic conventions of paradoxography, Phlegon does not attempt to explain how such a fantastical creature came to be.[33] Nevertheless, the details Phlegon gives about the centaur suggest that he is aware of medical-scientific objections to its existence, which he seeks to counter one by one:

> εὑρέθη ἐν Σαύνῃ τῆς Ἀραβίας πόλει ἱπποκένταυρος ἐπὶ ὄρους μάλα ὑψηλοῦ, ὃ ἔστιν γέμον φαρμάκου θανασίμου, καλεῖται δὲ τὸ φάρμακον ὁμώνυμον τῇ πόλει, ὀξύτατον δὲ καὶ ἀνυτικώτατον τῶν ὀλεθρίων καθέστηκεν. τὸν δὲ ἱπποκένταυρον συλλαβὼν ὁ βασιλεὺς ζωὸν ἀποπέμπει σὺν ἑτέροις δώροις πρὸς καίσαρα εἰς τὴν Αἴγυπτον. τροφὴ δὲ ἦν αὐτοῦ κρέα. οὐ φέρων δὲ τὴν μεταβολὴν τοῦ ἀέρος τελευτᾷ, καὶ οὕτως ὁ ἔπαρχος τῆς Αἰγύπτου ταριχεύσας ἀπέστειλεν εἰς Ῥώμην, καὶ πρῶτον ἐν τοῖς βασιλείοις ἀπεδείχθη, τὸ μὲν πρόσωπον ἀγριώτερον τοῦ ἀνθρωπίνου ἔχων, χεῖρας δὲ καὶ τοὺς τούτων δακτύλους τετριχωμένους, πλευρὰ δὲ συναφῆ τοῖς πρώτοις σκέλεσι καὶ τῇ γαστρί, ὁπλαὶ δὲ ἦσαν αὐτῷ ἵππου στερεαὶ καὶ ἐπίξανθοι χαῖται, καίπερ ὑπὸ τῆς ταριχείας συμμελαινόμεναι τῷ δέρματι. μέγεθος δὲ ἦν οὐχ οἷοιπερ οἱ γραφόμενοι, οὐδ' αὖ πάλιν μικρόν. ἐν δὲ τῇ προειρημένῃ πόλει Σαύνῃ ἐλέγοντο καὶ ἕτεροι εἶναι ἱπποκένταυροι. τὸν δὲ πεμφθέντα εἰς Ῥώμην εἴ τις ἀπιστεῖ, δύναται ἱστορῆσαι· ἀπόκειται γὰρ ἐν τοῖς ὁρ<ρ>ίοις τοῦ αὐτοκράτορος τεταριχευμένος, ὡς προεῖπον
>
> (Phleg. *Mir.* 34–35).

> In Saune, a city in Arabia, a hippocentaur was found upon a very high mountain which is full of a deadly herb, and the herb is named after the city, and it is the sharpest and most effective of the deadly drugs. The king captured the hippocentaur alive and sent it to Egypt with other gifts for Caesar. And its nourishment was meat. But it could not tolerate the change of climate and died, and so the prefect of Egypt embalmed it and sent it to Rome, and it was at first displayed in the palace. Its face was more savage than a human one, and its hands and fingers were covered with hair. Its ribs were connected to its front legs and its stomach, and it had the hard hooves of a horse and a tawny mane, although this, along with the skin, had become quite dark from the embalming. Its size was not exactly like those that

33 In particular, he avoids any of the common stories about sexual unions between humans and horses as the origin of centaurs (e.g. Pind. *P.* 2.42–48; A.R. 2.1232–1241; D.S. 4.69–70; Apollod. 1.4; Plut. *Mor.* 149c–e); see further Carey 1981, 40–41.

> have been depicted, but it was not small either. In the aforementioned city of Saune there are also said to be other hippocentaurs. But if anyone disbelieves the one sent to Rome, it is possible to conduct enquiry: for it is stored away in the storehouses of the emperor, embalmed, as I have said before.

This centaur defies all potential objections to its existence by appearing at a definite place and time: it is in no way assumed to be a fiction or a myth. In fact, Phlegon takes great pains to prove that it really existed by telling the reader exactly where its physical remains can still be found.[34] This appeal to autopsy – any skeptical readers can go and see its mummy for themselves – can be read as an implicit counter to the fixity-of-species argument so frequently deployed against centaurs in the authors surveyed above. Palaephatus and Lucretius argued that if it were possible for centaurs to exist, they still would; Phlegon asserts that they do.

Several aspects of Phlegon's description of the centaur's anatomy show his awareness of debates about its allegedly impossible physiology. One is the anatomical detail Phlegon presents: he takes some care to describe the centaur's body parts and how they fit together, in ways that appear to answer exactly the common medical-scientific objections to centaurs. Phlegon makes sure to emphasize that the creature indeed has features of both human and horse despite the fact that this was allegedly impossible. He gives particular attention to the creature's midsection, the point where the horselike and humanlike sections of its body join together (the area also singled out for special attention by Heraclitus and Lucian), and describes specifically how ribs, stomach, and forelegs relate spatially to each other. Phlegon also gives attention to the creature's limbs. Although Galen objects that it is impossible for any creature to have both four legs and hands, that is exactly what Phlegon asserts his centaur has; the phrase τοῖς πρώτοις σκέλεσι implies the existence of a second pair of legs behind the first. Phlegon also makes sure to specify that those four legs terminate in a horse's hooves, but that the creature also has two hands (presumably on its arms, which are not explicitly described). Even the hands as Phlegon describes them are of a hybrid form that combine human and equine features:[35] they seem to be normal human hands in that they are explicitly stated to be divided into fingers (and are thus differentiated from the creature's solid hooves [ὁπλαὶ… ἵππου στερεαί]), but

34 See Shannon-Henderson forthcoming (a) on the issue of sources, citations, and proof in Phlegon.

35 Cf. Doroszewska 2016, 126: "When meticulously describing the creature he apparently takes as his point of reference human appearance." Cf. Paus. 9.21.1 for a similar description of a Triton, which highlights the combination of human and fish body parts.

in the centaur's case they are covered with hair (τετριχωμένους) as a horse's body is.[36] Galen also objected that a centaur would have to have two mouths, to consume the two kinds of food for man and horse; but Phlegon's centaur's face merely looks wilder than a human one (τὸ μὲν πρόσωπον ἀγριώτερον τοῦ ἀνθρωπίνου ἔχων);[37] it does not have fundamentally different features. It is not merely the anatomy of the creature's dead body that defies physiological objections, but the uses to which it put that anatomy while it was alive. While Galen argues that centaurs, if they existed, would not be able to negotiate steep hills well, Phlegon states explicitly that the centaur was found on an extremely high mountain, and was apparently suited to that habitat (so much so that it died when removed from it). In his careful description of the centaur, then, Phlegon is not merely trying to create a vivid picture of the creature for his reader; he is creating that picture in such a way that it explicitly responds to common physiological arguments against centaurs' existence by specifying how human and animal characteristics are combined.

Phlegon also counters the common objection to centaurs on dietary grounds when he makes a point of stating that the centaur ate meat;[38] apparently, despite what Galen and other writers in the medical-scientific tradition would claim, there is in fact one food – meat – that is able to sustain both the horselike and humanlike sections of its body. The fact that a carnivorous diet is the answer to this puzzle perhaps also reveals deeper aspects of Phlegon's conception of the centaur. The dietary question is only a problem for those who view a centaur as a hybrid of human and horse, since eating meat is something which horses do not do except in extreme, monstrous, or unnatural cases, as with the man-eating horses of Diomedes in myth.[39] But eating meat is not uncommon for mythological centaurs: they are "eaters of raw flesh" according to Theognis (542 ὠμοφάγους), and when the "good" centaur Pholus hosted the hero Heracles, "he gave Heracles roasted meat, but he himself ate it raw" (Apollod. 2.5.4 οὗτος Ἡρακλεῖ μὲν ὀπτὰ παρεῖχε τὰ κρέα, αὐτὸς δὲ ὠμοῖς ἐχρῆτο). This uncouth diet symbolizes centaurs' bestial nature, and also confirms that they are *not* conceived of as horses or horse-

---

36 Cf. Lucian's description of the male centaur in Zeuxis' painting, which is covered with hair not just on the horselike sections of its body, but also its humanoid ones (*Zeux.* 5). For the hairiness of centaurs as evidence of their bestial nature, see Morawietz 2000, 18–19.

37 Compare Lucian *Zeux.* 5 on the male centaur in Zeuxis' painting: "Its glance, although it was laughing, was entirely beastlike, something of the mountains, wild" (τὸ βλέμμα, καίτοι γελῶντος, θηριῶδες ὅλον ὄρειόν τι καὶ ἀνήμερον).

38 Cf. Grant 1952, 63.

39 Cf. Eur. *Alc.* 494–6; Hyg. *Fab.* 30.9. Kurtz 1975 gives further examples drawn from literature and art.

hybrids, but as utterly separate, more savage beings.[40] While he is writing about "real life" and not myth, Phlegon would seem to agree. For him a centaur is not a hybrid, but something else entirely: its own creature, which eats meat like a predatory animal (rather than like a human) to sustain its whole body. Note again that he does not explain how or why this is the case. Indeed, his assertion that the centaur has the hooves of a horse yet is a meat-eater is explicitly counter to what other physiological writers say about how animals' feet relate to their diets: both Galen and Aristotle note that hooved animals are herbivores, while carnivorous quadrupeds need toed feet so that they can grasp their prey.[41] Phlegon's insistence on a hooved, carnivorous centaur raises a question: How do centaurs kill their meat if hooves are not the type of foot appropriate for this task? Phlegon does not explain, but with his description of the centaur merely asserts that it is true.

One final significant feature of Phlegon's description of the centaur is the way he introduces it: by connecting it with a drug (φάρμακον) that grows in the same Arabian mountain it inhabits. While plants and their amazing properties are the stock-and-trade of traditional Callimachean paradoxography,[42] they are not otherwise part of Phlegon's subject matter; this is the only passage where Phlegon displays any interest in this traditional paradoxographical *topos*. That makes this reference to the φάρμακον somewhat perplexing on content-related grounds. I would like to suggest an alternative explanation for its presence here. Drugs and centaurs are associated with one another elsewhere in ancient literature: the mythological centaur Chiron is said to have been associated with healing herbs,[43] and to have trained several demigods and heroes in the art of medicine (including Asclepius, who went on to be the master healer *par excellence* of Greek mythology).[44] Like Chiron, Phlegon's centaur is associated with φάρμακα, but the deadly drugs growing in its mountainous home are the opposite of Chiron's healing medicines. By opening his account of the centaur with φάρμακα, Phlegon primes the reader to think in medical terms. Yet just as his wild meat-eating centaur is the

---

40 Cf. Kirk 1971, 161–162; see also Segal 1974, 299–300.

41 See Arist. *HA* 2.1.497b 18–21 and *PA* 659a 24–26, 687b18–21; Gal. *UP* 3.175K, who notes that if carnivores had hooves they could run faster, but would "lose some essential functions of their limbs" (τὰς δ' εἰρημένας χρείας τῶν σκελῶν).

42 Giannini 1964, 107–108; Schepens/Delcroix 1996, 381.

43 Plin. *Nat.* 7.196, Hyg. *Fab.* 274.9 (Chiron discovered pharmacy and botany); Plin. *Nat.* 25.32–34 (two panacaeas discovered by Chiron).

44 Chiron taught medicine to Achilles (Hom. *Il.* 11.831–2), Asclepius (Pind. *P.* 3.1–6, 45–46), and Asclepius' son Machaon (Hom. *Il.* 4.216–19). On Chiron and medicine, see further Dawson 1949, 273–275; Kirk 1971, 159–162; DuBois 1982, 29–30.

antithesis of the civilized healer-centaur Chiron, everything about it contradicts what scientific and medical knowledge asserts is possible. The reference to the deadly φάρμακον, in other words, could be read programmatically: to put readers in a "medical" frame of mind, but also to forewarn them that what they may see as universally applicable medical or physiological norms are going to be contradicted, if not proven entirely false, by the centaur which Phlegon claims so definitively has existed.

4 Conclusion: Marvel and Explanation as a Matter of Genre?

Even among the marvels Phlegon records, which have a high degree of strangeness even for paradoxography, his centaur stands out as perplexing: it seems to push the limits of his chosen subject matter (marvels related to the human body) by introducing the element of hybridity. A centaur, after all, is not merely an extreme example of human physiology, but a creature that appears to probe the boundaries that separate humans from other species. This is certainly the attitude to centaurs displayed in the rationalizing, scientific, and medical writings I have examined here. While Phlegon never explicitly acknowledges these writers or their arguments, the details he gives about his "real-life" centaur show clearly that he is aware of their objections, and has chosen to present the creature in such a way that his description responds to common critiques of it on physiological grounds. Phlegon not only shows himself to be aware of medical-scientific discourse, but implicitly argues against it, casting himself in a polemical role, albeit tacitly.

Why would Phlegon do this? Why not explicitly acknowledge that he is disproving the common objections to centaurs? Part of the answer, I suggest, has to do with the generic conventions of paradoxography which distinguish it from truly scientific texts. While medicine/science and paradoxography might occasionally overlap in their subject matter, their attitudes to marvels have usually been understood to be fundamentally different. Both types of text deal in θαύματα; the difference comes in how the sense of wonder these θαύματα create is presented to the reader. Medical and scientific discourse seeks to find an explanation for the unusual phenomena that are its subject: θαύματα exist to be explained and understood. For Aristotle, for example, wonder is a valuable part of scientific enquiry, but can only be the first step: "All [enquiries] begin, as we have said, by wondering (ἀπὸ τοῦ θαυμάζειν) that things should be as they are"

(Arist. *Metaph.* 983a 14). The initial sense of wonder should not be where one's consideration of a θαῦμα *stops,* but where it *begins*; it should motivate one to observe and investigate the θαῦμα in pursuit of a deeper understanding.[45] The end result of such enquiry should be, in a way, the *end* of wonder: once the causative principles behind a marvel are understood, it ceases to be marvellous. A similar attitude to θαῦμα can also be found in medical texts. For example, the writer of the Hippocratic *On the Sacred Disease* is critical of those who believe epilepsy is miraculous or caused by divine intervention simply because it manifests in strange ways: this affliction

> does not seem to me to be any more god-like or sacred than other diseases; it has a nature (φύσιν) and a cause (πρόφασιν), but people think it is something divine because of inexperience and because of its marvelousness (θαυμασιότητος) in that it is not similar to other diseases... But if it is thought to be "divine" because of being marvelous (τὸ θαυμάσιον), there will be many sacred diseases and not just one, since I shall show that other diseases which nobody says are "sacred" are no less marvelous or monstrous (θαυμάσια οὐδὲ τερατώδεα).
>
> (*Morb.Sacr.* 1 [6.352L])

Marvel here does not necessarily need to be dispelled, as it did for Aristotle's geometrical investigations; the Hippocratic writer does not deny that epilepsy is marvellous, but he tries to disarm θαῦμα of the power it has over readers so that their focus will be on understanding the causation of the disease, which he claims operates according to perfectly rational principles despite its perplexing manifestations.[46] Galen, too, frequently refers to "the wonders of the body which have to be seen to be believed," and compares the study of the body through medicine to being inducted into the Eleusinian or Samothracian mysteries.[47]

---

45 Cf. Arist. *GA* 760 b31–33 on the generation of bees, a process which he did not fully understand: "The facts have not been sufficiently ascertained; and if at any future time they are ascertained, then credence must be given to the direct evidence of the senses more than to theories (τότε τῇ αἰσθήσει μᾶλλον τῶν λόγων πιστευτέον), and to theories too provided that the results which they show agree with what is observed (ἐὰν ὁμολογούμενα δεικνύωσι τοῖς φαινομένοις)" (trans. A.L. Peck, Loeb Classical Library edition). On the issue of firsthand observation as a means of enquiry in Aristotle, see Lloyd 1987, especially 53–54, 57–58. On Aristotle's attitude to θαῦμα, see recently Kazantzidis 2018, 43–45.

46 Compare the similar sentiments expressed at *Aër.* 22 (2.76–78L), on the affliction of the Anaries; see Grant 1952, 11. Kazantzidis 2018, 38–41 has identified this attitude to θαῦμα as characteristic of the Hippocratic writers.

47 Grant 1952, 13. See, e.g., Gal. *UP* 3.583K, on the nerves of the larynx: "Before we see them, we are convinced they are impossible, but when we have seen them, we realize that our understand-

The traditional scholarly view of paradoxographical writers places them at the opposite pole from scientific texts in terms of the use they make of θαῦμα: for them, simply creating a sense of wonder in the reader appears to have been the highest goal, and they are notoriously loath to provide anything approaching an explanation for any of the wonders they catalog. As Schepens and Delcroix have noted in their classic article on the literary characteristics of paradoxography,

> θαῦμα is no match for 'explanation'; the sense of the marvellous cannot survive on a rational basis. It is imperative for the paradoxographer to concentrate on… the establishment and the recording of facts without explaining them.[48]

If the paradoxographer were to explain the wondrous phenomena he catalogs, they would no longer inspire the sense of wonder in the reader that it seems to have been the entire point of his text to create. As we have seen, Phlegon's account of the centaur, indebted as it is to natural-scientific discourse about such creatures, maintains this avoidance of explanation: Phlegon merely asserts that certain facts about centaurs (which may contradict what readers think they know about why such creatures are physiologically impossible) are true, without telling us how or why. If he had explicitly acknowledged that he was arguing against the common natural-scientific discourse about centaurs, he would have needed to introduce the explanatory element. In other words, it might not have been enough to say, "Palaephatus and Lucretius are wrong in their claim that centaurs cannot exist," without adding the reasons why. This would push Phlegon's text out of the realm of paradoxography and into medicine or natural science.

This refusal of paradoxography to explain the marvels it catalogs has given it a reputation as an intellectually bankrupt genre, an unsophisticated form of literature which cannibalizes examples of θαῦματα from other texts and presents them without context. Stählin and Schmid famously called paradoxography a "parasitic growth on the tree of historical and natural-scientific literature" for this reason.[49] Yet this avoidance of explanation does not inherently mean that Phlegon is merely attempting to be sensationalistic. A more charitable view is

---

ing was deficient" (trans. Tallmadge May 1968, 270); and *UP* 4.246K, on aspects of the construction of the lungs and blood vessels: "We do not even have any faith at all that a thing is possible, unless we have seen it plainly and often" (trans. Tallmadge May 1968, 671). Kazantzidis 2018, 42–43 observes a similar effect in the Hippocratic treatise *Cord*. 10 (9.86–8L), the only instance in the Hippocratic writings where θαῦμα is meant as a positive emotion.

48 Schepens/Delcroix 1996, 391.

49 Stählin/Schmid 1920, 237 ("ein Parasitengewächs am Baum der historischen und naturwissenschaftlichen Literatur").

that paradoxography like Phlegon's, while it has very different generic conventions from natural-scientific texts, is not prohibited by this fact from participating in debates raised by that more "serious" genre. Phlegon's account of the centaur is merely one example from his work where this is the case. As I have shown elsewhere, his discussions of spontaneous changes of sex from female to male (*Mir.* 4–9 and especially 6–9) is likewise indebted to medical discourse on sex differentiation. While Phlegon does not explicitly acknowledge this or offer any explanation for the rare and marvellous cases of women spontaneously becoming men, the intellectual underpinning of his reports is the opinion, expressed in medical writers, that female genitalia anatomically speaking are merely an "inside-out" version of the male, which could theoretically be extruded from the body if women's naturally "colder" constitution would allow it.[50] Likewise, Phlegon's reports of children born with birth defects, such as a child with four heads (*Mir.* 20), suggest implicit awareness of medical and natural-scientific discussions of conjoined twins.[51] He also discusses a woman who gives birth to a monkey (*Mir.* 22), a phenomenon recognized and variously explained by medical and scientific writers.[52] As with the centaur, Phlegon's presentation of these anecdotes reveals the unmistakable stamp of medical discourse, as if he is responding to critiques he anticipates from readers approaching his text with a medical-scientific, "explanation-focused" mode of thought, or building on the expectations that medical knowledge has created in such readers. A learned reader, aware of medical/scientific explanations of the marvels he reads in Phlegon, can connect these θαῦματα to the larger web of knowledge he has acquired from reading other texts; nevertheless, the fact that Phlegon does not explicitly acknowledge or refute them allows the sense of wonder to persist, even for an educated reader. And that overriding sense of wonder is even stronger in the case of the centaur than it is for the other physiological marvels in Phlegon's collection. In the cases of spontaneous female-to-male transitions and birth defects, Phlegon engages with natural-scientific discourse in a "positive" way, in that what he presents as θαῦμα is also medically viable. But the case of the centaur is an example of "negative" engagement, in that Phlegon insists on the reality of a being that medical writers would say cannot possibly exist. So we see that

---

50 See Shannon-Henderson forthcoming (b); Arist. *GA* 582b30–583a4 (women's "coldness"), with Dean-Jones 1994, 133–134 and King 1998, 56–57, 154–155, 163; Gal. *UP* 4.159–160K (on "inside-out" genitalia), with Laqueur 1990, 25–35 and Flemming 2000, 200. On the "paradoxographical" nature of the female body as an area of overlap between medical texts and Phlegon's brand of paradoxography, see Kazantzidis 2018, 45–55.

51 E.g. Arist. *GA* 4.769b 26–770a6; see also Dasen 1997, 58; Charlier 2008, 85–86.

52 Cf. Arist. *GA* 1.729a 9–703b 32 and 4.769b 11–13; Soran. *Gyn.* 1.39.

Phlegon can not only build on the expectations of his educated readers, but that he can also challenge them as well. The world is not always as we would like to think it is.

Bibliography

Bailey, C. (1947), *Lucretius, De Rerum Natura*, Oxford.

Baur, P.V.C. (1912), *Centaurs in Ancient Art: The Archaic Period*, Berlin.

Campbell, G. (2003), *Lucretius on Creation and Evolution: A Commentary on De Rerum Natura Book 5, Lines 772–1104*, Oxford.

Campbell, G. (2007), "Bicycles, Centaurs, and Man-Faced Ox-Creatures: Ontological Instability in Lucretius", in: S.J Harrison/S.J. Heyworth/P.G. Fowler (eds.), *Classical Constructions: Papers in Memory of Don Fowler, Classicist and Epicurean*, Oxford, 39–62.

Carey, C. (1981), *A Commentary on Five Odes of Pindar:* Pythian *2*, Pythian *9*, Nemean *1*, Nemean *7*, Isthmian *8*, New York.

Charlier, P. (2008), *Les monstres humains dans l'Antiquité: analyse paléopathologique*, Paris.

Dasen, V. (1997), "Multiple Births in Graeco-Roman Antiquity", *Oxford Journal of Archaeology* 16, 49–63.

Dawson, W.R. (1949), "Chiron the Centaur", *Journal of the History of Medicine and Allied Sciences* 4, 267–75.

Dean Jones, L. (1994), *Women's Bodies in Classical Greek Science*, Oxford.

Debru, A. (2008), "Physiology", in: R.J. Hankinson (ed.), *The Cambridge Companion to Galen*, Cambridge, 263–282.

Doroszewska, J. (2016), *The Monstrous World: Corporeal Discourses in Phlegon of Tralles' Mirabilia*, Frankfurt am Main.

DuBois, P. (1982), *Centaurs and Amazons: Women and the Pre-History of the Great Chain of Being*, Ann Arbor.

Flemming, R. (2000), *Medicine and the Making of Roman Women: Gender, Nature, and Authority from Celsus to Galen*, Oxford.

Furth, M. (1987), "Aristotle's Biological Universe: An Overview", in: A. Gotthelf /J.G. Lennox (eds.), *Philosophical Issues in Aristotle's Biology*, Cambridge, 21–52.

Giannini, A. (1964), "Studi sulla paradossografia greca II", *Acme* 17, 99–140.

Grant, M. (2000), *Galen on Food and Diet*, London.

Grant, R.M. (1952), *Miracle and Natural Law in Graeco-Roman and Early Christian Thought*, Amsterdam.

Hankinson, R.J. (2008), "The Man and His Work", in: R.J. Hankinson (ed.), *The Cambridge Companion to Galen*, Cambridge, 1–33.

Hansen, W.F. (1996), *Phlegon of Tralles' Book of Marvels*, Exeter.

Harris-McCoy, D.E. (2012), *Artemidorus' Oneirocritica: Text, Translation, and Commentary*, Oxford.

Hawes, G. (2014a), "Story Time at the Library: Palaephatus and the Emergence of Highly Literate Mythology", in: R. Scodel (ed.), *Between Orality and Literacy: Communication and Adaptation in Antiquity*, Leiden, 125–147.

Hawes, G. (2014b), *Rationalizing Myth in Antiquity*, Oxford.

Holmes, B. (2013), “The Poetic Logic of Negative Exceptionalism in Lucretius, Book Five”, in: D. Lehoux/A.D. Morrison/A. Sharrock (eds.), *Lucretius: Poetry, Philosophy, Science*, Oxford, 153–192.
Inwood, B. (2007), *Seneca: Selected Philosophical Letters*, Oxford.
Kazantzidis, G. (2018), “Medicine and the Paradox in the Hippocratic Corpus and Beyond”, in: M. Gerolemou (ed.), *Recognizing Miracles in Antiquity and Beyond*, Berlin, 31–61.
Kilpatrick, R.S. (1996), “‘Amicus Medicus’: Medicine and Epicurean Therapy in *De Rerum Natura*”, *Memoirs of the American Academy in Rome* 41, 69–100.
King, H. (1998), *Hippocrates’ Woman: Reading the Female Body in Ancient Greece*, London/New York.
Kirk, G.S. (1971), *Myth: Its Meaning and Function in Ancient and Other Cultures*, Cambridge.
Kurtz, D.C. (1975), “The Man-Eating Horses of Diomedes in Poetry and Painting”, *Journal of Hellenic Studies* 95, 171–172.
Laqueur, T. (1990), *Making Sex: Body and Gender from the Greeks to Freud*, Cambridge, MA.
Li Causi, P. (2005), “Generazione di ibridi, generazione di donne. Costruzioni dell’umano in Aristotele e Galeno (e Palefato)”, *Storia Delle Donne* 1, 89–114.
Lloyd, G.E.R. (1987), “Empirical Research in Aristotle’s Biology”, in: A. Gotthelf/J.G. Lennox, (eds.), *Philosophical Issues in Aristotle’s Biology*, Cambridge, 53–63.
Moraux, P. (1951), *Les listes anciennes des ouvrages d’Aristote*, Louvain.
Morawietz, G. (2000), *Der gezähmte Kentaur: Bedeutungsveränderungen der Kentaurenbilder in der Antike*, Munich.
Osborne, R. (1994), “Framing the Centaur: Reading Fifth-Century Architectural Sculpture”, in: R. Osborne/S. Goldhill (eds.), *Art and Text in Ancient Greek Culture*, Cambridge, 52–84.
Osmun, G.F. (1956), “Palaephatus, Pragmatic Mythographer”, *Classical Journal* 52, 131–137.
Pease, A.S. (1958), *M. Tullii Ciceronis De Natura Deorum*, Cambridge, MA.
Pease, A.S. (1963), *M. Tulli Ciceronis De Divinatione Libri Duo*, Darmstadt.
Pretzler, M. (2009), “Form over Substance? Deconstructing Ecphrasis in Lucian’s *Zeuxis* and *Eikones*”, in: A. Bartley (ed.), *A Lucian for Our Times*, Newcastle, 157–171.
Schepens, G./Delcroix, K. (1996), “Ancient Paradoxography: Origin, Evolution, Production and Reception”, in: O. Pecere/A. Stramaglia (eds.), *La letteratura di consumo nel mondo greco-latino: Atti del convegno internazionale, Cassino, 14-17 settembre 1994*, Cassino, 373–460.
Schörner, G. (2002) “Ἡ Θήλεια Ἱπποκένταυρος des Zeuxis: Familiarisierung des Fremden?”, *Boreas: Münstersche Beiträge zur Archäologie* 25, 97–124.
Schrijvers, P.H. (1983), “Sur quelques aspects de la critique des mythes chez Lucrèce”, in: *Συζήτησις. Studi sull’epicureismo greco e romano offerti a Marcello Gigante*, Naples, 353–371.
Schrijvers, P.H. (1999), *Lucrèce et les sciences de la vie*, Leiden.
Scobie, A. (1978), “The Origins of ‘Centaurs’”, *Folklore* 89, 142–147.
Segal, C. (1974), “The Raw and the Cooked in Greek Literature: Structure, Values, Metaphor”, *Classical Journal* 69, 289–308.
Shannon, K.E. (2013), “Authenticating the Marvellous: *Mirabilia* in Pliny, Tacitus, and Suetonius”, *Working Papers on Nervan, Trajanic and Hadrianic Literature* 1.9. http://arts.st-andrews.ac.uk/literaryinteractions/?p=573.
Shannon-Henderson, K.E. forthcoming (a), “Constructing a New Imperial Paradoxography: Phlegon of Tralles and His Sources”, in: A. König/R. Langlands/J. Uden (eds.), *Literature and Culture in the Roman Empire, 96–235: Cross-Cultural Interactions*, Cambridge.

Shannon-Henderson, K.E. forthcoming (b), "Life After Transition: Spontaneous Sex Change and Its Aftermath in Ancient Literature", in: A. Surtees/J. Dyer (eds.), *Exploring Gender Diversity in the Ancient World*, Edinburgh.
Spittler, J. (2016), "Apollonios (Uncertain Date) (1672)", *Die Fragmente der griechischen Historiker Part IV*. Leiden. http://referenceworks.brillonline.com/entries/fragmente-der-griechischen-historiker-iv/apollonios-uncertain-date-1672-a167.
Stählin, O./Schmid, W. (1920), *Geschichte der griechischen Literatur, zweiter Teil: Die nachklassische Periode der griechischen Litteratur*, Munich.
Stern, J. (1996), *Palaephatus, ΠΕΡΙ ΑΠΙΣΤΩΝ: On Unbelievable Tales*, Wauconda, IL.
Tallmadge May, M. (1968), *Galen, On the Usefulness of the Parts of the Body. Περι Χρείας Μορίων. De Usu Partium*, Ithaca, N.Y.

Jessica Lightfoot

Galen's Language of Wonder

Thauma, Medicine and Philosophy in *On Prognosis* and *On Affected Parts*

Abstract: This chapter explores the place of wonder (*thauma*) within the writings of Galen of Pergamon in relation to his own perception of the nature and function of medical practice. It demonstrates that Galen's attitude towards the place of wonder within medicine was complex and conflicted due to the important position which *thauma* occupied within his own contemporary Second Sophistic performance culture, within the Hippocratic tradition, and within the philosophical tradition. The significance of *thauma* in Galen's conception of the intersection between medicine and philosophy becomes particularly clear in two of his treatises, *On Prognosis* and *On Affected Parts*. In *On Prognosis* Galen presents us with numerous case histories from his first visit to Rome 162 CE, a crucially important moment in his career which establishes his position among the social and intellectual elite of the city. *Thauma* figures prominently in many of the case histories which are presented in this treatise and Galen's impressive manipulation of its power becomes one of the ways in which he demonstrates his adeptness within the realms of medical practice and philosophy, as well as allowing him to display his own superiority over other rival doctors in various complex ways. Galen's ability to control and modulate the power of *thauma* on patients and observers within his own medical practice is also made clear in another case history recounted in *On Affected Parts*, in which he recalls his treatment of a fellow doctor at the behest of his philosopher friend Glaucon. In this treatise Galen's understanding of the place of *thauma* within medical practice once again becomes a means to establish his own status as the best doctor and philosopher among his medical and philosophical peers. In both of these treatises the significant place afforded to wonder within case histories which represent some of the most consequential moments of Galen's career in Rome demonstrates that *thauma* occupies an essential (if ambivalent) role within the Pergamene's own conception of the nature and purpose of medicine and its relation to philosophical endeavour.

https://doi.org/10.1515/9783110661774-008

1 Introduction

The place of wonder within medical practice is a tricky matter in Galen's works. Three overlapping influences condition his response to the thorny issue of the potential power of *thauma*. The first influence is the high value placed on the ability to arouse *thauma* in an audience in his contemporary Second Sophistic performance culture. The second is the generally negative attitude towards *thauma* which is found in earlier Hippocratic texts. The third is the much more ambivalent position which *thauma* occupies in the philosophical tradition as an integral starting point for philosophical inquiry in general. At times these three influences cohere in Galen's work, yet more often they jostle each other in uneasy ways. Galen's response to and use of wonder within his own medical practice becomes, by necessity, multi-faceted and often seemingly contradictory. An examination of the navigation of the issue of *thauma* in his written work is of interest not only because it tells us about some of Galen's most deeply held beliefs about his own conception of the doctor's role, but also because it can be seen as emblematic of his wider negotiation of competing intellectual traditions.

There are two treatises which shed particular light on Galen's stance towards the place of wonder in medicine and philosophy: *On Prognosis* (*Praen.*) and *On Affected Parts* (*Loc. Aff.*). The former treatise is an unusual and highly autobiographical work, dated to 178 CE, which retrospectively presents numerous 'case histories' from Galen's first visit to Rome in 162 CE.[1] The cases described in this treatise demonstrate the importance of the success of this first visit for Galen's subsequent medical career. In Rome an opportunity to impress the empire's preeminent intellectual and social elite presented itself for the first time, and Galen certainly did not allow this chance to manoeuvre himself into the personal networks of power and prestige to pass by without making himself noticed.[2] Both of these treatises contain discussions of one area in which Galen quickly made a name for himself: prognosis. Wonder becomes a particularly pressing concern in relation to prognosis because it almost by definition seems to invite astonishment when performed correctly in the presence of those who have no knowledge of the

1 On the dating see Nutton 1979, 49–51. It is important to note that the 'case histories' found in *Praen.* are not easy to categorise generically: although they clearly draw on the Hippocratic tradition of medical case histories found in works such as the *Epidemics*, they differ greatly in both tone and content. On the nature of Galenic case histories see Nutton 1972, 50–62 and 1979, 59–63, Mattern 2008, 27–47 and Lloyd 2009, 115–131.

2 On the significance of Galen's early success at Rome see Hankinson 2008, 5–14, Mattern 2013, 99–186 and Boudon-Millot 2012, 121–166.

medical theories upon which the doctor's predictions are based. In *On Prognosis* we see time and time again that the doctor's ability to control and modulate his own and others' wonder is an integral aspect of prognostic ability and medical practice. We also see this principle in action in *On Affected Parts*, a much later treatise composed after 192 CE. In this treatise it is again a feat of wonder-inducing prognosis, this time in the presence of both a fellow doctor and a fellow philosopher, which allows Galen to make a name for himself in Roman society for the very first time.

In this chapter I will show that Galen's discussion of the place and effect of *thauma* in medicine is particularly nuanced in these two treatises for several reasons relating to the place of wonder in the medical and philosophical traditions. I will begin by outlining the wider cultural context of the notion of *thauma* in Galen in greater detail, before moving on to the presentation of *thauma* in relation to case histories which involve other philosopher and doctor figures to demonstrate the importance of wonder for Galen's conception of the art of medicine as a whole.

2 Three Contexts for *Thauma* in Galen: *Thaumatopoiia*, Hippocrates, Philosophy

Feats of astonishing prognosis differ from those other most striking moments in Galen's work when he discusses his own ability to astonish his audiences: displays of vivisection and dissection. In *On Anatomical Procedures* (*AA*) Galen describes performing spectacular acts of anatomical virtuosity to evoke *thauma* and *ekplēxis* deliberately in his audience. For example, one such display involves ligating the intercostal nerves of a pig to silence its cries and cause astonishment, before untying the ligatures to demonstrate that the pig regains its voice – and thereby astonishing the audience even more.[3] As Maud Gleason has demonstrated, such deliberate anatomical 'wonder-working' is vital in allowing Galen

3 Galen describes such a display at *AA* 8.4 = 2.669K: ἐπιδεικνυμένῳ δὲ βέλτιόν ἐστιν αὐτῷ παρεσκευάσθαι τοῖς νεύροις ἅπασι λίνον ὑποβεβλημένον ἄνευ τοῦ δεδέσθαι· κέκραγε γὰρ οὕτω παιόμενον, εἶτ' ἐξαίφνης ἄφωνον γινόμενον ἐπὶ τῷ σφιγχθῆναι τοῖς λίνοις τὰ νεῦρα τοὺς θεατὰς ἐκπλήττει· θαυμαστὸν γὰρ εἶναι δοκεῖ, νεύρων μικρῶν κατὰ τὸ μετάφρενον βροχισθέντων, ἀπόλλυσθαι τὴν φωνήν ... βουλόμενος δὲ εὐθέως λῦσαι, καὶ δεῖξαι φωνοῦν αὖθις τὸ ζῶον – οὕτω γὰρ μᾶλλον οἱ θεαταὶ θαυμάζουσι – ἀγκύλας τε κατὰ τοὺς βρόχους ἐπίβαλλε καὶ μετρίως σφίγγε.

to display his own technical pre-eminence in dissection while asserting a concomitant epistemological superiority over his watching medical rivals.[4] Moreover, the gaping wonder of the audience induced by this sort of spectacle has much in common with the idealised response provoked by other types of agonistic display in this period, especially public declamation.[5] Since the inducement of wonder is one of their primary aims, Galen's vivisections and dissections have much in common with the sorts of spectacles produced by 'marvel-makers' (*thaumatopoioi / thaumatourgoi*), para-theatrical performers whose sole aim is to produce astonishment in the audience through spectacle.[6] In fact, this potential similarity between the more spectacular aspects of the doctor's art and the activities of marvel-makers was picked up by Aelius Aristides, who compares the ability of the two in terms of astonishing spectators and customers in his oration *Regarding the Well in the Temple of Asclepius* (39.14):

> ὥσπερ γὰρ οἱ παῖδες οἱ τῶν ἰατρῶν τε καὶ τῶν θαυματοποιῶν γεγυμνασμένοι πρὸς τὰς διακονίας εἰσὶ καὶ συμπράττοντες ἐκπλήττουσι τοὺς θεωμένους καὶ χρωμένους, οὕτω τοῦ μεγάλου θαυματοποιοῦ καὶ πάντα ἐπὶ σωτηρίᾳ πράττοντος ἀνθρώπων εὕρημα τοῦτο καὶ κτῆμά ἐστι.
>
> For just as the sons of doctors and of marvel-makers have been trained to help out and aid in astonishing spectators and those making use of their services, so this well is the discovery and possession of the great 'marvel-maker' [i.e. Asclepius] who does everything for the salvation of men.[7]

Aristides here contrasts the natural wondrous powers of the healing well of Asclepius with the man-made wonder produced by *thaumatopoioi* and doctors, who similarly make use of assistants to aid in astonishing their onlookers. The implicit contrast between natural and artificial man-made wonder which Aristides posits here is significant. There is a similar sort of contrast to be found in Galen's anatomical demonstrations. The *thauma* and *ekplēxis* produced by his epideictic displays is artificially created, ensuing from the audience's ignorance and Galen's

4 See Gleason 2009, 98–102 on the importance of wonder in Galen's anatomical demonstrations.

5 See von Staden 1995, 59 and 1997, 51 on the similar responses of wonder which public declamation and public dissection elicited in this period. For general discussions of Galen's place within the context of contemporary Second Sophistic culture see Bowersock 1969, 59–75, Kollesch 1981, 1–12, Swain 1996, 357–379 and Debru 1995, 69–81.

6 For a discussion of *thaumatopoioi* in para-theatrical contexts see Milanezi 2004, 183–209; see also Lightfoot (2018) for a detailed discussion of the literal and metaphorical uses and meanings of *thaumatopoiia* and *thaumatourgia* in Greek culture.

7 All translations are my own.

superior understanding of animal bodies. A key cause of the wonder created is Galen's almost total control over his animal subjects, as if they are artificial objects, especially during vivisections when he is able to control how the bodies on display move or make noise.[8]

The wonder which ensues from Galen's feats of prognostic activity, however, is different – it involves human patients suffering from naturally occurring and unpredictable medical ailments. An equal sense of *thauma* and paradox might ensue from Galen's ability to predict the course of an illness accurately in front of spectators, but the physician's control over the body he is working with is not as absolute as it is in an anatomical demonstration involving animal bodies. To the ignorant observer, however, the differences may not be so obvious at first glance. The fact that prognosis involves real live human patients rather than animal bodies makes the sense of wonder which surrounds the successful prognosticator and his subject much more ambivalent and potentially troubling. It is on this point that we can see Galen's use of prognosis skirting some issues that arise concerning *thauma* in the Hippocratic Corpus. In Hippocratic writings *thauma* is almost always portrayed in a negative light, most often because it raises suspicions of the influence of the supernatural rather than the rational in relation to illness and its cure.[9] Perhaps the strongest and most well-known statement against *thauma* in the presence of illness and its treatment comes in at the beginning of *On the Sacred Disease*, where the Hippocratic writer declares that the so-called 'sacred' disease is nothing of the sort and that the wonder which it causes is misleading and unwarranted (οὐδέν τί μοι δοκέει τῶν ἄλλων θειοτέρη εἶναι νούσων οὐδὲ ἱερωτέρη, ἀλλὰ φύσιν μὲν ἔχει ἣν καὶ τὰ λοιπὰ νουσήματα, ὅθεν γίνεται. φύσιν δὲ αὐτῇ καὶ πρόφασιν οἱ ἄνθρωποι ἐνόμισαν θεῖόν τι πρῆγμα εἶναι ὑπὸ ἀπειρίης καὶ θαυμασιότητος, ὅτι οὐδὲν ἔοικεν ἑτέρῃσι νούσοισιν, 1.1–5 = 6.352 L). In the face of medical knowledge the need for *thauma* is supposedly reduced: once the causes of a disease can be rationally explained illness and its potential cure can be understood. Furthermore, the course of future illness can be potentially predicted on the basis of past experience. A moderate type of wonder at a physician's prognostic ability does seem to be encouraged in certain circumstances, as we see in the Hippocratic *Prognosticon*, where prognosis on the basis of a knowledgeable and correct interpretation of signs is said to be a just cause of wonder at the physician himself (οὕτω γὰρ ἂν θαυμάζοιτό τε δικαίως, καὶ ἰητρὸς

---

8 See Gleason 2009, 101–102 on the force of Galen's powers of immobilisation and reanimation during his demonstrations of vivisection.

9 For a detailed discussion see Kazantzidis 2018, 31–61; cf. also Jouanna 1992, 223–236.

ἀγαθὸς ἂν εἴη, 1.1 = 2.112 L). This type of wonder, however, must always be balanced with the potential for prognosis to seem supernatural and fundamentally misleading.[10]

The relationship of *thauma* to medical practice is complicated further by the role it plays in philosophical discourse. In the Platonic and Aristotelian tradition *thauma* does not assume an inherently negative role in conceptions of the discipline's own practice in the same way as it tends to in Hippocratic writings. Rather, *thauma* is seen as 'the beginning of philosophy' (μάλα γὰρ φιλοσόφου τοῦτο τὸ πάθος, τὸ θαυμάζειν· οὐ γὰρ ἄλλη ἀρχὴ φιλοσοφίας ἢ αὕτη, *Theaetetus* 155d; cf. Aristotle, *Metaphysics* 982b), an integral starting point for philosophical inquiry which either dissipates or morphs into new forms once the question at hand is investigated. Furthermore, there is a place for *thauma* in relation to the process of understanding the formation and composition of even the smallest, most familiar and most insignificant of animal bodies in the Aristotelian tradition. Wonder at the composition of familiar biological bodies becomes the initial starting point for greater biological endeavours in Aristotle's *Parts of Animals*, where it is declared that there is "something wonderful in all aspects of nature", even in the "study of the lowest animal" (διὸ δεῖ μὴ δυσχεραίνειν παιδικῶς τὴν περὶ τῶν ἀτιμοτέρων ζῴων ἐπίσκεψιν. ἐν πᾶσι γὰρ τοῖς φυσικοῖς ἔνεστί τι θαυμαστόν, 645a15–17).[11] The different status placed upon *thauma* in the work of Plato and Aristotle in comparison to its place within Hippocratic writings is a particularly pressing issue in Galen's work because of his persistent keenness to emphasise the inseparable nature of philosophy and medicine, and nowhere is this concern more apparent than in *On Prognosis*, the treatise in which Galen describes at length how he proved his credentials as both a philosopher and a doctor in Rome for the first time.

---

10 See Jouanna 2013, 3 on the crucial nature of the 'justness' of the wonder here, which contrasts with the doubtful wonder caused by the actions of quack doctors. This type of prognostic wonder is explicitly condemned in the opening words of *Prorrhetic* 2.1 = 9.6 L: τῶν ἰητρῶν προρρήσιες ἀπαγγέλλονται συχναί τε καὶ καλαὶ καὶ θαυμασταί, οἵας ἐγὼ μὲν οὔτ' αὐτὸς προεῖπον οὔτ' ἄλλου του ἤκουσα προλέγοντος.

11 Cf. Lennox 2001, 172, Poulakos and Crick 2012, 301–304 and Tipton 2014, 68–69 on Aristotle's defence of the inherent *thauma* to be found in the study of even the lowest animal. On the unusual nature of this passage in the *Part. an.* as a whole see Balme 1972, 122–124.

3 Astonishing Eudemus and Boethus: Philosophers, Doctors and *Thauma* in Rome

The importance of philosophy for Galen's conception of himself as a doctor figures strongly from the very beginning of the *On Prognosis*. The treatise's opening is Platonic in tone and presents the best doctor as a philosopher who inevitably faces the hostility of rival, inadequate doctors as a result of his superior knowledge and practice of medicine.[12] Rather than receiving praise and rightful wonderment, the true doctor instead provokes accusations of sorcery from the ignorant masses as a result of his successful prognoses.[13] Galen goes on to equate his own status as a good doctor with the Platonic model of a Socrates-like 'true philosopher' who faces the potential envy and hostility of professional rivals and the public alike. Galen even alludes to the *Republic* while explaining that the true doctor may occasionally have to retreat from the injustice of modern life by fleeing away from the public 'as though in a great storm and tempest of winds' (ὥσπερ ἐν χειμῶνι μεγάλῳ καὶ ζάλῃ πνευμάτων, *Praen.* 1.11 = 14.603–604K; cf. *Republic* 496d).[14] The frequent Platonic echoes of the treatise's opening help to reinforce Galen's main point: his rivals are not interested in philosophy, but only in financial and social gain – a huge mistake, since philosophy is an integral part of medicine.[15]

As we shall see, it is *thauma* which comes to play a key role in reinforcing Galen's argument that this is the case. After stating his credentials as a true philosopher as well as a doctor in the opening of *On Prognosis* we soon reach a description of Galen's first major case in Rome. This encounter happens to be with a prominent contemporary philosophical figure: Eudemus the Peripatetic. Eudemus has been suffering from bouts of fever which his usual doctors have been

---

12 Nutton 1979, 59–60, 147–157 notes the Platonising tone and use of Platonic phrases which pervade this treatise, especially in its opening sections.

13 *Praen.* 1.6 = 14.601K: ξένον τε καὶ τέρας τοῖς ἰδιώταις ὑπ' ἀηθείας φαίνεται καὶ τοσοῦτον ἀποδεῖ τοῦ θαυμάζεσθαι παρ' αὐτοῖς ὁ προειπὼν, ὥστ' ἀγαπήσειεν ἄν, εἰ μὴ καὶ γόης τις εἶναι δόξειεν. All Greek text of *Praen.* is from Nutton's 1979 edition. See Rothschild 2013, 107–142 on Galen's prognosis, the potential accusations of sorcery it provoked and other contemporary accounts of wondrous predictions and healing.

14 Galen goes on to refer explicitly to Plato's writings once more at the end of the treatise's proem (*Praen.* 1.16 = 14.605K) when he compares the lure of his ignorant medical rivals on the public to Plato's mention of the contest between the cook and the doctor before a jury of fools or children at *Gorgias* 464d–e.

15 *Praen.* 1.14–16 = 14.604–605K.

unable to treat correctly or predict. Galen arrives and stuns everyone by accurately predicting the next onset of fever. Even Eudemus himself is astonished when Galen's prediction of a coming paroxysm is fulfilled, in contrast to the predictions of all his other doctors (*Praen.* 2.25 = 14.612K):

> γενομένου δὲ κἀκείνου περὶ τὴν αὐτὴν ὥραν τοῖς προγεγενημένοις ὁ μὲν Εὔδημος ἐθαύμαζέ τε καὶ τοῖς ἐπισκοπουμένοις αὐτὸν ἅπασιν ἐδήλου τὰς ἐμὰς προρρήσεις – ἦσαν δ' οὗτοι σχεδὸν ἅπαντες οἱ κατὰ τὴν Ῥωμαίων πόλιν ἀξιώματί τε καὶ παιδείᾳ προὔχοντες.
>
> And when that paroxysm also took place at the same time as the previous ones, Eudemus marvelled and made my predictions clear to all the people who were paying him a call – these people present were nearly all of the foremost worthy and educated men in the city of Rome.

At this point Galen immediately becomes an object of envy and wonder to his rivals not only because of his medical skill, but even because of his dignified way of life (ἐμοὶ δ' ἀρχὴ φθόνου τότε πρῶτον ἐγένετο θαυμαζόμενος ὡς ἐπί τε βίου σεμνότητος καὶ τοῖς κατὰ τὴν τέχνην ἔργοις, *Praen.* 3.4 = 14.614K). He goes on to emphasise even more explicitly how the jealousy of his contemporaries, and his own success with patients, were inherently connected with his ability to provoke wonder through prognosis in the case of Eudemus (ἐκ γὰρ τῶν τριῶν τεταρταίων τὸν μὲν πρῶτον ἀρξάμενον ἐν τῇδε παύσασθαι τῇ ἡμέρᾳ προειπὼν ἐθαυμάσθην· ἐπεὶ δὲ καὶ τοῦ δευτέρου τὴν προθεσμίαν τῆς λύσεως ἠλήθευσα ἅπαντες μὲν ἐξεπλάγησαν, *Praen.* 3.5 = 14.614K). Furthermore, the nature of his astonishing prognostic skill does not go unnoticed by one of the biggest medical names of his day: Martianus the famous anatomist is extremely annoyed that Eudemus is now declaring that Galen justly deserves to be an object of *thauma* as well as praise (ἀνιαθεὶς δὲ καὶ αὐτὸς ἐφ' οἷς Εὔδημος οὐ μόνον ἐπαινεῖσθαι χρῆναί με πρὸς ἅπαντων δικαίως ἀλλὰ καὶ θαυμάζεσθαι δεῖν ἔφασκεν, *Praen.* 3.7 = 14.615K).

Throughout this description of the treatment of Eudemus Galen takes great pains to stress how his own actions provoked *thauma* in both his patient and his rival doctors. But Eudemus himself is left in no doubt that wonder at the correct prognosis is in fact unwarranted when Galen reveals the medical knowledge underlying his seemingly supernatural predictions at the end of his account. He explains to Eudemus that his prognosis has in fact arisen logically from an examination of his pulse. It transpires that by following logical deductions in a step by step fashion Galen's method here is not so different from that of any other branch of philosophical inquiry. Eudemus recognises this: he now understands his affliction and is able to say to Galen that he has made an account of how he reached this conclusion "in a way which is skilled in logical argument" (διαλεκτικῶς, ἔφη, συνελογίσω τὴν εὕρεσιν τοῦ γενησομένου, *Praen.* 3.16 = 14.618K). By demonstrating to this philosopher patient that medicine can also begin in (prognostic) wonder Galen proves that his art is not so different from philosophy after all – in fact, it brings the added practical benefit of saving Eudemus' life. In the case of Eudemus we can thus understand why Galen's occlusion of his initial theories here is quite deliberate: it results in a prolonged sense of wonder at his prognostic abilities which brings Eudemus the philosopher round to medical as well as philosophical thinking, cementing Galen's position as the best doctor and philosopher in Rome. In this way Galen is able to use *thauma* 'justly' to become and be seen as a good doctor – as advocated in the Hippocratic *Prognosticon*.

As *On Prognosis* progresses we begin to see a pattern arise: a (seemingly) marvellous Galenic prediction is followed by a rational explanation of the theoretical grounding behind each prognosis. Galen reinforces the importance that his ability to induce *thauma* through prognosis possesses by relating two more case histories which show how his impressive prognostic talents allowed him to convince another prominent philosopher to take an interest in his own medical theories and practice. The philosopher in question this time is Flavius Boethus, a senator and ex-consul who is a friend of Eudemus and an Aristotelian philosopher taught by Alexander of Damascus.[16] Galen describes how he impressed Boethus with the treatment of his sick son, who is suffering from a mystery illness (*Praen.* 7.1–18 = 14.635–641K). For some reason the boy repeatedly suffers from sudden relapses of fever whenever his mother, who is tending him, leaves the sick room. In this case Galen quickly works out what the problem is through logical deduction: the relapses take place when the boy eats hidden food when left alone. Boethus, however, fails to notice what Galen has observed and is amazed when he announces that he knows the cause of the illness after taking the boy's pulse because it seems as if the pulse itself has revealed the answer to him (ὁ δ' οὖν Βοηθὸς ὑπὲρ πάντας γελῶν ἐθαύμαζε πῶς ὁ σφυγμός, εἰ καὶ τὸ κατακεκρυμμένον ἐδώδιμον, ἱκανός ἐστι δηλοῦν, *Praen.* 7.14 = 14.639K). But the explanation makes all clear: the increase in pulse rate only reveals that the boy is psychologically worried about something – in this case, the discovery of the food. From the boy's worried state Galen works out that he must be indulging in some sort of forbidden activity which is causing the symptoms. Galen thus reveals to his philosopher friend that he possesses superior powers of logic by deducing what the issue is likely to be

16 Galen emphasises Boethus' philosophical credentials when first mentioning him at *Praen.* 2.24 = 14.612K: Φλάβιος <Βοηθός>, ὑπατικὸς μὲν ὢν ἤδη καὶ αὐτός, ἐσπευκὼς δὲ περὶ τὴν Ἀριστοτέλους φιλοσοφίαν. Cf. also *Praen.* 5.9 = 14.627K, which mentions that Alexander of Damascus instructed Boethus in Peripatetic doctrine, and *On My Own Books* (*Lib. Prop.*) 19.13K, where Galen tells us again that Boethus practised Aristotelian philosophy.

and then using the measurement of the pulse to confirm his hypothesis, once again showing himself able to combine philosophical reasoning and medical knowledge in a way which produces a positive and practical clinical outcome. Boethus' wonder then switches from misplaced amazement at the diagnostic potential of the pulse, to wonder at Galen himself: he cannot believe that other doctors are so ignorant in comparison to him (ἀκούσας οὖν ὁ Βοηθὸς ταῦτα, νὴ τοὺς θεοὺς ἔφη θαυμάζειν εἰ οὕτως εὔγνωστα φάρμακα τῶν ἰατρῶν οὐδεὶς οἶδεν. εὔδηλον γὰρ ὅτι μήτ' αὐτοὶ τοιοῦτον ἔργον ἐπεδείξαντο πώποτε καὶ σὲ πάντα μᾶλλον ἢ ἐξ ἰατρικῆς τέχνης αὐτὰ πράττειν φασίν, *Praen.* 7.17 = 14.640K).

Galen's superiority is reinforced further when he goes on to astonish Boethus even more, this time in relation to his treatment of his wife, who is suffering from a mysterious female flux. This case is much more clinically difficult than the previous one and Galen's successful treatment confirms his position as a superior practitioner even further, to the extent that he gains the name 'wonder-worker' and 'wonder-teller' because of it (ἓν οὖν ὄντως θαυμάσιον πραχθὲν ὃ οὐ μόνον με παραδοξολόγον ὡς ἔμπροσθεν οἱ πολλοὶ τῶν ἰατρῶν ὠνόμαζον ἀλλὰ καὶ παραδοξοποιὸν ἐποίησε κληθῆναι, *Praen.* 8.1 = 14.641K). In this case Galen relies on his knowledge of medical theory, and a process of trial and error, to hit upon the correct cure. He first refutes the woman's midwives by realising that Boethus' wife is not pregnant, as they suspect. After trying out various drying substances Galen eventually cures the illness by remedying the levels of moisture in the woman's body and allowing the correct amount of purging to occur. At this point Galen's status as the pre-eminent philosopher-doctor is assured, his superiority demonstrated by his ability to help the philosophers Eudemus and Boethus with medical issues which they struggled to think their way through logically. Moreover, their wonder at Galen's medical art seems to serve as a protreptic to further study of medicine in the future, especially in the case of Boethus, who becomes Galen's most important patron in Rome and to whom several of the later treatises discussing medical and philosophical matters are dedicated, including the first six books of *On the Doctrines of Hippocrates and Plato* (*PHP*) and the first book of *On the Utility of the Parts* (*UP*).[17]

17 For Galen's account of the numerous treatises which he dedicated to Boethus see *Lib. Prop.* 19.13–16K.

4 Bodies and Texts: Knowledge, Ignorance and *Thauma* in *On Prognosis*

As we have seen then, the production of medical *thauma* becomes one of the most powerful ways in which Galen is able to claim that medicine and philosophy are not so different after all. But as well as positively drawing wealthy, powerful and philosophical patrons into the path of Galen's medical thought, *thauma* also has the potential to be wielded as a much more aggressive weapon in the face of more mundane medical rivals, such as those doctors who see no place for philosophy in medicine who are the target of Galen's opening complaints in *On Prognosis*. By causing fellow doctors to marvel at his ability to understand the nature of any given ailment and its cures, Galen is able to flaunt his own superior medical knowledge. In the account of the treatment of Boethus' son, Galen has already emphasised the importance of his superior knowledge and its relation to wonder: the account begins with the claim that Boethus' astonishment at the nature of the successful treatment of his son soon transforms into wonder at the very *ignorance* of every other doctor once Galen has explained his own logical deductions (ἓν οὖν ἔτι προσθεὶς ἐφ' οὗ παραχρῆμα μὲν ἐξεπλάγη Βοηθὸς ἀκούσας δ' ὅπως εὑρέθη θαυμάζειν οὐκέτι ἔφασκεν ἀλλὰ τῶν ἀγνοούντων τὸ θεώρημα καταγινώσκειν ὡς ἀμαθῶν, ἐπ' ἄλλο τι μεταβήσομαι, *Praen.* 7.1 = 14.635K).

The ignorance of other doctors when it comes to basic Hippocratic theories is also a weakness which Galen exposes through the use of *thauma*. This is a point which is increasingly emphasised in the treatise's last few case histories, at a point when Galen has convincingly demonstrated that he is a successful practitioner and is now engaged in the task of directing us to his works on specific medical issues, especially relating to the pulse – an area of knowledge which he had particularly developed. The case of Sextus Quintilius Condianus (*Praen.* 10.13–22 = 14.655–657K), a young man suffering from a feverish illness, is a particularly good example of this rhetorical manoeuvre. Once Galen predicts that Sextus' fever will increase temporarily before abating quickly, the fellow doctors present at Sextus' bedside, who seem to have picked up on his reputation for marvel-making, soon make fun of Galen's 'wonderful prophecy' (ἡ θαυμαστὴ μαντεία τοῦ Γαληνοῦ, *Praen.* 10.18 = 14.657K). But, as usual, the patient's symptoms follow Galen's predicted course, to the envy and amazement of the other assembled doctors. At this point Galen quickly presses his advantage and turns the language of *thauma* against his rivals, claiming that if only the other doctors had read Hippocrates, and his own works, they would have understood that the prediction was correct and never wasted any time in wondering at the prognosis or its results

(καὶ ταῦτα τῆς προγνώσεως οὐδὲν ἐχούσης θαυμαστὸν, ὡς ἔδειξά σοι διά τε τῶν Εἰς <τὸ> πρῶτον <τῶν> Ἐπιδημιῶν ὑπομνημάτων ἔτι τε τὴν Περὶ τῶν κρίσεων πραγματείαν. τούτοις μέντοι τοῖς ἰατροῖς οὐ μόνον ἀγνοεῖν ὑπάρχει τὰ γεγραμμένα τοῖς παλαιοῖς ... αὕτη μὲν οὖν ἡ πρόρρησις, ὡς ἔφην, [ὡς] εἰ καὶ θαυμαστὴ τοῖς πολλοῖς τούτοις ἰατροῖς ἔδοξεν, *Praen.* 10.19–22 = 14.656–657K).

This insistence on the need for an understanding of the medical texts of the past and present in order to dispel the potential wonder of prognosis is reinforced even more insistently as the treatise progresses. For example, in the case of the illness of the emperor's young son Commodus the imperial chamberlain Peitholaus is at first amazed by Galen's claim that an inflammation of the tonsils could alter the boy's pulse (καὶ ταῦτ' ἀκούσας ὁ Πειθόλαος θαυμάζειν ἔφησεν εἰ τῶν παρισθμίων ἡ φλεγμονὴ τὸν σφυγμὸν ἠλλοίωσε τοῦ παιδὸς, *Praen.* 12.1 = 14.661–662K). But Galen reveals that he knows precisely what to do because his reading of Hippocrates, not to mention his own voluminous written work on pulses, has allowed him to read the pulse correctly – unlike the Methodist doctors who are present (διὰ τοὺς τοιούτους ἰατροὺς ἔναγχος ἔγραψα τρεῖς πραγματείας, μίαν μὲν τὴν Περὶ τῆς διαφορᾶς τῶν πυρετῶν, ἑτέραν δὲ τὴν Περὶ τῶν κρισίμων ἡμερῶν καὶ τρίτην τὴν Περὶ τῶν κρίσεων, ἐπιδεικνὺς ὑφ' Ἱπποκράτους γεγράφθαι τὴν θεωρίαν ἀφ' ἧς ἄν τις προγινώσκοι τὰ γενησόμενα περὶ τοὺς ἀρρώστους, *Praen.* 12.10 = 14.664K). In fact, these doctors cannot even read and learn from Galen's treatises on pulses correctly, such is their ignorance, never mind 'read' and understand the ailments of a sick body (οἱ δ οὕτως εἰσὶν ἀφυεῖς ὥστε μηδὲ μετὰ τῆς ἐμῆς ἐξηγήσεως δύνασθαι αὐτὰ μαθεῖν, *Praen.* 12.11 = 14.665K). In the next case Epigenes, the treatise's addressee, is himself present when an ill young man suffers from an unexpected haemorrhage. Galen, using his knowledge of Hippocratic texts, predicts that the young man will have a nosebleed on the fifth day of his illness; the assembled doctors are once again astonished (οἱ μὲν <οὖν> ἰατροὶ ταῦτ' ἀκούσαντες ἐθαύμαζον δῆθεν, *Praen.* 13.5 = 14.666K). But, as Galen explains in response to Epigenes' inquiry, there is no wonder in this case which could not be dispelled by a sound knowledge of Hippocrates' own works (ἐγὼ δ' ἐρομένῳ σοι τὴν θεωρίαν τῆς προγνώσεως ἐδήλωσα πᾶσαν ἐκ τῶν ὑφ' Ἱπποκράτους εἰρημένων δεδιδαγμένος, ἔτι δὲ καὶ τοῦτο προσέθηκα σφοδρὰν ἔσεσθαι προσδοκᾶν τὴν αἱμορραγίαν, *Praen.* 13.10 = 14.668K). Finally, in the case of a steward with an irregular pulse, Galen again describes how his prognosis astonished many people (ἔναγχος <δέ>, ὡς οἶσθα, καὶ τοιόνδε τι προειπόντος μου τοὺς πολλοὺς ἐξέπλησσεν ἡ πρόγνωσις, *Praen.* 14.1 = 14.670K). But once more he reveals (*Praen.* 14.4 = 14.671K) that there is nothing astonishing about his prediction, since all doctors might know how to understand pulses if only they read Galen's own works on the matter: his three treatises *Diagnosis by*

Pulses (*Dig. Puls.*), *Causes of Pulses* (*Caus. Puls.*) and *Prognosis by Pulses* (*Praes. Puls.*). If only the doctors present had read these works, Galen claims, they would have known about the natural differences between pulses (γνώσεσθε δὲ, ἔφην, ὅσαι παρὰ φύσιν εἰσὶν ἐν τοῖς σφυγμοῖς διαφοραὶ, τουτὶ τὸ βιβλίον ἀναγνόντες, *Praen.* 14.10 = 14.673K) – but unfortunately they are again incapable of even reading and gaining the knowledge which has already been provided for them by his own medical skill.[18]

As these final case histories suggest, Galen increasingly instructs the reader to turn first to Hippocrates, then to his own works by using the ignorant wonder of other doctor figures in *On Prognosis* as a negative paradigm of what a successful doctor should be. Once again, we see that Galen skirts the boundaries between the two contrasting attitudes towards *thauma* found in the philosophical and medical traditions. For Galen, there is certainly a place for *thauma* in medicine. Ideally, however, *thauma* must be turned to good use by acting as a motivation for inquiry into the workings of the human body, thus avoiding the state of continued ignorance which rival doctors are castigated for throughout *On Prognosis*.

5 *Thauma* and the Emperor: The Wonder of Marcus Aurelius

There is, however, one case in which *thauma* retains its power even in the face of a doctor’s knowledge: the illness of Marcus Aurelius. While all other cases in the *On Prognosis* fail to deserve wonder intrinsically and are marvelled at for prolonged periods only by the hopelessly ignorant, the illness and treatment of the emperor is somehow different. This difference is articulated several times in the description of the imperial ailment and its cure (*Praen.* 10.22–11.1 = 14.657–658K):

> αὕτη μὲν οὖν ἡ πρόρρησις, ὡς ἔφην, [ὡς] εἰ καὶ θαυμαστὴ τοῖς πολλοῖς τούτοις ἰατροῖς ἔδοξεν, ἀλλ’ οὐ τοιαύτη γε κατ’ ἀλήθειαν ἦν, ὥσπερ οὐδ’ ἡ μετὰ γνώσεως τῶν ἐνεστώτων θεραπεία τοῦ παιδὸς αὐτοῦ Κομ<μ>όδου κατὰ τὴν ἐπιδημίαν ἐκείνου γενομένη. θαυμαστὴ

18 Cf. the similar account at *On Recognizing the Best Physician* (*Opt. Med. Cogn.*) 3.17, a treatise which has survived in Arabic translation, in which Galen treats a man with an ulcer in the eye and exposes the ignorance of his fellow doctors (tr. Iskandar 1988): “Not a single day has passed without me showing skill in the art in cases of such dimensions or in similar ways. The majority of physicians who saw these (performances) did not know where to find written material on this or on other subjects. Some, upon witnessing this performance, nicknamed me ‘wonder-worker’, others ‘wonder-teller’”.

δ' ὄντως ἡ νῦν ἐπ' αὐτοῦ τοῦ βασιλέως συμβᾶσα δόξαντος μὲν καὶ αὐτοῦ καὶ τῶν ἀμφ' αὐτὸν ἰατρῶν ὅσοι συναπεδήμησαν αὐτῷ παροξυσμόν τινα πυρεκτικὸν ἄρξασθαι, σφαλέντων δὲ πάντων καὶ τῆς δευτέρας καὶ τρίτης ἡμέρας ἕωθεν καὶ περὶ τὴν ὀγδόην ὥραν.

Therefore, as I have said, this prognosis [i.e. of Sextus' illness], even if it seemed wondrous to the majority of these doctors, was not truly so. In the same way the cure of the emperor's son Commodus when he was present in Rome was not wondrous after an inquiry into the circumstances. But the cure which occurred in the case of the emperor himself really was wondrous. Both he himself and all those doctors who were with him when he went on campaign thought that a feverish paroxysm had begun, but they were all tripped up by what happened on the second and third day at dawn and at around the eighth hour.

The anticipation of the great wonder which will ensue from the following description of the emperor's illness and treatment is soon undercut: it turns out that Marcus is suffering only from indigestion, easily alleviated by the application of warm nard ointment and a cup of Sabine wine. Nevertheless, Galen insists that it is *this* case alone which retains its wonder in the face of his knowledge and medical skill, reiterating this fact again once more after he describes Marcus' increased esteem for him after his successful diagnosis of an unfortunate bout of over-eating (*Praen.* 11.8–9 = 14.660K):

καὶ τῷ Πειθολάῳ μετὰ τὸ πιεῖν <εἰπὼν> ὡς ἰατρὸν ἔχομεν ἕνα καὶ τοῦτον ἐλεύθερον πάνυ διετέλει [τε] περὶ ἐμοῦ λέγων ἀεὶ, καθάπερ οἶσθα καὶ σὺ, τῶν μὲν ἰατρῶν πρῶτον εἶναι, τῶν δὲ φιλοσόφων μόνον· ἐπεπείρατο γὰρ ἤδη πολλῶν οὐ μόνον φιλοχρημάτων ἀλλὰ καὶ φιλονείκων καὶ φιλοδόξων καὶ φθονερῶν καὶ κακοήθων. ὅπερ οὖν ἔφην ἐγὼ, ταύτης τῆς ἐπισκέψεως οὐδεμίαν ἄλλην ἡγοῦμαί μοι γεγονέναι θαυμαστοτέραν.

And after drinking the wine he said to Peitholaus, "We have one doctor, and this man has very much lived a life full of learning". As you know he was always speaking of me as first among doctors and unique among philosophers. For he had already had experience of many who were not only lovers of money, but also lovers of quarrels and lovers of fame, jealous and malicious men. And as I said, I think that no other investigation of mine was more marvellous than this one.

This is not the final time Galen emphasises the continuing wonder of the investigation into Marcus' indigestion. The importance of *thauma* to medical practice throughout this treatise is made clear by the decision to leave the treatise's internal addressee Epigenes (and, by extension, the reader) with his final thoughts on the issue of the relationship between illness, medical treatment and the experience of wonder at the very end of the work in the final sentences of *On Prognosis* (*Praen.* 14.11–12 = 14.673):

τοῦτ' οὖν, ὦ Ἐπίγενες, ἀξιόλογον ἔργον ἰατρικῆς προγνώσεώς ἐστιν, ὥσπερ καὶ τὸ κατὰ τὸν αὐτοκράτορα τῆς δοκούσης αὐτῷ εἰσβολῆς γεγενῆσθαι τοῦ παροξυσμοῦ. τῶν δ' ἄλλων ὅσα

> θαυμάζουσιν οἱ πολλοὶ τῶν ἰατρῶν, οὐδὲν οὐδ' ἐγγὺς ὅμοιόν ἐστι τοῖσδε. θαυμαστὸν γὰρ εἶναι φαίνεται διὰ τὴν τῶν πολλῶν ἄγνοιαν, οὐ δι' ἑαυτά, τοῖς νομίμως ἠσκηκόσι τὰ κατὰ τὴν τέχνην οὐκ ἔχοντα δύσκολον τὴν πρόγνωσιν.
>
> And so this [i.e. Galen's successful treatment of a steward suffering from an intermittent pulse], Epigenes, is a work of medical prognosis worth mentioning, just as the case concerning the emperor who believed that he had suffered an attack of feverish paroxysm was. But out of all of the other cases which the majority of doctors wonder at, none is in any way like that one. For the other cases seem to be wondrous because of the ignorance of the majority, though they are not inherently wondrous, at least to those who have rightly practised medicine without difficulty in respect of prognosis.

Two questions arise from this unusual emphasis on wonder: is the marvellous nature of this case being stressed simply because the emperor's high social status renders his indigestion inherently wonderful? Or is the imperial body inherently deserving of wonder, and if so, what does that have to do with medicine and philosophy?

Given the complex nature of the status of wonder in both medicine and philosophy and Galen's careful use of *thauma* elsewhere in the treatise it seems unlikely that the emperor's case remains marvellous solely because of his social status – though of course, the emperor's power and influence do make Galen's successful treatment here a marvellous opportunity for his own social advancement. It is worth considering other aspects of the figure and role of the emperor which might explain the continuing wondrous spell which the emperor's body is able to cast. As Rebecca Flemming has pointed out, the concept of a provident demiurge figure which Galen develops in his writings on philosophy and physiology is influenced by contemporary political as well as philosophical thinking: just as the emperor maintains the order, integrity and systematicity of the empire, so does Nature/the demiurge maintain the order of the cosmos itself.[19] In the treatise which describes the workings of Galen's demiurge figure in relation to the structure and functionality of the human body in the greatest detail, *On the Utility of the Parts*, we find that *thauma* is frequently and repeatedly connected to provident Nature/the figure of the demiurge.[20] It is this order and systematicity which the emperor replicates in the political realm, and it is this which contributes to the continued wonder of both the emperor's body and Galen's treatment of it in *On Prognosis*. Just as Galen presents himself as the only person capable of

19 Flemming 2009, 59–84.

20 For more examples of the explicit wondrousness of nature in *UP* see e.g. 3.134K, 3.225K, 3.252K, 3.254K, 3.288K, 3.335K, 3.426K, 3.508K, 3.530K, 3.545K, 3.566K, 3.589K, 3.601K, 3.792K, 3.883K, 3.884K, 3.885, 3.939K, 4.5K, 4.15K, 4.58K, 4.61K, 4.197K, 4.243K.

properly systematising human physiology and understanding Nature's works in *On the Utility of the Parts*, so too is he the only doctor capable of understanding the workings of the imperial body itself in *On Prognosis*. The implacable wonder surrounding the figure of the emperor is thus related to the fact that *thauma* lies at the heart of Galen's conception of nature and the natural order itself.

6 *Thauma*, Philosophy and Medicine in *On Affected Parts*: The Case of Glaucon's Friend

As we have seen, the repeated presence of *thauma* at key moments of Galen's account of his first and most influential cases in Rome can be accounted for to some extent by the peculiar nature of the *On Prognosis* as a treatise in which he is particularly keen to emphasise his credentials as not only the best doctor in Rome at that time, but as the best philosopher as well. The importance of the use of *thauma* as a means of positioning himself in Rome in relation to both fields can be seen from the fact that the issue is still one which exercises Galen many years later in *On Affected Parts*. Within a wider discussion of diseases affecting the chest and abdomen in this treatise we come across an unexpected and lengthy reminiscence of the use of prognosis to treat an unknown liver problem during Galen's first visit to Rome. Since this work was composed at some time after 192 CE, long after his first encounter with the centre of the empire in 162 CE, Galen explicitly tells the reader why he is harking back to this long-distant event at the beginning of his account: he advises us that remembering the signs which attend various diseases, and the correct prognosis which results from this remembrance, will lead to the wonder of patients, as well as their praise (οὕτως γὰρ οὐ μόνον ἐπαινεῖσθαι πρὸς τῶν χρωμένων ἡμῖν, ἀλλὰ καὶ θαυμάζεσθαι γενήσεται, 5.8 = 8.361K).

The notion of wonder which is introduced here is again crucial to the following account of one of Galen's earliest successes. The scene is set carefully: Galen retrospectively notes that his conduct in this case concerning the diagnosis of liver disease at the very beginning of his Roman sojourn had the specific effect of inducing a great sense of wonder in his friend Glaucon the philosopher (ἐγὼ γοῦν, ὁπότε πρῶτον εἰς Ῥώμην ἀνῆλθον, ὑπὸ Γλαύκωνος τοῦ φιλοσόφου μεγάλως ἐθαυμάσθην ἐπὶ τοιᾷδέ τινι διαγνώσει, 5.8 = 8.361K). Glaucon informs Galen that a friend of his, a Sicilian doctor, has fallen ill. He invites him to demonstrate his powers of prognosis and diagnosis, for he has heard from others that Galen's predictions are more like prophecy than medical art (διαγνώσεις τε καὶ προγνώσεις πεποιῆσθαί σε μαντικῆς μᾶλλον ἢ ἰατρικῆς ἐχομένας, 5.8 = 8.362K). Galen accepts the challenge and sets off: the stage for a demonstration of his astonishing prognostic skill is duly set.

Before entering the sick doctor's room, however, it again becomes clear that there is much more to the art of prognosis than examining the patient directly. Before even reaching the patient, Galen notices an attendant carrying a bowl full of thin bloody liquid like that which freshly slaughtered meat gives out: a definite sign, he tells us, of liver disease (ἔχουσαν οἷον κρεῶν νεοσφαγῶν πλύμα, λεπτὸν αἵματος ἰχῶρα, βεβαιότατον σημεῖον ἥπατος πάσχοντος, 5.8 = 8.362K). But Galen does not let on that he has already formed an opinion about the patient's affliction from this sign and deliberately avoids telling Glaucon about what he has noticed (ὡς οὖν μηδ' ὅλως ἑωρακὼς αὐτὸ εἰσῆλθον ἅμα τῷ Γλαύκωνι πρὸς τὸν ἰατρὸν, 5.8 = 8.362–63K). Galen's decision to conceal his knowledge from those around him at this stage is crucial for the deliberate evocation of *thauma* and *ekplēxis* during the upcoming face-to-face encounter with the Sicilian doctor. He performs the same trick again upon entering the sick room itself. After approaching the Sicilian and taking his pulse Galen notices a pot full of hyssop in water and honey and deduces from this that his patient has been feeling pain around his false ribs and believes that he is suffering from pleurisy (5.8 = 8.363K). Galen again fails to mention what he has noticed, and astonishment ensues (5.8 = 8.363–64K):

> τοῦ δ' ὁμολογήσαντος ὁ Γλαύκων ἐκ τοῦ σφυγμοῦ μόνου τὴν διάγνωσιν τοῦ πεπονθότος τόπου νομίσας γεγονέναι, καταφανὴς ἦν μοι θαυμάζων. ὅπως οὖν αὐτὸν μᾶλλον ἐκπλήξαιμι, προσετίθην καὶ ταῦτα· καθάπερ, ἔφην, ὡμολόγηκας ἐνταυθοῖ ἀλγεῖν, προσομολόγησον ὅτι καὶ τοῦ βῆξαι γίγνεταί σοι προθυμία, καὶ βήττεις ἐκ διαστημάτων μειζόνων βηχία σμικρὰ ξηρά, μηδενὸς ἀναπτυομένου. ταῦτα λέγοντος ἐμοῦ, κατὰ τύχην ἔβηξε τοιοῦτον εἶδος βηχὸς, ὁποῖον ἔλεγον· ὥστε τὸν Γλαύκωνα μεγάλως θαυμάσαντα μὴ κατέχειν ἑαυτὸν, ἀλλ' ἐπαινεῖν κεκραγότα μεγάλῃ τῇ φωνῇ.
>
> And when the patient admitted that this was the case Glaucon believed that I had made the diagnosis of the affected part from the pulse alone and was evidently marvelling at me. And in order to astonish him more I added these words: "In the same way," I said, "that you have admitted that you feel pain here, admit too that an urge to cough has come over you, and that you cough briefly and drily at great intervals, spitting nothing out." After I said this he coughed by chance in the way I described: as a result Glaucon marvelled greatly and did not contain himself, instead he called out praising me in a loud voice.

Galen does not stop here: he goes on to astonish the patient so much with his correct description of his symptoms that he cries out and marvels aloud (ἐπὶ τούτοις οὐδ' αὐτὸς ὁ νοσῶν ἔτι ἡσύχαζεν, ἀλλὰ θαυμάζων ἐκεκράγει μετὰ τοῦ

Γλαύκωνος, 5.8 = 8.364–65K). The language of wonder and astonishment continues to suffuse this passage as Galen proceeds to prey upon the ignorance of his interlocutors, first informing his patient that he will no doubt feel his collarbone being pulled downward, and even appearing to be able to read the Sicilian's mind by telling him what disease he has mistakenly thought himself to be suffering from, a final flourish which assures the sick doctor's sense of wonder for Galen himself (θεασάμενος ἐγὼ τὸν κάμνοντα θαυμαστῶς ἐκπεπληγότα … ὁ νοσῶν ἐπὶ τῷ παραδόξῳ τῆς ὑποσχέσεως ἐκπεπληγὼς ἐνέβλεπέν μοι δριμὺ … ὁ μὲν ἐμαρτύρησεν θαυμάζων, 5.8 = 8.365K).

The fact that the interlocutors involved are a philosopher and a doctor is once more at the heart of the persistent use of wonder for effect in this case. The philosopher Glaucon, like Eudemus and Boethus in *On Prognosis*, is alerted by his wonder to medicine's potential as a form of philosophical inquiry. According to Galen the effect on Glaucon after witnessing the Sicilian's treatment was immediate and caused him to hold a high opinion of the medical art as a whole, despite the fact that he did not think highly of it beforehand (ὁ δὲ Γλαύκων ἐξ ἐκείνου περί τε ἡμῶν καὶ ὅλης τῆς ἰατρικῆς ἔσχεν ἀξιόλογον ὑπόληψιν, ἔμπροσθεν οὐδὲν μέγα τὴν τέχνην ἔχειν οἰόμενος, 5.8 = 8.366K). This newfound medical interest seems to have been sustained on Glaucon's part, since Galen goes on to dedicate a treatise, *Therapeutics to Glaucon* (*MMG*), to his philosopher friend. The wonder of the anonymous Sicilian doctor, however, is less positive. In his case, it points to his ignorance of the medical teachings which Galen is basing his treatment upon and an inability to think through his own empirical observations in a logical manner. This inability has catastrophic practical effects as the Sicilian is unable to help himself in any way, despite supposedly being a doctor – who knows how ill he would have become if Galen had not turned up on time?

Once again, the potential importance of wonder and its effects in Galen's case histories is made apparent. It is clear from the multiple case histories in *On Prognosis*, and from the account of the treatment of Glaucon's Sicilian friend in *On Affected Parts*, that the complex role which wonder plays in both medicine and philosophy as a potential incentive to further study, or as a distraction, means that Galen must frame the potentially wondrous aspects of his own medical practice very carefully. When used against his medical opponents, the ability to create wonder proves Galen's own professional superiority and medical knowledge and allows him to condemn the ignorance of rival doctors. At the same time, Galen's work takes account of the negative aspects of the use of *thauma* in medicine and its potential to distract which are outlined in the Hippocratic corpus – though he certainly does not banish wonder completely from contemporary medical practice. For Galen, a complete dismissal of *thauma* from medicine is undesirable for three main reasons. The first is that in the hands of the right practitioner, the evocation of *thauma* confirms medicine's essential compatibility with philosophical inquiry. The second is that *thauma* has the potential to enable the best type of doctor to turn others towards the future practice of medicine as a worthy philosophical endeavour. Finally, in the right hands, *thauma* even has the ability to reveal the fundamental wonder which lies at the heart of the natural order itself. For Galen, it is these three reasons which make *thauma* an essential aspect of his own medical art.

Bibliography

Balme, D.M. (1972), *Aristotle: De partibus animalium I and De generatione animalium I*, Oxford.

Boudon-Millot, V. (2012), *Galien de Pergame: un médecin grec à Rome*, Paris.

Bowersock, G.W. (1969), *Greek Sophists in the Roman Empire*, Oxford.

Debru, A. (1995), "Les démonstrations médicales à Rome au temps de Galien", *CM* 27, 69–81.

Flemming, R. (2009), "Demiurge and Emperor in Galen's World of Knowledge", in: C.Gill/T.Whitmarsh/J. Wilkins (eds.), *Galen and the World of Knowledge*, Cambridge, 59–84.

Gleason, M.W. (2009), "Shock and Awe: The Performance Dimension of Galen's Anatomical Demonstrations", in: C. Gill/T. Whitmarsh/J. Wilkins (eds.), *Galen and the World of Knowledge*, Cambridge, 85–114.

Hankinson, R.J. (2008), "The Man and his Work", in: R.J. Hankinson (ed.), *The Cambridge Companion to Galen*, Cambridge, 1–33.

Iskandar, A.Z. (1988), *Galen: On Examinations By Which the Best Physicians Are Recognized.* (Corpus Medicorum Graecorum, Supplementum Orientale 4), Berlin.

Jouanna, J. (1992), "Le statut du thauma chez les médecins de la Collection hippocratique", in: A. Thivel (ed.), *Le miracle grec*, Nice, 223–236.

Jouanna, J. (2013), *Hippocrate 3.1: Pronostic*, Paris.

Kazantzidis, G. (2018), "Medicine and the Paradox in the Hippocratic Corpus and Beyond", in: M. Gerolemou (ed.), *Recognizing Miracles in Antiquity and Beyond*, Berlin/Boston, 31–61.

Kollesch, J. (1981), "Galen und die Zweite Sophistik", in: V. Nutton (ed.), *Galen: Problems and Prospects*, London, 1–12.

Lennox, J.G. (2001), *Aristotle: On the Parts of Animals*, Oxford.

Lightfoot, J. (2018), *Wonder and the Marvellous from Homer to the Hellenistic World*, DPhil thesis, University of Oxford.

Lloyd, G.E.R. (2009), "Galen's un-Hippocratic Case-Histories", in: C. Gill/T. Whitmarsh/J. Wilkins (eds.), *Galen and the World of Knowledge*, Cambridge, 115–131.

Mattern, S.P. (2008), *Galen and the Rhetoric of Healing*, Baltimore.

Mattern, S.P. (2013), *The Prince of Medicine: Galen in the Roman World*, Oxford.

Milanezi, S. (2004), "À l'ombre des acteurs: les amuseurs à l'époque classique" in: C. Hugoniot/F. Hurlet/S. Milanezi (eds.), *Le statut de l'acteur dans l'Antiquité grecque et romaine*, Tours, 183–209.

Nutton, V. (1972), "Galen and Medical Autobiography", *PCPhS* 18, 50–62.

Nutton, V. (1979), *Galen: On Prognosis* (Corpus Medicorum Graecorum 5.8.1), Berlin.

Poulakos, J./Crick, N. (2012), "There is Beauty Here, Too: Aristotle's Rhetoric for Science", *Ph&Rh* 45.3, 295–311.
Rothschild, C.K. (2013), "Hocus Pocus, Galen's *On Prognosis* and the Gospel of Mark" in: T. Nicklas/J.E. Spittler (eds.), *Credible, Incredible: the Miraculous in the Ancient Mediterranean*, Tübingen, 107–142.
von Staden, H. (1995), "Anatomy as Rhetoric: Galen on Dissection and Persuasion", *JHM* 50, 47–66.
von Staden, H. (1997), "Galen and the 'Second Sophistic'", in: R. Sorabji (ed.), *Aristotle and After*, London, 33–54.
Swain, S.C.R. (1996), *Hellenism and Empire: Language, Classicism, and Power in the Greek World, AD 50–250*, Oxford.
Tipton, J.A. (2014), *Philosophical Biology in Aristotle's Parts of Animals*, Heidelberg.

Georgia Petridou

Literary Remedies and Rhetorical Prescriptions in Aelius Aristides

Medical Paradoxography or Common Practise?

Abstract: This chapter surveys examples of two types of literary therapy in Aelius Aristides' *Hieroi Logoi*: a) the 'rhetorical remedies', b) the 'poetic prescriptions'. It engages closely with the discourse of medical paradoxography in the *Hieroi Logoi* and the ways these remedies were received in the blooming Aristides-related scholarship of the last decade or so, and finishes with some general thoughts on declaiming, writing and narrating as a basic modality of therapy in the second sophistic. The aim is twofold: to demonstrate that Aristides is in fact far more mainstream in using rhetoric, literature and music to cure bodily ailments than we have previously thought, while simultaneously showcasing how exceptional Aristides' use of these particular remedies really is. Although Aristides works with previously well-attested healing practises (e.g. in Plutarch, Galen, Antyllus) and commemorative discourses, he elevates them to a whole new level of efficacy and embeds them firmly into his rhetorical oeuvre.

1 Introduction

In chapter 8 of Aristides' *An Address Regarding Asclepius* (*Or.* 42 Keil), we read:

> In fact, there is very much that is paradoxical in the remedies of the god (καὶ μὴν τό γε παράδοξον πλεῖστον ἐν τοῖς ἰάμασι τοῦ θεοῦ), for example one man drinks gypsum, another hemlock, and another undresses and bathes in cold water with no need of warmth, as one would expect. Indeed, he has also honoured us in this way, by stopping catarrhs and colds with baths in rivers and the sea, by curing our inability to lay in bed with long walks, by adding indescribable purgatives (καθάρσεις) to frequent fasting, and by commanding me to speak and write when I found it difficult to breathe (ἀναπνεῖν δὲ ἀποροῦντι λέγειν καὶ γράφειν προστάττων), so that if people cured in this way can boast a little bit about it, we have too our share of boasting.

This passage introduces two groups of remedies: on the one hand, we have the prescriptions which candidly contradict contemporary mainstream medical approaches based on the so-called 'humoural medicine' and medical ideas about regulated exercise and dietary control, and hence could feature easily in medical

https://doi.org/10.1515/9783110661774-009

paradoxographical accounts; and on the other hand, we have the more nuanced rhetorical therapies, which perhaps would suit more an aristocratic man of letters. [1] This passage is significant for two reasons: a) it gives us an insight into Aristides' conceptualisation of the two groups, which were traditionally kept apart, as one and the same; and b) it introduces neatly the main theme of this chapter: literature and oratory, writing and reading, as healing practises in the work of Aelius Aristides.

In particular, we are told that among the rich gamut of mind-blowing medicaments and eye-catching dietary and exercise regimes, Asclepius commands Aristides to write and perform his writings, not only despite the apparent breathlessness of his patient, but *precisely because of that*: "the god commended me to perform orally and write, when I could not even breathe" (ἀναπνεῖν δὲ ἀποροῦντι λέγειν καὶ γράφειν προστάττων), he says.[2] This last-mentioned remedy exemplifies a particular kind of therapy which can be termed 'literary therapy', and can be further distinguished in the following three sub-types: a) the 'rhetorical remedies', b) the 'poetic prescriptions' and 'music medicaments', and finally, c) the 'epistolary endorsements'. Due to space constraints, this paper focusses on the first two categories.[3] In a nutshell, this study surveys some examples of literary therapy in the *Hieroi Logoi*, their reception in the blooming Aristides-related scholarship of the last decade or so, and finishes with some general thoughts on declaiming, writing, and narrating as a basic modality of therapy in the second sophistic. My main aim is twofold: on the one hand, I would like to demonstrate that Aristides is in fact far more mainstream in using rhetoric, literature, and music to cure his bodily ailments than we have previously thought; on the other hand, I would like to showcase how exceptional Aristides really is precisely because, although he works with previously well-attested healing practises and commemorative discourses, he elevates them to a whole new level of efficacy.

---

1 This paper has benefited from comments and suggestions from audiences at Max-Weber Kolleg, Universität Erfurt, University of Patras, and Université de Reims Champagne-Ardenne. I am grateful to George Kazantidis for all his pertinent comments on an earlier draft of the paper. I am indebted to Jörg Rüpke and the Max-Weber Kolleg for a generous research fellowship under the auspices of the DFG and FWF-funded International Research Training Group "Resonant World Relations in Ancient and Modern Socio-Religious Practices" project (shared between the University of Erfurt, Germany and Karl-Franzens University, Graz, Austria), which allowed me to work on the revisions of this paper. The text follows Keil's edition. All translations are mine, unless otherwise stated.

2 On the importance of voice in the formation of Aristides' rhetorical career and identity, see Gleason 1995, chs. 3 & 4.

3 The third category is discussed in Petridou 2017a.

2 Rhetorical Remedies

When in section 8 of his *An Address Regarding Asclepius* (quoted above), Aristides refers to Asclepius ordering him to press on with the writing and performing of his rhetorical declamations despite his apparent inability to breathe, he is clearly cross-referencing chapters 15–18 from his fourth book of the *Hieroi Logoi*, where he describes luridly his incredible transformation from a panting patient to a powerful orator.[4] In this passage, Aristides' difficulty to perform basic respiratory functions is treated by a 'rhetorical remedy', i.e. a divine prescription which centres on scripting and publicly performing an oration:[5]

> While I rested in Pergamum because of divine summons and my supplication, I received from the god a command and exhortation (γίγνεται παρὰ τοῦ θεοῦ πρόσταγμα καὶ παράκλησις) not to abandon rhetoric. (15) It is impossible to say through the length of time which dream came first, or the nature of each of these dreams on the whole. But those which occurred at the very beginning were exhortatory dreams. "It befits you to speak in the manner of Socrates, Demosthenes, and Thucydides. And one of the distinguished personages, who were older than I, was pointed out, in order that I would be especially moved to speak. And the god commanded me to go to the Temple Stoa, which is at the Theatre, and to offer to him the very first fruits of these improvised and competitive orations (καὶ τό γε σφόδρα πρῶτον ἀπάρξασθαί με ἐκέλευεν ἑαυτῷ προσελθόντα εἰς τὴν στοὰν τοῦ ἱεροῦ τὴν πρὸς τῷ θεάτρῳ τῶν αὐτοσχεδίων δὴ τούτων λόγων καὶ ἀγωνιστικῶν)." And so it happened. (16) There was a very magnificent spectacle in the city, either a bull hunt, I think, or some such thing. All those from the temple had rushed down, and the city was engaged in these things. We had been left alone in the Temple, two of the more distinguished worshippers, I and a Nicean, a man of praetorian rank, called Sedatius, but originally Theophilus. We were sitting in the temple of Hygieia, where the statue of Telesphoros was, and we were asking one another, as we were accustomed, whether the god had prescribed anything new. For in a way certain of our diseases were also similar. (17) I said that I did not know what I should do, for the prescription was like an order to fly, the practice of rhetoric, for one who could not breathe, and this here (ἔφην οὖν ἐγὼ μὴ ἔχειν ὅ τι χρήσομαι, προστετάχθαι γάρ μοι ἴσα καὶ πέτεσθαι, μελέτην λόγων ἀναπνεῖν οὐ δυναμένῳ, καὶ ταύτην ἐνταυθοῖ) – I mean the Stoa – and I recounted the dream to him. And when he heard it, he said, "What will you do, and how do you feel about it?" "What else", I said "than I shall do whatever I can? Arrange on my clothes, stand so, make a note of the problem to myself, begin some little thing, and then I shall stop. And so my obligation has

4 As a whole, *An Address Regarding Asclepius* (*Or.* 42 Keil) contains two more cross-references to the *Hieroi Logoi* (42.4 and 11), where the title of the work is mentioned explicitly.

5 In *Or.* 50.14, i.e. in what proceeds immediately before our passage, Aristides tells his reader that he could not vouch for either the right narrative order or the exact content of these exhortatory dreams because there were so many of them.

been fulfilled". "Not at all", he said "not so. But you have me here as a listener. Then contend with all zeal. Strength will be the God's concern. How do you know whether your dream pertains to more than this?" And at the same time, he told me a marvellous deed of the god, how he commanded some sick man to compete in this way, and by causing him to perspire through the exercise, brought an end to the whole disease (καὶ ἅμα διηγεῖταί μοι ἔργον τοῦ θεοῦ θαυμαστὸν, ὥς τινι κάμνοντι προστάξας οὕτω διαγωνίσασθαι συμβάντος ἱδρῶτος δι' ἀγωνίαν λύσειε τὸ νόσημα πᾶν). It seemed necessary to do this. (18) And while we were talking and taking counsel, Maximus the African entered in the third place, a worshipper of the ancients, and in a fashion zealous about oratory (θεραπευτὴς τῶν παλαιῶν καί τινα τρόπον πρόθυμος περὶ λόγους). It was he who proposed the problem. And the problem was as follows, for I remember it, since it was the first I received: "While Alexander", he said, "is in India, Demosthenes advises that it is time to act". I immediately accepted the omen of Demosthenes speaking again and of the subject, which was about empire. And pausing a little, I competed, and my new strength was such as is of the god's devising, and the year seemed not to have passed in silence, but in training (καὶ μικρὸν ἐπισχὼν ἠγωνιζόμην, καὶ τά τε δὴ τῆς ἄλλης δυνάμεως ἦν οἷα θεοῦ παρασκευάζοντος, καὶ ἔδοξεν ὁ τοῦ ἐνιαυτοῦ χρόνος οὐ σιωπῆς, ἀλλ' ἀσκήσεως εἶναι).[6]

As expected, this is not the only case where Asclepius prescribes a rhetorical declamation against purely physical ailments. In chapters 59–60 of the first book of his *Hieroi Logoi*, for example, Aristides lists numerous divine prescriptions for writing, performing, and correcting his oratory amongst a sheer mountain of purgations, enemas, phlebotomies, endless fasting or strictly regulated food-intake, and abstinence from bathing;[7] while in chapter 50 of book four, a rhetorical remedy is prescribed by the god to treat Aristides' toothache and mouth ulceration. This lastly mentioned passage is worth quoting in length:[8]

And once I happened to have a toothache, and was unable to open my mouth, and was in terrible difficulty. But he commanded me to summon a gathering of my friends and to read

6 Trans. Behr with emendations. There are some problems with the Greek in this passage and Keil's edition, which I discuss in detail in Petridou 2017b.

7 Aristid. *Or.* 47.60: ἀλλὰ τάς γε ἀσιτίας αὐτὰς ἁπάσας καὶ τὰς ἔτι τούτων πρότερον καὶ μετὰ τοῦτο γενομένας ἡμῖν ἐν τῷ χειμῶνι τούτῳ σχεδὸν διημερεύσαμεν περὶ λόγους, γράφοντές τε καὶ λέγοντες καὶ τὰ γεγραμμένα ἐξετάζοντες και παρετείντες οὐκ ἔλαττον ἢ εἰς μέσας νύκτας τὰ πλείω, 'But despite all this fasting, both happening even before those things and afterwards, we spent the whole period, almost to this winter, in writing and speaking and correcting that which had been written. And mostly we worked on at least until the middle of the night'.

8 One may be tempted to read all those physical ailments which concern the upper respiratory system and mouth as revealing of Aristides' wounded ego, fragmented professional identity as an orator, and his thwarted ambitions of a celebrated public speaker.

> them one of the speeches which I had written. Then I had in hand the third of the speeches to him. I read this through, and before I had completed all of it, I was free from the pain.[9]

The attentive reader of the passage would be quick to remark that the emphasis of this divine prescription lies equally on prompting Aristides to perform in public and on devising a performance enhancement technique for his rhetorical declamations: our Mysian patient is ordered to comfortably surround himself by a well-predisposed audience who were bound to boost his confidence and self-esteem.

Performance enhancement is also intrinsic in the rhetorical remedy recounted in chapters 15–18 from the fourth book of the *Hieroi Logoi*. The same passage deserves our attention for many reasons, not least because it marks out unequivocally the beginning of Asclepius' attentiveness in reconstructing Aristides' rhetorical career during his period of professional inactivity in Pergamum, to which he refers as the *Cathedra*.[10] Although Aristides appears to have forgotten most of the details of the oneiric prescription itself, he seems to remember vividly how the god ordered him to go to the temple of Hygeia. It was there that he found his fellow-patient Sedatius and revealed to him, not without a certain degree of incredulity, that the god's remedy for his breathing difficulty consisted in urging him to proceed with a full-fledged rhetorical declamation. While narrating his divine prescription, Aristides did not conceal his initial surprise and discontent when faced with the enormity and the difficulty of the task at hand, which did not seem to measure up to his limited ability to engage even with the most basic of biological functions, such as breathing:

> I said that I did not know what I should do, for this prescription to practice oratory for one who could not breathe was the equivalent of ordering a man to fly (ἔφην οὖν ἐγὼ μὴ ἔχειν ὅ τι χρήσομαι, προστετάχθαι γάρ μοι ἴσα καὶ πέτεσθαι, μελέτην λόγων ἀναπνεῖν οὐ δυναμένῳ).[11]

In truth, what Asclepius urged him to do was to go to the Temple Stoa, which was at the theatre, and make a sacrificial offer to him out of the very first fruits of his extemporaneous, competitive orations (καὶ τό γε σφόδρα πρῶτον ἀπάρξασθαί με

---

9 Aristid. *Or.* 50.30: καὶ δὴ καὶ ὀδόντας ἀλγῶν ποτε ἔτυχον καὶ οὔτε διᾶραι τὸ στόμα οἷός τ' ἦν, ἀπορίᾳ τε εἰχόμην δεινῇ· ὁ δὲ προστάττει τῶν λόγων τινὰ ἀναγνῶναι τῶν πεποιημένων μοι τοῖς φίλοις ἐπαγγείλαντα συνουσίαν. εἶχον δὲ τότ' ἐν χερσὶ τὸν τρίτον τῶν εἰς αὐτὸν λόγων· τοῦτον ἀνέγνων διὰ τέλους, καὶ πρὶν ἅπαντα διελθεῖν, τῆς ὀδύνης ἀπαλλάγμην.

10 This was a particularly important dream not only for Aristides' rhetorical career, but also for his relationship with the god himself, since it was the god himself who by ordering him to abide in Pergamum in the first place thwarted his professional ambitions.

11 *Or.* 50.17.

ἐκέλευεν ἑαυτῷ προσελθόντα εἰς τὴν στοὰν τοῦ ἱεροῦ τὴν πρὸς τῷ θεάτρῳ τῶν αὐτοσχεδίων δὴ τούτων λόγων καὶ ἀγωνιστικῶν·)".[12] Although written down several decades after the original event, the Greek implies that the sacrificial language, whereby Aristides' rhetorical speeches are portrayed as sacrificial ἀπαρχαί, was part of the original dream. But it is not until he receives a thumbs-up from his fellow-patient Sedatius that Aristides finally proceeds with executing the divine prescription. Sedatius, the praetor from Nicaea, generously offers to be the audience of Aristides' rhetorical *agōn* and encourages him to overcome his initial disinclination. To be more precise, Sedatius emboldens him by recounting a parallel *diēgēsis* of another patient's successful treatment of a physical ailment by means of competitive rhetorical performance:

> And at the same time, he told me a wondrous deed of the god, how he commanded a patient to compete in this way in rhetorical display, and by causing him to perspire through the exercise, brought the whole disease to an end" (καὶ ἅμα διηγεῖταί μοι ἔργον τοῦ θεοῦ θαυμαστὸν, ὥς τινι κάμνοντι προστάξας οὕτω διαγωνίσασθαι *συμβάντος ἱδρῶτος* δι' ἀγωνίαν λύσειε τὸ νόσημα πᾶν).

At this point, we should note that the term ἀγωνία can denote the mental or the physical struggle, the agony, the striving for victory in an athletic contest or a rhetorical competition, and that both meanings are indeed appropriate to our context.[13] Essentially, Sedatius' *comparandum* reaffirms the efficacy of the 'wondrous' (*thaumaston*) rhetorical remedy Asclepius prescribes, and further elucidates it by intersecting a more widely accepted medical explanation for the recommended course of action: namely, the rhetorical remedy works because it sets in motion a type of mental and/or physical anguish, which in turn causes perspiration. It hardly needs pointing out that perspiration, along with bleeding, vomiting, and excretion, is viewed, at least in the so-called humoural medicine, as a potentially helpful outlet for evacuating excess fluids, and thus as means of reinstating the fragmented equilibrium of humours and elemental qualities in the body of the sufferer.[14]

12 *Or.* 50.15.

13 'Contest, struggle for victory': Hdt. 2.91; Eur. *Hec.* 314, *Tro.* 1003; esp. in athletic games: Pi. *O.* 2.52, *P.* 5.113; 'gymnastic exercise': Hp. *Art.* (CMG I 1, 28) 11 = VI 238 Littré; Plat. *Men.* 94b, *Lg.* 765c; 'mental struggle, agony, anguish': Dem. 18.33, Arist. *Pr.* 869b6; Chrysipp. Stoic. 2.248; Nic. Dam. *Vit.Caes.* 9.

14 Cf. Mattern 2008, 64–75, esp. n. 63 and Wilkins 2016.

3 Poetic prescriptions and music medicaments

Asclepius' divine favour and patient supervision with regards to Aristides' literary production was not restricted to rhetoric, as we can see in chapters 11–13 of his *An Address Regarding Asclepius*:[15]

> (11) But it is even said that the god revealed boxing tricks to a certain boxer of our day in his sleep, which if he used, he must of necessity have defeated one of his famous opponents. But the god has revealed to us means of study, lyric poetry, subjects of speeches, and in addition to this, the actual ideas and the style, like those who teach boys to write (μαθήματα δὲ ἡμῖν γε καὶ μέλη καὶ λόγων ὑποθέσεις καὶ πρὸς τούτοις ἐννοήματα αὐτὰ καὶ τὴν λέξιν, ὥσπερ οἱ τοῖς παισὶ τὰ γράμματα). Since I have put, as it were, the finishing touch to the god's benefits, I shall close my speech on this point. (12) For I have received, O Lord Asclepius, as I have said, many, various gifts from your generosity, but the greatest, the one deserving the most gratitude, and nearly, one might say, the most wholesome, is oratory. You have changed what happened to Pindar, for Pan danced out his paean, as the story goes. But if it is proper to express it, *I say that I am the performer of your compositions*. For you yourself have exhorted me to oratory and have guided my literary exercises (μέγιστον δὲ καὶ πλείστης χάριτος ἄξιον καὶ σχεδὸν ὡς εἰπεῖν οἰκειότατον οἱ λόγοι. τὸ γὰρ τοῦ Πινδάρου μετέβαλες. ἐκείνου μὲν γὰρ ὁ Πὰν τὸν παιᾶνα ὠρχήσατο, ὡς λόγος, ἐγὼ δὲ, εἰ θέμις εἰπεῖν, *ὧν ὑποκριτὴς εἶναι·* προὔτρεψάς τε γὰρ αὐτὸς ἐπ' αὐτοὺς καὶ τῆς ἀσκήσεως κατέστης ἡγεμών). (13) And this was not enough for you. But you also were concerned with what was likely to come next, that your work would be famous. And there is no city, no private citizen, no official, who after a brief association with us did not salute us and praise us as extensively as possible, and it was not, I think, the effect of my oratory, but the effect of you my Lord.[16]

In fact, as Aristides informs us in the same extract, Asclepius' favour extended to a wide-ranging and all-encompassing career coaching strategy, which provided our Mysian orator not only with study models (μαθήματα), but also with the subject matter for both his rhetorical and hymnic composition (καὶ μέλη καὶ λόγων ὑποθέσεις), as well as meticulous instruction, which extended well beyond the realm of ideas into the area of their precise linguistic construction (καὶ πρὸς

---

15 Aristid. *Or.* 42.12: ἐμοὶ γάρ, ὦ δέσποτα Ἀσκληπιέ, πολλὰ καὶ παντοῖα, ὥσπερ ὑπεῖπον, παρὰ σοῦ καὶ τῆς σῆς φιλανθρωπίας γεγένηται, μέγιστον δὲ καὶ πλείστης χάριτος ἄξιον καὶ σχεδὸν ὡς εἰπεῖν οἰκειότατον οἱ λόγοι. 'For I have received, O lord Asclepius, as I have said, many, various gifts from your generosity, but the greatest, the one deserving the most gratitude, and nearly, one might say, the most wholesome is oratory.'

16 Trans. Behr with emendations.

τούτοις ἐννοήματα αὐτὰ καὶ τὴν λέξιν). On numerous occasions in the *Hieroi Logoi*, the very process of composing poetry has an unmistakable healing effect on Aristides' bedridden body.

This is precisely what we referred to as 'poetic prescriptions' in the introductory section of the paper. The following extract from the first book of the *Hieroi Logoi* (*Or.* 47.73) is yet another fitting example:

> When I was faint (λιποψυχοῦντα) and wholly at a loss (παντελῶς ἀπορούμενον), I wrote a poem about the marriage of Coronis and the birth of the god, and I stretched the strophe to great lengths. And thus I wrote the verses peacefully and in solitary reflection, and I was entirely oblivious of all difficulties (καὶ ἐποίησα τὰ ᾆσματα ἐφ' ἡσυχίας οὑτωσὶ καὶ κατ' ἐμαυτὸν ἐνθυμηθεὶς, καὶ πάντων ἤδη λήθη ἦν τῶν δυσχερῶν).

The participle λιποψυχοῦντα (73) denotes 'leaving life', either temporarily, in which case it means 'fainting', or permanently, in which case it is used as a synonym for 'dying'. The participle picks up the general idea of chapter 69 of the same book, where Aristides literally describes himself as being on the brink of death (καὶ σύμπαντος τοῦ σώματος οὕτως ἔχειν ὥστε ἐπ' ἔσχατον ἐλθεῖν), and conveys roughly the same meaning of extreme pain, fatigue, utter desolation and hopelessness. Composing here a hymn to Asclepius becomes the remedy not of a specially localised ailment, but of a generalised, life-threatening condition. Furthermore, it paves the way for a more 'invasive' medical procedure, which comes in the form of an enema, and limited dietary sustenance, which revolves around having a wild lettuce for dinner. In short, this poetic prescription is essential for the patient's bodily recovery.

Asclepius continued initiating and moulding Aristides' *ars poetica* and *ars rhetorica*, providing instruction on both style and content, and even managed to regulate the performative context of his oratory and poetry by ordering him to act as a *chorēgos*, namely as the leader and trainer of choruses which consisted of both boys and men.[17] Those choruses were trained to sing Aristides' choral and lyric compositions, and it was these choral performances of boys in particular that the local attending physician Theodotus utilised in order to provide immedi-

---

17 *Or.* 50.38–42. More importantly, as Aristides believed, Asclepius even made decisive interventions to secure an enthusiastic reception of Aristides' oratory and poetry. Cf. *Or.* 50.43–47. On the difference between initiating and moulding *ars poetica* in the cases of theophilic poets, seers, and prophets, see Petridou 2015, ch. 4; on Aristides' theophilic aspirations, see Petridou 2018.

ate and effective treatment to Aristides' breathlessness, asthma attacks, and possibly his stomach ulcers too, as the colourful narration in chapter 38 of his fourth book of the *Hieroi Logoi* has it:

> Tale follows tale, and let us say again that along with other things, Asclepius, the Saviour, also commanded us to spend time on songs and lyric verse, and to relax and maintain a chorus of boys. There would be no end of saying in how many other ways we benefited from this advice in contentment and self-sufficiency. But the children sang my songs; and whenever I happened to choke, if my throat were suddenly constricted, or my stomach became disordered, or whenever I had some other troublesome attack, the doctor Theodotus, being in attendance and remembering my dreams, used to order the boys to sing some of my lyric verse. And while they were singing, there arose unnoticed a feeling of comfort, and sometimes everything that pained me went completely away (ὅσα μὲν δὴ καὶ ἄλλα τῆς συμβουλῆς ταύτης ἀπελαύσαμεν εἰς εὐθυμίαν καὶ τὸ ἀνταρκεῖν ἀπέραντον ἂν εἴη λέγειν, τὰ δ' ᾄσματα ᾖδον οἱ παῖδες, καὶ ὁπότε ἢ πνίγεσθαι συμβαίνοι, τοῦ τραχήλου ταθέντος ἐξαίφνης ἢ τοῦ στομάχου καταστάντος εἰς ἀπορίας, ἤ τις ἄλλη γένοιτο ἄπορος προσβολή, παρὼν ἂν Θεόδοτος ὁ ἰατρὸς καὶ μεμνημένος τῶν ἐνυπνίων ἐκέλευε τοὺς παῖδας ᾄδειν τῶν μελῶν, καὶ μεταξὺ ᾀδόντων λάθρα τις ἐγίγνετο ῥᾳστώνη, ἔστι δ' ὅτε καὶ παντελῶς ἀπῄει πᾶν τὸ λυποῦν.).

This and other similar passages, which are telling of Aristides' poetic prescriptions, along with some of the other passages, which contained the rhetorical remedies Aristides received, have been expertly discussed by Laurent Pernot in his 2006 article entitled 'Rhetoric of Religion'.[18] According to Pernot, in employing literary therapies in his health regime, Aristides draws primarily on his professional identity, his idiosyncrasies, and his extreme proximity to his divine healer. In short, literary therapy was a 'tailor-made' therapy for this rather extraordinary individual.[19] While there is certainly truth in this suggestion, this is not the whole of it. Narrative therapy in general and literary therapy in particular was not exceptional measures taken exclusively in Aristides' case. They may sound peculiar to us, they may seem like perfect additions to the blossoming genre of medical paradoxography;[20] nonetheless, literary therapies and rhetorical prescriptions

---

18 The piece was published in the *Rhetorica* journal subsequently reprinted in the second volume of *New Chapters in the History of Rhetoric*, which was also edited by Pernot.

19 Pernot 2009, 344: "Because he was an orator and a sophist, Aristides drew on his rhetorical culture in his relationship with Asclepius, which led him to link rhetoric with every stage of his medical-religious adventure, through devices of great literary and psychological complexity, whose importance is crucial to our understanding of the mentalities of antiquity".

20 On paradoxography and the discourse of miracle in both the context of Asclepian healing and second-century literary and epigraphical production, see Petsalis-Diomidis 2010, 151–166 and 238–275. One need not to look further than Galen's *On Prognosis* to see how many times the

were common practice in the temples of Asclepius, or at least this is what Galen has us believing when in his *de sanitate tuenda*, his treatise on hygiene, he embeds literary therapy in the wide range of remedies given to the occupants of the Pergamene Asclepieion in order to regulate their bodily warmth and deal with both physical and psychological disorders:

> No mean witness of this opinion is our ancestral divinity Asclepius (ὁ πάτριος ἡμῶν θεὸς Ἀσκληπιός), who caused not a few odes to be written and humorous mimes and songs to be composed (οὐκ ὀλίγας μὲν ᾠδάς τε γράφεσθαι καὶ μίμους γελοίων καὶ μέλη τινὰ ποιεῖν ἐπιτάξας) by those in whom the excessive activity of passion made the constitution of the body hotter than normal. And others, not a few also, he caused to hunt, ride, and exercise in arms.[21]

Patricia Cox-Miller aptly summarises the gist of the passage: "Thus whether one was hot-headed or depressive, Asclepius had remedies ready to prescribe in dreams and, interestingly, they connected psychic therapy with physical activity – the quiet sitting of literary authorship for the overly passionate, and the vigorous pursuits of hunting and riding for those lacking in emotional drive".[22]

Crucially, declaiming in private or in public, as well as writing and/or reading literary texts, were not restricted as therapeutic strategies to the realm of sacred medicine. Indeed as a passage from Plutarch's *On Advice on keeping well* (Ὑγιεινὰ παραγγέλματα – *De tuenda sanitate*) amply shows, regular reading and performing rhetorical exercises was firmly embedded in the recommended health regime of Plutarch's contemporaries (130a–d). Rhetorical exercises or simply reading aloud literary texts was apparently as essential for the well-being of the *philologoi*, the intellectuals which constituted Plutarch's target audience, as physical exercise was for wrestlers. The homology between rhetorical exercises and physical exercises culminates in coupling "passionate and convulsive vociferations" (κραυγὰς περιπαθεῖς καὶ σπαραγμώδεις) with violent and sudden bodily movements. The first may cause just as much harm to the men of letters as the latter can to professional athletes. More significantly, a course of *apotherapy* and massage is recommended after a rhetorical session to distribute evenly the vital spirit (*pneuma*) which the intellectual and physical workout has produced and to ease the body and mind back to a less excitable position.

---

verb *thaumazō* and its cognates appear in Galen's depiction of both his patients and his rivals reactions' to his outstanding ability for *prognosis*.

21 Galen *San. Tu.* (CMG V 4,2) 1.8.17–23 = Kühn VI 40–42. On this passage, see Pietrobelli 2017.

22 Cox-Miller 1994, 108. On the close correlation of body and mind in Galen, see von Staden 2000, 105–116. On Galen's extensive literary knowledge, see von Staden 1998 and Pietrobelli 2013.

What is more,as Antoine Pietrobelli has convincingly argued,[23] the idea of reading aloud rhetorical and/or literary texts as breathing exercise was at least as old as the Hippocratic *De Victu*, where we learn that this sort of therapy was prescribed to treat illnesses caused by excessive moisture. To cast our net more widely, the rhetorical practise of *anaphōnēsis* (ἀναφώνησις, often rendered in Latin as *clamor* or *vociferatio*) was popular with physicians from both the sect of the Pneumatists (such as Archigenes) and that of the Methodists (such as Thessalus), as well as with other eminent doctors of the calibre of Soranus, Caelius Aurelianus, and Galen.[24] Pietrobelli rightly argues, however, that nowhere is *anaphōnēsis* more accurately described than in Antyllus, a second-century CE physician and medical author whose fragments Pietrobelli has edited.[25] *Anaphōnēsis* was thought of as a rhetorical exercise that regulates the body's natural heat (φυσικὴ θερμασία) and features both as a means of therapy and as part of a health regime.[26] More significantly, it was prescribed as a remedy against all sorts of vocal pathologies and illnesses of the upper and lower respiratory system such as asthma or excessive accumulation of phlegm in the lungs, as well as in cases of patients who suffered from digestive discomfort.[27] Section 6.10.17–18 of Antyllus' writings is of special interest here because it provides us with a detailed medical explanation of how reading aloud helps the evacuation of excess bodily

---

23 Pietrobelli 2017. See also his introduction to the volume (7–20) and the annex (141–153). Pietrobelli identifies the following passages: *Vict.* (CMG I 2.4) 26.3 = VI 498 Littré and 87.3 = VI 642 Littré as of particular interest. Cf. esp. *Vict.* (CMG I 2.4) 61.2 = VI 576 Littré, where we read: "Ὅσοι δὲ πόνοι φωνῆς, ἢ λέξιες ἢ ἀνάγνωσιες ἢ ᾠδαί, πάντες οὗτοι κινέουσι τὴν ψυχήν· κινεομένη δὲ ξηραίνεται καὶ θερμαίνεται, καὶ τὸ ἐν τῷ σώματι ὑγρὸν καταναλίσκει." Cf. also Gleason 1995, 88–91.

24 E.g. Galen, *San. Tu.* 2, 11.4 (Kühn VI 147 = CMG V 4.2, 65) and 5, 10.40–43 (Kühn VI 358–359 = CMG V 4.2, 158); *MM* IV, 4 (Kühn X 261–265 = Johnston and Hosley I, 394–402).

25 Antyllus' work is preserved in a fragmentary state in Oribasius' compilations of earlier famous medical authors (*Collectionum Medicarum Reliquiae*, I. Libri I–VIII; II; IX–XVI. Raeder (CMG VI.1.1–2) Leipzig & Berlin, Teubner 1928–9). Oribasius (320–390/400 AD) is known to the historians of medicine for being a doctor and a prolific medical compiler, and of course, the personal physician to the emperor Julian (361–363 AD). To the historians of religion, however, Oribasius is more well-known for allegedly receiving the last prophecy from Delphi. More on the topic in Pietrobelli 2017. See also the extremely useful annex to the same volume of *Métis* Pietrobelli has edited (pp.141–153).

26 Remedies: Orib. *Coll. Med.* 6.8.1–5 Raeder; as part of what we would call today 'preventive medicine': Orib. *Coll. Med.* 6.9.1–15 Raeder. I am indebted to Antoine Pietrobelli for these references.

27 The gamut of illness for which *anaphōnēsis* could be prescribed is extremely wide. Suffice to say, it extends to pregnant women. Cf. 6.8.1–5.

fluids through perspiration (δι' ἱδρώτων), which brings to mind the medical explanation Sedatius offers to Aristides to encourage him to proceed with Asclepius' recommended course of rhetorical declamation in book four (*Or.* 50.15–18). Of course, I am not arguing that Aristides and his fellow-incumbants were familiar with this specific extract from the work of this specific author. What I hope to have shown is that Aristides operated within a wider cultural tradition that considered rhetorical and literary exercises as therapies for an array of respiratory problems and vocal disorders.

4 Conclusion

To pull the threads together, this study has shown that Aristides' therapeutic use of rhetoric, literature, and music was far more mainstream and far less controversial than we had previously thought. Aristides was not alone in having been prescribed rhetorical declamations to treat his breathing difficulties. Other *literati* before him as well as physicians of the calibre of Galen did employ rhetorical declamations and literary therapy to cure bodily ailments, especially those related to the upper respiratory system. In other words, in Aristides' paradoxical and sacred world, there are elements which, though wondrous and marvellous at first sight, are also attested in secular medicine. This suggests an overlap between sacred and secular medicine and brings out very well the difficulty (and the anachronism) in drawing a straight line of distinction between so-called paradoxography and medicine. In this light, Aristides appears far less exceptional than portrayed in the secondary literature. Nonetheless, in the Aristidean corpus these previously well-attested healing practises pertaining to books, rhetoric, music, and poetry composition are elevated to a whole new level of efficacy. Although not alone, Aristides was unique in conceptualising these rhetorical remedies as unambiguous signs of divine favour.

Bibliography

Behr, C.A. (1968), *Aristides and the Sacred Tales*, Amsterdam.
Behr, C.A. (1978), "Aristides and the Egyptian Gods", *Hommages à Maarten J. Vermaseren*, vol. 1, Leiden, 13–24.
Behr, C.A. (1981–1986), *P. Aelius Aristides: The Complete Works*. 2 Vols., Leiden.
Brockmann, C. (2013), "Galen und Asklepios", *Zeitschrift für Antikes Christentum* 17, 51–67.

Busine, A. (2012), "The Discovery of Inscriptions and the Legitimation of New Cults", in: B. Dignas/R.R.R. Smith (eds.), *Historical and Religious Memory in the Ancient World*, Oxford, 241–253.
Coulehan, J. (2003), "Metaphor and Medicine: Narrative in Clinical Practice", *Yale Journal of Biology and Medicine* 76, 87–95.
Cox Miller, P. (1994), *Dreams in Late Antiquity*, Princeton, NJ.
Downie, J. (2009), "A Pindaric Charioteer: Aelius Aristides and his Divine Literary Editor (*Oration* 50.45)," *CQ* 59, 263–269.
Downie, J. (2008), "Proper Pleasures: Bathing and Oratory in Aelius Aristides' *Hieroi Logoi* I and Oration 33", in: W.V. Harris/B. Holmes (eds.), *Aelius Aristides between Greece, Rome and the Gods*, Leiden, 117–130.
Downie, J. (2013), *At the Limits of Art. A Literary Study of Aelius Aristides'* Hieroi Logoi, Oxford.
Eliasoph, N./Lichterman, P. (2003), "Culture in Interaction", *American Journal of Sociology* 108, 735–794.
Frankfurter, D. (2008), "The Interpretation of Ritual Spaces in Late Antique Religions: An Overview", *Archiv für Religionsgeschichte* 10, 211–222.
Gladigow, B. (1995), "Anatomia Sacra: Religiös motivierte Eingriffe in menschliche oder tierische Körper", in: P.J. van der Eijk *et al.* (eds.), *Ancient Medicine in its Socio-Cultural Context*, Amsterdam, 345–331.
Gleason, M.W. (1995), *Making Men: Sophists and Self-Presentation in Ancient Rome*, Princeton.
Gleason, M.W. (2009), "Shock and Awe: the Performance Dimensions of Galen's Anatomy Demonstrations", in: C. Gill/T. Whitmarsh/J. Wilkins (eds.), *Galen and the World of Knowledge*, Cambridge, 85–114.
Gourevitch, D. (1984), *Le Triangle Hippocratique dans le Monde Gréco-Romain: Le Malade, sa Maladie et son Médecin*, BEFAR 251, Rome.
Hughes, I. (2008), "Fragmentation as Metaphor in the Classical Healing Sanctuary", *Social History of Medicine* 21, 217–236.
Holmes, B. (2008), "Aelius Aristides' Illegible Body", in: W.V. Harris/B. Holmes (eds.), *Aelius Aristides between Greece, Rome and the Gods*, Leiden, 81–113.
Hoof van, L. (2011), "Plutarch's 'Diet-Ethics'. Precepts of Healthcare. Between Diet and Ethics", in: G. Roskam/L. van der Stockt (eds.), *Virtues for the People: Aspects of Plutarchan Ethics*, Leuven, 109–129.
Israelowich, I. (2012), *Society, Medicine and Religion in the Sacred Tales of Aelius Aristides*, Leiden.
Johnson, L.T. (2009), *Among the Gentiles: Greco-Roman Religion and Christianity*, New Haven/London.
Johnson, W.A. (2010), *Readers and Reading Culture in the High Roman Empire: A Study of Elite Communities*, Oxford/New York.
King, H. (1999), "Chronic Pain and the Creation of Narrative", in: J.I. Porter (ed.), *Constructions of the Classical Body*, Ann Arbor, 269–286.
King, H. (2006), "The Origins of Medicine in the Second Century AD", in: S. Goldhill/R. Osborne (eds.), *Rethinking Revolutions through Ancient Greece*, Cambridge.
Κούκη, Ε. (2012), *Ἱεροὶ Λόγοι. Σώμα και γλώσσα στα όνειρα ενός ρήτορα*, Αθήνα.
Mattern, S. (1999), "Physicians and the Roman Imperial Aristocracy: The Patronage of Therapeutics", *Bulletin of the History of Medicine* 73, 1–18.
Mattern, S. (2008), *Galen and the Rhetoric of Healing*, Baltimore.

Moog, F.P., (2001), "Im Auftrag des Asklepios: die wundersame Mission der Anyte von Tegea", *Schriftenreihe der Deutschen Gesellschaft für Geschichte der Nervenheilkunde* 7, 197–212.
Mylonopoulos, I. (2006), "Greek Sanctuaries as Places of Communication through Rituals: An Archaeological Perspective", in: E. Stavrianopoulou (ed.), *Ritual and Communication in the Greco-Roman World*, Kernos Supplements, Liège, 69–110.
Pearcy, L. (1988), "Dream, Theme, and Narrative: Reading the Sacred Tales of Aelius Aristides", *Transactions of the American Philological Association* 118, 377–391.
Pernot, L. (1998), "*Periautologia*. Problèmes et méthodes de l'éloge de soi-même dans la tradition éthique et rhétorique gréco-romaine", *Revue des Études Grecques* 111, 101–124.
Pernot, L. (2006), "The Rhetoric of Religion", *Rhetorica* 24, 235–254 [reprinted in (2009), *id.* ed. *New Chapters in the History of Rhetoric*, Leiden/Boston, 327–346].
Petridou, G. (2015), *Divine Epiphany in Greek Literature and Culture*, Oxford.
Petridou, G. (2017a), "Poésie pour l'esprit, rhétorique pour le corps: Remèdes littéraires et cautions épistolaires dans les *Hieroi Logoi* d'Aelius Aristide", *Mètis* 15, 69–94.
Petridou, G. (2017b), "Contesting Religious and Medical Expertise in the *Hieroi Logoi*: The *therapeutai* of Pergamum as Religious and Medical Entrepreneurs", in: R.L. Gordon/ G. Petridou/J. Rüpke (eds.), *Beyond Priesthood: Religious Entrepreneurs and Innovators in the Roman Empire*, Berlin/New York, 183–208.
Petridou, G. (2018), ""One has to be so terribly religious to be an artist": Divine Inspiration and theophilia in Aelius Aristides' Hieroi Logoi", *Archiv für Religionsgeschichte* 20, 253–268.
Petsalis-Diomidis, A. (2006), "Sacred Writing, Sacred Reading: The Function of Aelius Aristides' Self-presentation as Author in the Sacred Tales", in: B. McGing/J. Mossman (eds.), *The Limits of Ancient Biography*, Swansea, 193–211.
Petsalis-Diomidis, A. (2010), *Truly Beyond Wonders: Aelius Aristides and the Cult of Asclepius*, Oxford.
Pietrobelli, A. (2013), "Galien Agnostique: Un Texte Caviardé Par La Tradition", *Revue des Études Grecques* 126, 103–135.
Pietrobelli, A. (2017), "Déclamer pour soigner son corps. L'anaphonèse chez Antylle et Oribase", *Mètis* 15, 95–122.
Platt, V.J. (2011), *Facing the Gods: Epiphany and Representation in Graeco-Roman Art, Literature and Religion*, Cambridge.
Rapp, C. (1998), "Storytelling as Spiritual Communication in Early Greek Hagiography", *Journal of Early Christian Studies* 6, 431–448.
Remus, H. (1996), "Voluntary Association and Networks: Aelius Aristides at the Asclepieion in Pergamum", in: J.S. Kloppenborg/S.G. Wilson (eds.), *Voluntary Associations in the Graeco-Roman World*, London/New York, 146–175.
Renberg, G.H. (2010), "Incubation in Saqqâra", in: Proceedings of the Twenty-Fifth International Congress of Papyrology, Ann Arbor 2007, *American Studies in Papyrology*, 649–662.
Renberg, Gil H. (2017), *Where Dreams May Come. Incubation Sanctuaries in the Greco-Roman World*, 2 vols., Leiden.
Rutherford, I.C. (2009), "Aristodama and the Aetolians: An Itinerant Poetess and her Agenda", in: I.C. Rutherford/R. Hunter (eds.), *Travel, Locality and Panhellenism*, Cambridge, 237–248.
Silverberg, L.I. (2003), "Bibliotherapy: The Therapeutic use of Didactic and Literary Texts in Treatment, Diagnosis, Prevention, and Training", *Journal of the American Osteopath Association* 103, 131–135.

Sluiter, I. (2010), "Textual Therapy: On the Relationship Between Medicine and Grammar in Galen", in: H.F.J. Horstmanshoff (ed.), *Hippocrates and Medical Education*, Leiden, 25–52.
Skinner, M.B., (2001), "Ladies' Day at the Art Institute: Theocritus, Herodas, and the Gendered Gaze", in: A. Lardinois/L. McClure (eds.), *Making Silence Speak: Women's Voices in Greek Literature and Society*, Princeton/Oxford, 210–222.
Steger, F. (2016²), *Asklepios. Medizin und Kult*, Stuttgart.
Sokolowski, F. (1974), "Propagation of the Cult of Sarapis and Isis in Greece", *Greek Roman and Byzantine Studies* 15, 441–448.
Staden von, H. (1992), "The Discovery of the Body: Human Dissection and Its Cultural Contexts in Ancient Greece", *The Yale Journal of Biology and Medicine* 65, 223–241.
Staden von, H. (1997), "Galen and the Second Sophistic", *Bulletin of the Institute of Classical Studies* 41, 33–35.
Staden von, H. (1998), "Gattung und Gedächtnis: Galen über Wahrheit und Lehrdichtung", in: W. Kullmann/J. Althoff/M. Asper (eds.), *Gattungen wissenschaftlicher Literatur in der Antike*, Tübingen, 65–94.
Staden von, H. (2000), "Body, Soul, and Nerves: Epicurus, Herophilus, Erasistratus, the Stoics, and Galen', in: J.P. Wright/P. Potter (eds.), *Psyche and Soma: Physicians and Metaphysicians on the Mind-Body Problem from Antiquity to Enlightenment*, Oxford, 79–116.
Wilkins, J.M. (2016), "Treatment of the Man: Galen's Preventive Medicine in the *De Sanitate* Tuenda', in: G. Petridou/C. Thumiger (eds.), *Homo Patiens: Approaches to the Patient in the Ancient World*, Leiden, 411–431.
Winkler, J.J. (1985), *Auctor and Author: A Narratological Reading of Apuleius's Golden Ass*, Berkeley.

Michiel Meeusen

Unknowable Questions and Paradoxography in ps.-Alexander of Aphrodisias' *Medical Puzzles and Natural Problems*

Abstract: The *Medical Puzzles and Natural Problems* transmitted under the name of Alexander of Aphrodisias, but probably spurious, deals with a wide range of particular and often quite peculiar questions pertaining to ancient medicine and natural science. In line with the *Natural Problems* attributed to Aristotle, these questions are commonly introduced with "Why?" (Διὰ τί;) by which the author inquires specifically into the physical causes of the problems at hand. The 228 problem chapters gathered in the collection are subdivided into two books, each one opening with a preface. In the preface to the first book, ps.-Alexander provides a classification of several kinds of problems based on criteria of difficulty and solubility. An extensive list of paradoxical phenomena is given to illustrate what he means by "unknowable questions" (ἄποροι ζητήσεις). By examining the broader medical and philosophical backdrop of (a selection of) these phenomena, the present chapter aims to contribute to a better understanding of the medical-naturalist research project undertaken by ps.-Alexander, and the context, methods and conceptual limits that define it.

I am grateful for the useful feedback I received from my colleagues at King's College London, esp. Michael Trapp, on an earlier version of this paper, read at a departmental work in progress seminar. An updated version was read at the 12th London Ancient Science Conference: thanks are due to the audience for their stimulating remarks. I would like to extend thanks to George Kazantzidis and Kenneth Yu for their insightful comments on the penultimate version. All translations are mine, unless otherwise indicated.

https://doi.org/10.1515/9783110661774-010

1 Introduction

The *Medical Puzzles and Natural Problems* (ἰατρικὰ ἀπορήματα καὶ φυσικὰ προβλήματα)[1] transmitted under the name of Alexander of Aphrodisias, but probably spurious,[2] deals with a wide range of particular and often quite peculiar questions pertaining to ancient medicine and natural science. In line with the *Natural Problems* attributed to Aristotle, these questions are commonly introduced with 'Why?' (Διὰ τί;) by which the author inquires specifically into the physical (that is, material and efficient) causes of the problems at hand. Typical examples include: "Why do some people, when they feel shame, sweat from the armpits?", "Why do people, when they feel fear, become pale?", "Why do they also shiver?", "Why do people, when they are drunk, often die?", "Why is mincemeat difficult to digest?", "Why do stupid people often bear highly intelligent children, and highly intelligent people very stupid ones?", "Why do people when they see someone yawning, yawn in return?", "Why, when wood is being cut, do we see the blow immediately from afar, but hear the sound later, although the sound arises together with the blow?" etc.[3]

The 228 problem chapters gathered in the collection are subdivided into two books, each one opening with a preface. The preface to the first book is particularly intriguing as it outlines the types and general method of medical-naturalist problem research, indicating which topics of investigation are of interest for medical-scientific education, how they can be approached and what are the conceptual limits of this type of research. The preface has a clear protreptic function since it is designed to instruct the reader – who is identified as a student

1 Ed. Ideler 1841, 3–80. A new edition is currently being prepared by Carl-Gustaf Lindqvist of Gothenburg University (the forthcoming of which is still "eagerly awaited", to use the words of Kapetanaki/Sharples 2006, 1 n. 1). Katerina Oikonomopoulou, Luigi Silvano and I are currently collaborating on a paper about the medical and philosophical sources and traditions that ps.-Alexander relies on in the two prefaces (the paper will also include an English translation and critical edition of these texts). See also Silvano 2017 and 2018.

2 For speculation about the authorship of the *Medical Puzzles*, see Sharples 2005, 53–56, who on the basis of epigraphical evidence suggests attributing the work (and part of the *Supplementary problems* and the *On fevers*) to the Commentator's father, whose name was also Alexander and who was also a philosopher – a theory as intriguing as it is tentative.

3 Ps.-Alex., *Med. Puzz.* 1.1;11; 12; 13; 17; 22; 28; 34; 38 respectively.

(διδασκόμενος) – about the proper method and procedures of 'problematic' research.[4] To this end, the author provides a classification of several kinds of problems based on criteria of difficulty and solubility, emphasizing the intermediate nature of the medical-naturalist problems he will be concerned with. The author, thus, aims to regulate the reader's reception of the work by setting out the classificatory and methodological standards for this kind of inquiry.[5]

2 Classifying problems

Ps.-Alexander first makes a basic distinction between problems that are soluble and those that are not. The kind of questions that are soluble, or to be more precise "immediately credible and comprehensible (πιστὰ καὶ γνώριμα), and without the savour of any ambiguity or investigation (πάσης ἀμφιβολίας καὶ ζητήσεως ἄγευστα)" (*Med. Puzz.* 1.*Praef.* 1–2), are of the following type: "Why do birds have feathers?", or "Why did some animals receive horns, others stings, and still others sharp claws or the like?". The answers ps.-Alexander provides for these questions are of a teleological kind and support his belief in a goal-oriented design of the natural world, which applies also to the anatomy of animals (feathers are for the sake of heat and beauty, and horns, stings, claws etc. for the sake of defence).[6] Notably, this type of explanation is generally absent from the problems discussed in the collection itself, where the introductory Διὰ τί; mostly inquires into the physical principles at work in the phenomena under discussion, rather than their inherent teleology.[7] Yet it does underline the idea, as developed further on, that nature relies on a providential ordering.

---

4 Ps.-Alex., *Med. Puzz.* 1.*Praef.* 93–96: "since the student should not be satisfied only with the general method but should also be guided by means of particular cases, we shall commence the (collection of) solutions" (ἐπειδὴ δὲ οὐ μόνον ἀρκεῖσθαι χρὴ τῇ καθόλου μεθόδῳ, ἀλλ' ἤδη τοῖς κατὰ μέρος χειραγωγεῖν τὸν διδασκόμενον, ἀρξόμεθα τῶν λύσεων).

5 The work as a whole is explicitly linked to ancient medical education, providing numerous topics for intellectual training of aspirant doctors. For the idea that the first preface promotes an "active reading" of the problem chapters by activating the reader's attentiveness to the strategies that are employed both in raising and in solving such problems, see Meeusen 2018.

6 The topic of horns being designed by nature for the sake of defence recurs in ps.-Alex./Arist., *Sup. Pr.* 2.158, which asks: "Why do boars have tusks?". After providing a material explanation, the author continues: "Or is it that as nature has given horns for the sake of defence and assistance (ἀλκῆς χάριν καὶ βοηθείς), so it has given tusks to boars?" (transl. Kapetanaki/Sharples).

7 Final causation is rare also in the Aristotelian *Problems*: see Stoyles 2015.

Ps.-Alexander is straightforward in suggesting that this type of problems do not really trigger any inquiry, since they do not pose any considerable difficulty (*Med. Puzz.* 1.*Praef.* 24–30). In so doing, he alludes to Aristotle's *Topics* (105a3–9), where we find a similar account (*mutatis mutandis*) of the topics of investigation, which are unsuitable for dialectical training (γυμναστική):

Ps.–Alex., *Med. Puzz.* 1.*Praef.* 24–30	**Arist., *Top.* 105a3–9**
ὅσοι μὲν τοιαῦτα γνωστὰ καὶ σαφῆ προτείνουσιν, ἄντικρυς δέονται νοῦ· ὅσοι δὲ διχοστατοῦσιν, εἰ σύμφυτος τῷ πυρὶ σύνεστιν ἡ θερμότης, ἁπτικῆς αἰσθήσεώς εἰσιν ἐνδεεῖς. ὅσοι δέ, πότερον φύσις καὶ λόγος προνοητικὸς προμυθεύεται τὰ ἐν γενέσει καὶ φθορᾷ, τὴν τάξιν, τὴν κίνησιν, τὴν θέσιν, τὴν διάπλασιν, τὰς χρόας, τὰ παραπλήσια, κολάσεσιν τυγχάνουσιν ἔνοχοι.	Οὐ δεῖ δὲ πᾶν πρόβλημα οὐδὲ πᾶσαν θέσιν ἐπισκοπεῖν, ἀλλ' ἣν ἀπορήσειεν ἄν τις τῶν λόγου δεομένων καὶ μὴ κολάσεως ἢ αἰσθήσεως· οἱ μὲν γὰρ ἀποροῦντες "πότερον δεῖ τοὺς θεοὺς τιμᾶν καὶ τοὺς γονεῖς ἀγαπᾶν ἢ οὔ" κολάσεως δέονται, οἱ δὲ "πότερον ἡ χιὼν λευκὴ ἢ οὔ" αἰσθήσεως. οὐδὲ δὴ ὧν σύνεγγυς ἡ ἀπόδειξις, οὐδ' ὧν λίαν πόρρω· τὰ μὲν γὰρ οὐκ ἔχει ἀπορίαν, τὰ δὲ πλείω ἢ κατὰ γυμναστικήν.
All those who propose such well-known and clear problems are completely lacking in intelligence, and anyone who doubts whether heat is innate to fire, lacks the sense of touch. Then again, those who feel doubt, whether nature and a providential reason predict the processes of generation and corruption, the order of things, their motion, position, formation, complexions and things closely related to them, should be punished.	One should not examine every problem and every thesis but the one about which people might be puzzled – people who require reason and do not need punishment or sensation. For those who are puzzled as to whether or not the gods should be honoured and parents loved, need punishment, while those who doubt whether snow is white or not, need sensation. We should not discuss matters of which the demonstration is too near at hand or too far-off, for the former raise no difficulty, while the latter raise more than is appropriate to dialectical training.

Flashar interprets the concept of κόλασις in ps.-Alexander's text as referring to the phrasing of the problems themselves, some of which would require "correction" as to how they should be formulated ("Korrektur in ihrer Fragestellung"); as the passage from the *Topics* shows, however, it is the people who ask such 'tabooed' questions that require "Korrektur", presumably because of their godlessness.[8]

8 Flashar 1962, 365. See also Meeusen 2018, 99.

Although the allusion is to Aristotle's logic and his contemplation of what constitutes a proper dialectical πρόβλημα, ps.-Alexander continues his argument in a rather Platonic vein. As regards the insoluble (ἄλυτα) questions, he notes that these are known only to God (θεῷ μόνῳ γνώριμα), who created the world in a providential way.[9] He did so after the manner of a craftsman (τεχνίτης), who assembles the material bits and pieces to form compound substances (ὑποστήσαντι), and has detailed causal knowledge of how the world's machinery works.[10] In sum, there are specific epistemological limits to ps.-Alexander's 'problematic' research. Some problems are too difficult to solve, while others raise no difficulty at all; therefore, neither of these two categories is of interest to the type of research ps.-Alexander has in mind.[11]

3 Unknowability and paradoxography

An extensive list of paradoxical phenomena is provided to illustrate what ps.-Alexander considers "unknowable questions" (ἄποροι ζητήσεις). These questions are ἄποροι not in the sense that they are very difficult to solve, but – according to the author – they are fundamentally insoluble, hence unknowable. The passage runs as follows (*Med. Puzz.* 1.*Praef.* 35–57):

> ἄποροι δὲ ζητήσεις εἰσὶν αἱ τοιαίδε· τίνος ἕνεκεν οἱ γαργαλιζόμενοι μαχάλας ἢ πέλματα ἢ πλευρὰς γελῶσιν; ἢ τίνος χάριν ἀκούοντές τινες μαρμάρων παρατριβομένων ἢ πριζομένων ἢ τρίζοντος ἢ ῥινουμένου σιδήρου τοὺς ὀδόντας εὐθέως μαρκῶσιν; ἢ διὰ τί τὴν ἀπὸ τῶν ψυχρῶν ὀπωρῶν προσγινομένην αἱμωδίαν τοῖς ὀδοῦσιν ἀνδράχνη ψυχρὰ πεφυκυῖα θεραπεύει καὶ οὐκέτι τὰ ἐναντία τῶν ἐναντίων ἰάματα, ἀλλὰ τὰ ὅμοια; ἢ διὰ τί λίθος ἡ μαγνῆτις ἕλκει μόνον τὸν σίδηρον, ὑπό τε τῶν τούτου ῥινημάτων ζῳοποιεῖται ἡ λίθος, ἥ τε ἤλεκτρος λεγομένη μόνα τὰ κυρήβια καὶ τὰ κάρφη συνανασπᾷ κολλωμένη τούτοις; καὶ λέων ἀλεκτρυόνα δέδοικε μόνος, ὄρνις δὲ κατοικίδιος ᾠὸν τεκοῦσα τοῖς κάρφεσιν ἑαυτὴν ἀποκαθαίρει πανταχόσε τοῦ σώματος· ὄρτυγές τε σιτοῦνται τὸν ἐλλέβορον τοῖς ἀνθρώποις

9 Rose 1863, 219 speaks of Neoplatonist influence in the *Medical Puzzles*. At any rate, Galen's *On the Utility of the Parts* is just around the corner (see below).

10 *Med. Puzz.* 1.*Praef.* 32–34: "after all, a craftsman, after constructing a mechanical device, knows all the causes of its activities, whereas a layman is completely bereft of causal insight" (καὶ γὰρ ὁ τεχνίτης ἔργον τι μηχανικὸν κατασκευάσας οἶδεν αὐτοῦ πάσας τῶν ἐνεργειῶν τὰς αἰτίας, ἰδιώτης δὲ παντελῶς ἄμοιρος τῶν αἰτιῶν ἐστιν).

11 As we learn further on, the type of problems that *are* of interest for further inquiry "have a middle position" (μέσην ἔχοντα φύσιν): they are situated between those that "are quite clear and understood by everybody" (εὔδηλα πᾶσι γινωσκόμενα) and those that "are altogether obscure and admit no solution" (πάντα κεκρυμμένα λύσιν οὐχ ὑποδεχόμενα) (*Med. Puzz.* 1.*Praef.* 82–84).

δηλητήριον ὄντα· ψάροι δὲ τὸ κώνειον· ἀσκαμωνία δὲ μᾶλλον χολὴν ξανθὴν ἕλκει· κολοκυνθὶς δὲ καὶ ἀγαρικὸν καὶ λευκὸς ἐλλέβορος εὐφόρβιόν τε καὶ κόκκος Κνίδιος φλέγμα· μέλας δὲ ἐλλέβορος καὶ ἐπίθυμον μέλαιναν χολήν; τινὲς δὲ ὑπὸ μὲν τῶν καθαιρόντων στεγνοῦνται τὴν κοιλίαν, ὑπὸ δὲ τῶν στελλόντων καθαίρονται μᾶλλον. καὶ ἄλλος πρὸς τήνδε πλέον ἥδεται τὴν τροφήν, ῥᾷον αὐτὴν μεταβάλλων. οὐδεὶς δὲ καὶ τὴν θαλασσίαν νάρκην ἀγνοεῖ· πῶς δὴ τῆς μηρίνθου τὸ σῶμα ναρκοῖ; τρίγλη δὲ κρατουμένη ἀντιπαθεῖ τῇ νάρκῃ.

Unknowable questions are as follows: why do people laugh when one tickles their armpits, soles or ribs? Or why do some people immediately grind their teeth when they hear the sound of marble blocks being rubbed against each other or being sawn, or when they hear iron creaking or being filed? Or why does purslane, which is cold by nature, heal bleeding gums caused to the teeth by cold fruits, and why do not now opposite but similar qualities cure each other? Or why does the magnet only attract iron, and is it brought to life by the iron filings, or why does the so-called amber stone only draw up husks and straws when conjoined to them? And the lion fears only the cock, and when domestic fowls have laid an egg they cleanse off their entire body with dry straws. Quails eat hellebore, which is poisonous to men, while starlings eat hemlock. Scammony draws up yellow bile more, whereas gourd, tree fungi, white hellebore, spurge and Cnidian berries draw up phlegm more, and black hellebore and hell-weed draw up black bile more. Some people become costive in their bowels by purgative drugs, whereas by astringent drugs they are purged more. And others enjoy this food more, digesting it more easily. In addition, there is nobody who does not know the electric sea-eel. Well, how does it benumb the body of the fishing-line? Whereas a red mullet, when kept in the hand, counteracts the electric eel.

By virtue of their arousing a certain feeling of amazement the problems listed in this passage have a lot in common with ancient paradoxography and *mirabilia* literature.[12] The Stoic notions of sympathy and antipathy appear to be central here (cf. ἀντιπαθεῖ at the very end of the passage): in combination, they reveal a permanent interaction of specific phenomena in the cosmos around us, either in a positive or a negative way (viz. by the processes of attraction and repulsion respectively).[13] In what follows, I will examine the broader intellectual context of these paradoxical phenomena, with the aim of contributing to a better understanding of the medical-naturalist research project advanced by ps.-Alexander. It should be pointed out in advance that there are many parallels for these paradoxes in ancient literature. Therefore, I will be selective in my approach, focusing only on the most relevant cases.

---

12 Some parallels can be found in the paradoxograpical literature (e.g., Antig., *Mir.* 48 on the electric sea-eel). For further parallels, see Röhr 1923, 97.

13 See Röhr 1923, 96–98. Both concepts recur throughout the collection (for συμπάθεια, see *Med. Puzz.* 1.13; 33; 35; 77; 152; 2.35; for ἀντιπάθεια, see *Med. Puzz.* 1.152; 2.64). Paradoxes did not escape the attention of the Stoics since they provided evidence of the workings of providence or of the unity of all things in the universe.

4 Wonder and ir/rationality

Paradoxical phenomena, such as those listed by ps.-Alexander, are open to a proper explanation that would take away the strangeness and enigma of the (alleged) facts at hand; however, given that our author identifies them as 'unknowable', they are not really of interest to his research project. This is much in line with what a marvel-writer like Aelian (ca. 175–235 CE) states in a parallel passage about the lion (and the basilisk) fearing the cock (as well as the elephant's fear of the pig) at the end of Book 8 of his *Nature of Animals* (8.28), where we read:

> φύσεως δὲ ἀπόρρητα ἐλέγχειν οὐκ ἐμόν, καὶ εἰκότως, ἐπεὶ καὶ ἀλεκτρυόνα δέδοικε λέων καὶ τὸν αὐτὸν βασιλίσκος καὶ μέντοι καὶ ὗν ἐλέφας· τὰς δὲ αἰτίας ὅσοι σχολὴν ἄγουσι πολλὴν ζητοῦντες τοῦ μὲν χρόνου καταφρονήσουσιν, οὐ μὴν ἐς τέλος ἀφίξονται τῆς σπουδῆς.
>
> To examine the mysteries of nature is of no concern to me, and for good reason, since the lion fears the cock, and so does the basilisk, furthermore the elephant fears the pig. But those who have much leisure to look for the causes of these things will lose track of time and will truly never reach the end of their effort.[14]

By censuring any attempt at a scientific explanation of the "mysteries of nature" (φύσεως ἀπόρρητα – note the rather mystical formulation), the wonder (θαῦμα) which Aelian experiences – and before him other paradoxographers in general – is not rationally founded, since it does not lead to an examination of the causes of natural phenomena. It is rather an emotional reaction towards the unfamiliar and the bizarre. Especially striking is the contrast with the way in which natural scientists, including a physician like Galen, write about how they experience wonder/marvel and what this means to them.

For a medical scientist like Galen, as Tieleman points out, the wonder and awe inspired by natural scientific research, especially anatomical research, "results precisely from gaining insight into nature's rationality, not from accepting things as mysteries ... Thus Galen uses the term *thauma* (θαῦμα, "wonder," "marvel") not for things that defy causal explanation but that inspire awe and admiration for Nature's (or the Demiurge's) clever arrangements. This response, then, typically follows from acquiring knowledge, in particular about the facts revealed through dissection".[15]

14 On the lion fearing the cock, see also Ael., *NA* 3.31; Aesop., *Fab.* 84.1–3; S.E., *P.* 1.58.

15 Tieleman 2013, 104 with n. 10 for further references. See also *ibid.* 112: "For Galen, the experience of something amazing signifies ignorance of its true causes on the part of the person who

In his work *On the Utility of the Parts*, Galen repeatedly claims to admire the wonderful organisation of the human body and the artful way in which the Demiurge arranged it. In so doing, he fashions the text as a "hymn of praise to the Creator" (τοῦ δημιουργήσαντος [...] ὕμνον), and invites the reader to become skilful in Nature's art (τέχνη) too, so that he can be called "a natural philosopher and no longer a layman" (ἄγε δή μοι καὶ σὺ περὶ φύσιν γίγνου δεινός, ἵνα σε μηκέτ' ἰδιώτην, ἀλλὰ φυσικὸν ὀνομάζωμεν).[16] This is reminiscent of the point ps.-Alexander is making, namely that the τεχνίτης (in that case, God) has knowledge whereas the ἰδιώτης (us mortal beings) has not (see n. 10 above). Ps.-Alexander, however, reconfigures this idea within a rather mystical framework, which is also present in Aelian, whose concern is not to explore the ἀπόρρητα of nature. By emphatically excluding paradoxical phenomena from his research on the basis that they produce unknowable questions known only to the prime cosmic τεχνίτης, ps.-Alexander seems to place himself more in the camp of irrational marvel writers (like Aelian), who assume that there are certain things in the world that cannot be fully accounted for, than that of the rational admirers of divine providence in nature (like Galen).[17]

5 Polemics and methodology

Interestingly, a common feature of paradoxographical literature has to do with the fact that it is not concerned with formulating explanations for the natural *mirabilia* it collects. On the contrary, ancient paradoxographers were mostly preoccupied with simply listing wonder-inducing phenomena and with preserving their wondrous nature by intentionally abandoning any attempt at formulating a reasonable explanation for them. In many cases, they even omit the explanations

experiences it. For those who, on the basis of the art of medicine, do know, the astonishment has been replaced by admiration."

16 *UP* III 237–9 (cf. also III 41; 154; 696; 698–699; 875; IV 198; 248; 301; 361). The topic goes back directly to Aristotle's *Parts of Animals* 645a7–10 (a passage discussed by Oikonomopoulou in this volume).

17 Notably, the only kind of problems that Galen – much unlike ps.-Alexander, as we will see further on – considers unanswerable are those that *cannot* be settled on the basis of empirical testing (πεῖρα): e.g., whether the universe is created or not, whether there is an extra-cosmic void, whether god is corporeal or not, whether the soul is (or is not) corporeal or mortal, and what its substance is. See Gal., *Prop.Plac.* 2 Boudon-Millot/Pietrobelli; *PHP* V 766; *Pecc.Dig.* V 67; 98–102. See Hankinson 2009, 228–230.

that had already been provided in the scientific literature, from which the material is mostly drawn.[18] Whether ps.-Alexander in the passage at hand is directly relying on such paradoxographical literature or not is difficult to say. Notably, however, for some of the phenomena he considers unknowable other authors did come up with explanations. This is the case, for instance, with the link between tickling and laughter (a pressing issue, indeed, at least in view of Aristotle's claim that only human beings laugh when tickled).[19] An explanation is provided in the Aristotelian *Problems*,[20] where the phenomenon is ascribed to the thinness of the skin and because these parts of the body are not accustomed to being touched.[21] The Aristotelian *Problems* provide an explanation also for the question of purslane curing αἱμωδία ('bleeding gums'):[22] this is due to the fact that the viscous moisture from the purslane, which contains acidity, draws out the acidity from the gums, being συγγενής to it ('like attracts like').[23]

Ps.-Alexander may well have been aware of the fact that some of the questions which he claims to be unknowable were not considered to be so by others, although he forcefully opposes those who advocate that they can be answered (*Med. Puzz.* 1.*Praef.* 58–76):

> καὶ μυρίων ἄν σοι τοιούτων προκαταβαλοίμην κατάλογον, πείρᾳ μόνον γινωσκομένων, ἃ παρὰ τοῖς ἰατροῖς ἰδιότητες ἄρρητοι λέγονται· τὸ γὰρ ἴδιον ἑκάστου προφορόμενον ἄῤῥητον ὑπάρχει πρὸς ἀπόδοσιν τῶν αἰτίων. κακῶς γὰρ ἔνιοι λύσεις ἀθρόας τούτων παραβάλλουσι, ἀσυμφόρους δὲ καὶ ἀπιθάνους. φασὶ γὰρ τὰ καθαρτήρια θερμότατα τοὺς χυμοὺς ἕλκειν. ὅπερ

18 For more background and further literature on ancient paradoxography, see Schepens/Delcroix 1996, esp. 390–394. Jacob 1983 appropriately speaks of "la fabrication du merveilleux" as a main preoccupation of the genre (see esp. 133, *sub* "Le privilège du fait brut. La disparition des causes"). The genre flourished in the time of the Imperial Era: see, e.g., Naas 2011, Beagon 2011, and Meeusen 2014.

19 *PA* 673a2–10 (cf. *EN* 1150b22).

20 On the paradoxical nature and formulation of the *Problems*, see Flashar 1962, 299 and 342–343. Apollonius the paradoxographer (2nd century BCE) references the *Problems* relatively frequently: *Mir.* 7 (~ *Pr.* 21.24; 38.10); 9 (= fr. 234 Rose); 21 (= fr. 230 Rose); 22 (~ *Pr.* 10.44); 23 (= fr. 219 Rose ~ *Pr.* 38.7); 28 (= fr. 237 Rose); 37 (~ *Pr.* 13.10); 42 (= fr. 239 Rose); 45 (= fr. 228 Rose); 51 (= fr. 232 Rose).

21 *Pr.* 35.2.964b30–2; cf. also 35.8.965a23–32, where it is ascribed to a sudden exit of breath, dissolved from moisture, a result, in turn, of warming in the region that is being tickled.

22 This concept refers, more precisely, to "the sensation of having the teeth set on edge" (LSJ, s.v.), "irritation of the teeth" (BrillDAG, s.v.). See Hipp., *Morb.* 2.16 and particularly Galen's discussion in *Loc.Aff.* VIII 86–110 where he associates the usage with Archigenes.

23 *Pr.* 1.38.863b11–8; virtually identical to 7.9.887b1–7.

ψεῦδος. ἔδει γὰρ πᾶν θερμὸν εἶναι καὶ καθαρτήριον· οὕτω γὰρ τὸ πέπερι θερμὸν ὂν οὐχ ἑλκτικόν ἐστιν, ἀλλὰ πεπτικὸν καὶ τονωτικόν. ὡσαύτως δὲ καὶ μαστίχη καὶ ἀλόη. φαμὲν δὲ μὴ ἀντιστρέφειν τὸν λόγον. πᾶν γὰρ καθαρτήριον θερμὸν μὲν τῇ κράσει, κενωτικὸν δὲ τῇ δυνάμει. οὐ πᾶν δὲ θερμὸν ἤδη καὶ τὴν δύναμιν καθαρτήριον. λέγουσι δὲ τὸν στρουθοκάμηλον σίδηρον πέττειν, οὐκ ἰδιότητί τινι, μᾶλλον δὲ θερμότητι· ὅπερ ἄτοπον. λέων γὰρ τούτου τοῦ ζῴου θερμότερος ὢν οὐ πέττει τὸν σίδηρον. οὐ μόνον δὲ παρὰ τοῖς ἰατροῖς ἐστιν ἰδιώματα μόνοις, ἀλλ' ἤδη καὶ παρὰ φιλοσόφοις καὶ γραμματικοῖς, πάθη λεγόμενα καὶ σεσημειωμένα ταῖς χρήσεσι.

I could present to you a catalogue of thousands of such phenomena that are known only by experience, which amongst physicians are called 'unsayable properties': for when the peculiar character of each of these phenomena is presented it is un–sayable in view of an explanation of the causes. Some people do offer a flood of solutions for those problems, albeit in a bad way, and the solutions are unsuitable and implausible. For they claim that purgatives that are very hot draw up the humours, but this is a lie, because, in that case, anything hot would also necessarily have to be purgative. So the pepper, although it is hot, is not fit for drawing up humours, but is digestive and strengthening. The same is true for mastics and bitter aloes. We are saying that the terms are not convertible, since every purgative is, indeed, hot in its composition and depletive in its power. But everything that is hot does not also have a purgative power. They say that the ostrich concocts iron not by means of some property, but rather by heat, which is absurd. For the lion, which has a hotter temperament than that animal, does not concoct iron. There are properties not only in the doctors alone, but also in the philosophers and grammarians, where they are called modifications in form and noted as exceptions by their use.

The rhetorical and polemical undertone of this passage is striking, which is not at all unsuitable for a prefatory text.[24] It surely helps to convey the message to the target audience in a clear way, although perhaps more forcefully than is strictly needed. It should not come as a surprise therefore that whether a question is strictly unknowable or not remains open to debate, as is shown by the fact that for some of the problems collected in the *Medical Puzzles* ps.-Alexander adduces the principle of 'unsayable properties' (ἰδιότητες ἄρρητοι) only as a possible alternative to several other explanations (thus implicitly demonstrating what happens to theory when put to practice).[25]

Whether ps.-Alexander with the ἔνιοι who do provide explanations for unknowable questions has real adversaries in mind or imagined ones is difficult to say. As the question about tickling and the one about purslane treating αἱμωδία suggest, he may be taking an anti-Aristotelian/Peripatetic position, but then

24 Note, e.g., the hyperbolic *praeteritio* "I could present to you a catalogue of thousands of such phenomena", and the emphatic ψεῦδος ('liars!').

25 For a separate analysis of the notion of 'unsayable properties' (ἰδιότητες ἄρρητοι) in ps.-Alexander's *Medical Puzzles*, see Meeusen (forthcoming).

again some problems were considered insoluble also by the Peripatetics. For instance, Theophrastus mentions the chicken cleaning itself after laying an egg as an example of "those things we cannot give the reason for" (fr. 362A.20 FHSG: ὧν οὐκ ἔχομεν λόγον ἀποδοῦναι).[26] In this light, ps.-Alexander's claim about paradoxical unknowability may have more general methodological implications, serving as a direct criticism of people *in general* who set no formal limits to their scientific research, since they do not acknowledge their intellectual limitations, in comparison to God.[27]

If it is true that ps.-Alexander's main argument is primarily of a methodological kind, aimed at clearly delineating and defending the envisaged research project for his intended readership (i.e., his students), it is worthwhile to take a closer look at how some of the paradoxical phenomena listed therein become topic of debate elsewhere in parallel passages about the proper method of medical–scientific research. That at least some of these phenomena had become common topics for debate in philosophical milieus at the time (i.e., in the Imperial Era) is suggested by the commentary of Alexander of Aphrodisias (the 'real' one) on the passage from Aristotle's *Topics* quoted earlier on. Alexander there categorises the problem of magnetic stones attracting iron as a natural problem of which the causes are unknown, as distinct from dialectical problems on physical topics (*in Top.* 1.8.62.30–63.19 = Arist., fr. 112 Rose: ὧν γὰρ φυσικῶν ὄντων τὰ αἴτια ἀγνοεῖται, ταῦτα φυσικὰ προβλήματα). In so doing he references Aristotle's *On*

26 Passage originating from Theophrastus' *Creatures that are said to be grudging* (see Phot., *Bibl.* 528a40–b26: Περὶ τῶν λεγομένων ζῴων φθονεῖν). Cf. Arist., *HA* 6.2.560b7–9; Plin., *Nat.* 10.116 (who interprets it as an act of religious purification); Plut., *QC* 7.2.1.700CD (referencing a work by Theophrastus ἐν οἷς πολλὰ συναγήοχεν καὶ ἱστόρηκεν τῶν τὴν αἰτίαν ἀνεύρετον ἡμῖν ἐχόντων – presumably the aforementioned title). Some questions Theophrastus finds absurd to ask, e.g., why fire burns and snow chills (fr. 159.10–1 FHSG; see Silvano 2018, 92, n. 14). The former is mentioned as an evident problem also by ps.-Alexander, *Med. Puzz.* 1.*Praef.* 25–27: "anyone who doubts whether heat is innate to fire, lacks the sense of touch (ἁπτικῆς αἰσθήσεως)".

27 With regard to such epistemic restrictions, it is noteworthy that Polybius (12.26c) denounces the Academic Sceptics (followers of Arcesilaus and Carneades) for their excessive interest in useless παραδοξολογία (e.g., whether or not it is possible for those in Athens to smell eggs being roasted in Ephesus). See Silvano 2018, 94, n. 23. The allusion is to their 'contradictory discussion' (ἐπιχείρησις εἰς ἑκάτερον, *disputatio in utramque partem*), where topics are argued from both sides, eventually leading to suspension of judgement (ἐποχή). But whereas the Sceptics, thus, "abound in plausibilities" (εὐποροῦσι πιθανότητας), ps.-Alexander, by contrast, does not ascribe any plausibility to the explanations people provide for paradoxical phenomena; he rather attributes their cause to the principle of 'unsayable properties' (ἰδιότητες ἄρρητοι).

Problems (Περὶ προβλημάτων), but this work is now lost – one may wonder if this was also one of ps.-Alexander's sources.[28]

An important point from the perspective of medical-scientific methodology is ps.-Alexander's claim (stated at the beginning of the quoted passage) that insoluble, paradoxical phenomena "are known only by experience" (πείρᾳ μόνον γινωσκομένων), which implies that such phenomena can only be empirically tested but cannot be explained in scientific parlance. This directly relates to the question of the role of experience in the development of medicine, and more broadly to the debates between Rationalist and Empiricist doctors about the proper method of healing. There are a number of striking parallels in the medical literature. For instance, the problem of purslane treating αἱμωδία recurs in the ps.-Galenic *On the Best Sect*, where it serves to illustrate the Empiricist tenet that observation (τήρησις) can lead to treatment "without knowledge of the productive causes" ([*Opt. Sect.*] I 127,14: ἄνευ τῆς καταλήψεως τῶν ποιούντων αἰτίων).[29] In Galen's *On Sects for Beginners* we find Erasistratus' objection that experience (ἐμπειρίας) is only useful for the discovery of simple remedies such as purslane curing αἱμωδία, but not for complex ones. Therefore experience is capable to make some discoveries but insufficient to find all of them (*S.I.* I 75,15–6: οὐ μὴν εἰς ἅπαντά [sc. ἐξευρίσκειν] γ' ἱκανὴν εἶναι [sc. τὴν ἐμπειρίαν]). It is perhaps not so surprising, in this regard, that the various pharmaceutical substances ps.-Alexander lists among the unknowable phenomena are all simple, that is, non-compound, drugs.[30]

---

28 See Mansfeld 2009, 43 n. 34. The same entry is listed among Aristotle's writings by D.L. 5.23, nr. 51 (see Moraux 1951, 88; Louis 1991, xx n. 50). Potential evidence that the *On Problems* circulated more widely in the Imperial Era is provided by the fact that the same title is listed in the *Lamprias Catalogue* (nr. 193), a list of writings by Plutarch of Chaeronea containing many spuria (see Irigoin 1986).

29 Repeated in [*Opt.Sect.*] I 139,9; 141,3; 142,6–9; 146,6. See also Gal., *Alim.Fac.* VI 634,10–3 (referencing a work by Galen *On Readily Available Medicines*: cf. *Rem.* XIV 430,3–6); *SMT* XI 830–1 (mentioning the coldness of purslane; cf. also *Temp.* I 679); *Comp.Med.Loc.* XII 874,1–2. Cf. also Dsc., *Eup.* 1.72; Paul. Aeg., *Ep. Med.* 3.26.9.2; 7.3.1.216–9; Orib., *ad Eunap.* 4.62.4.1.

30 A great many parallels can be found in the literature for the beneficent effects of these simple drugs for drawing up humours from the body. These are found especially in Galen's pharmacological writings. Cf. *Comp.Med.Loc.* XII 383 on hell-weed and black hellebore's power to clear black bile (cf. also *MM* X 977; [*Ther.Pis.*] XIV 223); XII 857 on gourd attracting phlegm; [*Ther.Pis.*] XIV 223 on Cnidian berries attracting phlegm (cf. also *Nat.Fac.* II 42,10; *Loc.Aff.* VIII 153,11; *SMT* XI 610–2) and scammony's ability to attract yellow bile (cf. also *Comp.Med.Loc.* XII 382). On hellebore attracting phlegm, cf. [*Int.*] XIV 757. On quails feeding on hellebore, and starlings on hemlock, cf. *Temp.* I 684,2; *Alim.Fac.* VI 567; *SMT* XI 382; 551–552; 600–601; 612; [*Ther.Pis.*] XIV 227;

Certain therapeutic data were empirical and at the same time considered unknowable, because the doctors and philosophers could not entirely account for them in terms of their constitutive elements and sensible qualities. Some substances (e.g., medicines, foodstuffs, antidotes, amulets etc.) were held to work partly because of their material constituents but also partly because of their "unsayable properties" (ἰδιότητες ἄρρητοι) as ps.-Alexander calls them, that is, properties deemed beyond description.[31] In a similar vein, Galen uses the electric sea-eel along with the magnet (and the scorpion) as examples of the "great power" (ἰσχυροτάτην […] δύναμιν) that can be exerted by a small thing, to make plausible his medical theory that the unwonted retention of semen may be a cause of many ills (*Loc. Aff.* VIII 421–422).[32] He does not specify this any further. But the ability of the magnetic stone to attract iron recurs in the (presumably)[33] ps.-Galenic *On Theriac to Piso* (XIV 225)[34] in the wider context of the divinity of nature, where it serves as a parallel example for the ability of simple drugs to draw up humours from the body. The magnet's attractive power is emphatically considered divine there (θείας δυνάμεις).

6 Conclusion

What passages like these illustrate is that some substances were deemed to be packed with preternatural, God-infused healing powers that did not need to be

---

Hipp.Epid. XVIIB 307. On the role of λόγος and ἐμπειρία in Galen's pharmacology, see Vogt 2008, 314–317.

31 The concept of 'unsayable properties' in itself was considered a valid category of explanation by ps.-Alexander (see Meeusen forthcoming). These are the occult properties (the *qualitates occultae*) of medieval physicians that pertained to a brand of magical thought that remained influential well until the Scientific Revolution. See Röhr 1923, 96–106 and Copenhaver 1991 (esp. 380–1 on ps.-Alexander and Galen; and nn. 22–23 for other medical texts).

32 Cf. also Gal., *Ut.Resp.* IV 497–498; *Alim.Fac.* VI 737; *Caus.Symp.* VII 108–9; 143–144; *Loc.Aff.* VIII 70–73. Galen also suggests that a live electric sea–eel could cure headache: *SMT* XII 365. On the magical properties attributed to the electric sea–eel from Antiquity to the Scientific Revolution, see Copenhaver 1991.

33 For a convincing case against the authenticity of *On Theriac to Piso*, see (most recently) Boudon-Millot 2016, lxxiv–lxxx.

34 Cf. also, e.g., Arist., fr. 112 Rose (see n. 28); Thphr., *Lap.* 4; Gal., *SMT* XI 612. As to the attractive power of the so-called amber stone, cf., e.g., Thphr., *Lap.* 28 (citing Diocles, fr. 239a van der Eijk); Clem.Al., *Strom.* 2.6.26.2.

understood scientifically in order to be used. The same idea is present in ps.-Alexander, but in his case we find an exceptionally systematic account of the methodological and epistemic repercussions such a theological motivation has for medical-scientific research (or rather *should* have, so as to avoid κόλασις).[35] What we also learn is that ps.-Alexander's research project, including his contemplation about its scope and procedures, was firmly rooted in the ancient medical debate about the proper method to be followed for treating patients. The search for the hidden causes of diseases was a procedure common to the Rationalist school of medicine, whereas the Empiricist school put its faith in observation and testing.

Although unknowable, the paradoxical phenomena ps.-Alexander lists are very significant for illustrating the conceptual and intellectual limits that shape his medical-scientific research project. This has specific religious motivations, as we saw. In fact, the working of divine providence in nature should not be questioned, and those who do question it deserve punishment. In comparison to the prime cosmic τεχνίτης who gave substance to the world and has clear causal insight of how everything works, we human beings are mere ἰδιῶται. Whether this is proof of scientific ignorance or of religious devotion on the author's side (or both) seems less important than the fact that the implied reader (the medical διδασκομένος) now has an explanatory *carte blanche* up his sleeves when confronted with problems he finds difficult to solve, that is, the concept of 'unsayable properties' (ἰδιότητες ἄρρητοι).

35 Compare, for instance, Galen's criticism of Archidamus (reported by Diocles of Carystus in a work named after him; frs. 185–186 van der Eijk) for not examining the causes of the facts he states (viz. the properties of oil) by formulating them in the form of natural problems, "as Aristotle, Theophrastus and other philosophers" did (*SMT* XI 474,12–4 = fr. 223 Rose: δέον δὲ ὥσπερ ὁ Ἀριστοτέλης καὶ Θεόφραστος, ἕτεροί τέ τινες ἄνδρες φιλόσοφοι, τὰ τοιαῦτα τῶν προβλημάτων ἐν τοῖς φυσικοῖς ζητήμασιν προβάλλουσί τε καὶ λύουσι). He says that "one should always clearly postulate the phenomenon first and examine its cause afterwards" (XI 474,18–475,2: τὸ μὲν γὰρ φαινόμενον ἐναργῶς ἀεὶ χρὴ τίθεσθαι πρῶτον, ἐπισκέπτεσθαι δὲ ἐφεξῆς, εἴ τις ἐθέλοι, τὴν αἰτίαν αὐτοῦ). But for some problems the experts have no explanations (e.g., why oil is a remedy for fatigue). The same is true for the working of some simple drugs (e.g., why white hellebore purges upwards, whereas black hellebore purges downwards, or why safflower attracts phlegm, or hellweed black humours). Although they do not know how these drugs work exactly, doctors use them for the purposes for which experience (πεῖρα) has shown them useful and they laugh with those who furnish the opposite drugs using logic (XI 477,4–5: τῷ λόγῳ). Moreover, the solutions to some problems are "very difficult" to find (XI 482,16–7: εἰσὶ δὲ τῶν τοιούτων ἁπασῶν ἀποριῶν αἱ λύσεις, εἰ μὲν ὡς φυσικὰ προβλήματα προβάλλοιντο, παγχάλεποί τινες).

Bibliography

Beagon, M. (2011), "The Curious Eye of the Elder Pliny", in: R. Gibson/R. Morello (eds.), *Pliny the Elder: Themes and Contexts*, Leiden/Boston, 71–88.

Boudon-Millot, V. (2016), *Galien. Œuvres*. Tome VI: *Thériaque à Pison*, Paris.

Copenhaver, B.P. (1991), "A Tale of Two Fishes: Magical Objects in Natural History from Antiquity through the Scientific Revolution", *Journal of the History of Ideas* 52, 373–398.

Flashar, H. (1962), *Problemata Physica*, Berlin.

Hankinson, R.J. (2009), "Galen on the Limitations of Knowledge", in: C. Gill/T. Whitmarsh/J. Wilkins (eds.), *Galen and the World of Knowledge*, Cambridge, 206–242.

Ideler, J.L. (1841), *Physici et Medici Graeci Minores*, vol. 1, Berlin.

Irigoin, J. (1986), "Le Catalogue de Lamprias: tradition manuscrite et éditions imprimées", *REG* 99, 318–331.

Jacob, C. (1983), "De l'art de compiler à la fabrication du merveilleux. Sur la paradoxographie grecque", *Lalies* 2, 121–140.

Kapetanaki, S./Sharples, R.W. (2006), *Pseudo-Aristoteles (Pseudo-Alexander): Supplementa Problematorum*, Berlin.

Louis, P. (1991), *Aristote, Problèmes*, vol. 1, Paris.

Mansfeld, J. (2009), "*Physikai doxai* and *problêmata physika* in Philosophy and Rhetoric: From Aristotle to Aëtius (and Beyond)", in: J. Mansfeld/D.T. Runia (eds.), *Aëtiana. The Method and Intellectual Context of a Doxographer, vol. 3: Studies in the Doxographical Traditions of Ancient Philosophy*, Leiden/Boston, 33–97.

Meeusen, M. (2014), "Plutarch and the Wonder of Nature. Preliminaries to Plutarch's Science of Physical Problems", *Apeiron* 47, 310–341.

Meeusen, M. (2018), "An Interpretation of the Preface to *Medical Puzzles and Natural Problems* 1 by Ps.-Alexander of Aphrodisias in Light of Medical Education", in: P. Bouras-Vallianatos/S. Xenophontos (eds.), *Greek Medical Literature and its Readers: From Hippocrates to Islam and Byzantium*, London, 94–109.

Meeusen, M. (forthcoming), "Ps.-Alexander of Aphrodisias on Unsayable Properties in *Medical Puzzles and Natural Problems*", in: M. Meeusen/E. Gielen (eds.), *Where Does it Hurt? Ancient Medicine in Questions and Answers*, Leiden.

Moraux, P. (1951), *Les listes anciennes des ouvrages d'Aristote*, Louvain.

Naas, V. (2011), "Imperialism, *mirabilia* and Knowledge: Some Paradoxes in the *Naturalis Historia*', in: R.K. Gibson/R. Morello (eds.), *Pliny the Elder: Themes and Contexts*, Leiden/Boston, 57–70.

Oikonomopoulou, K./Meeusen, M./Silvano, L. (forthcoming), "The Prefaces to Pseudo-Alexander of Aphrodisias' *Medical Puzzles and Natural Problems*, Books 1 and 2: Relationship, and Background".

Röhr, J. (1923), *Der okkulte Kraftbegriff im Altertum*, Philologus Supplementband 17.1, Leipzig.

Rose, V. (1863), *Aristoteles Pseudepigraphus*, Leipzig.

Schepens, G./Delcroix, K. (1996), "Ancient Paradoxography: Origin, Evolution, Production, and Reception", in: O. Pecere/A. Stramaglia (eds.), *La Letteratura di Consumo nel Mondo Greco–Latino*, Cassino, 375–460.

Sharples, R.W. (2005), "Implications of the New Alexander of Aphrodisias Inscription", *BICS* 48, 47–56.

Silvano, L. (2017), "Un'edizione da rifare: i *Problemata* dello Pseudo-Alessandro di Afrodisia", *Philologia Antiqua* 10, 19–29.
Silvano, L. (2018), "Studiare la natura per problemi: il proemio al primo libro dei *Dubbi medici e problemi fisici* dello Pseudo-Alessandro di Afrodisia", *Seminari Romani di Cultura Greca* 7, 89–106.
Stoyles, B.J. (2015), "Material and Teleological Explanations in *Problemata* 10", in: R. Mayhew (ed.), *The Aristotelian Problemata Physica: Philosophical and Scientific Investigations*, Leiden/Boston, 124–150.
Tieleman, T. (2013), "Miracle and Natural Cause in Galen", in: S. Alkier/A. Weissenrieder (eds.), *Miracles Revisited. New Testament Miracle Stories and their Concepts of Reality*, Berlin, 101–115.
Vogt, S. (2008), "Drugs and pharmacology", in: J. Hankinson (ed.), *The Cambridge Companion to Galen*, Cambridge, 304–322.

List of Contributors

Julia Doroszewska is affiliated with the University of Warsaw and works as Research Associate in the *Cult of Saints in Late Antiquity* Research Project (ERC Advanced Grants). Her main scholarly interests include ancient paradoxography, ancient novels, and late-antique collections of miraculous stories which she examines with the use of anthropological approaches, particularly with the concept of liminality. She has published on paradoxography, especially on Phlegon of Tralles to whom she devoted her book *The Monstrous World. Corporeal Discourses in Phlegon of Tralles' Mirabilia*. Her other publications concern space, as well as the senses in ancient literature and culture.

Lucia Floridi is Senior Assistant Professor in Classical Philology at the University of Bologna. She has studied Classics in Florence and Udine (PhD: 2004), and held research fellowships in Classics at the Harvard Center for Hellenic Studies (2009), at the University of Cincinnati (Margo Tytus Research Fellow: 2010) and at the University of Milan (Research Fellow: 2010-2018). She works mainly on Greek Literature of the Hellenistic, Imperial and Late Antique periods, particularly on epigrams and Greek prose of the Second Sophistic. Her publications include annotated critical editions of two major epigrammatists of the Imperial Age, Strato of Sardis (*Stratone di Sardi. Epigrammi*, Hellenica 24, Edizioni dell'Orso, Alessandria 2007) and Lucillius (*Lucillio. Epigrammi*, TuK 47, De Gruyter, Berlin / Boston 2014), and a number of articles on authors such as Palladas, Ausonius, Longus, and Lucian.

Maria Gerolemou is a Leventis Postdoctoral fellow at the Classics and Ancient History Department of the University of Exeter. Her research focuses on Ancient Greek drama, Wunderkultur and, more recently, ancient sciences. She is the author of the book *Bad Women, Mad Women: Gender und Wahnsinn in der Griechischen Tragödie* (2011) and the editor of the collective volumes *Recognizing Miracles in Antiquity and Beyond* (De Gruyter, 2018) and *Mirrors and Mirroring: From Antiquity to the Early Modern Period* (with L. Diamantopoulou, Bloomsbury, forthcoming 2019).

George Kazantzidis (BA Thessaloniki; DPhil Oxford) is Assistant Professor of Latin Literature at the University of Patras. He has recently completed a first draft of a monograph on Lucretius (*On the Morbid Nature of Things: Disease in Lucretius' De rerum natura*) and is currently working on a new project on 'Greek and Roman Paradoxography: Science, Horror, the Sublime'. In collaboration with Dimos Spatharas, he is co-editing the series *Ancient Emotions* (*Trends in Classics*, De Gruyter).

Jessica Lightfoot is Junior Research Fellow in Classics at Trinity College, Cambridge. She has recently completed a PhD thesis entitled *Wonder and the Marvellous from Homer to the Hellenistic World* at the University of Oxford.

Michiel Meeusen (PhD KU Leuven, 2013) is a British Academy Postdoctoral Research Associate at King's College, London. He specialises in ancient science, medicine and the literature and culture of the Early Roman Empire. Among his publications are a monograph on Plutarch's *Quaestiones Naturales* (Leuven, 2016) and a co-authored edition of the text in the CUF (Paris,

2018). He also published on the broader genre of natural-medical *problems* after the model of the Aristotelian *Natural Problems* with specific attention to the circulation of this work in the Early Imperial period.

Katerina Oikonomopoulou is Assistant Professor of Ancient Greek Literature at the University of Patras. Her research focuses on Graeco-Roman imperial encyclopaedic and compilatory writing, as well as on the ancient literature of *problems*. Her publications include book chapters on the pseudo-Aristotelian *Problemata Physica* and on Plutarch's *Quaestiones*-collections, and a volume of essays on Plutarch's *Table Talk* (*The Philosopher's Banquet: Plutarch's 'Table Talk' in the Intellectual Culture of the Roman Empire*, co-edited with Frieda Klotz, Oxford University Press 2011). Current projects include a monograph on Greek miscellanistic writing in the Second Sophistic (in progress) and the *Companion to the Reception of Plutarch* (co-edited with Sophia Xenophontos, Brill, forthcoming 2019).

Floris Overduin is tenured Assistant Professor of Greek Language and Literature at the Radboud University in Nijmegen (The Netherlands). His interest lies in Hellenistic and Imperial Greek literature, particularly didactic and pharmacological poetry. Among his publications are articles on Marcellus of Side, Eudemus, Philo of Tarsus, Aglaias of Byzantium, Andromachus the Elder, and Nicander of Colophon. A literary commentary on Nicander's *Theriaca* was published by Brill in 2015.

Georgia Petridou is Lecturer in Ancient Greek History at the University of Liverpool in the UK. She works on Classical Literature, History of Greek and Roman Religion, and Ancient Medicine in its socio-political context. She is the author of *Divine Epiphany in Greek Literature and Culture* (OUP, 2015) and the co-editor (with Chiara Thumiger) of *Homo Patiens. Approaches on the Patient in the Ancient World* (Brill, 2016), as well as (with Richard Gordon and Jörg Rüpke) of *Beyond Priesthood. Religious Entrepreneurs and Innovators in the Imperial Era* (De Gruyter, 2017).

Kelly E. Shannon-Henderson holds a BA in Classics from the University of Virginia and a DPhil in Greek and Latin Languages and Literature from Oxford University. She is currently Assistant Professor of Classics in the Department of Modern Languages and Classics at the University of Alabama. She is the author of a monograph entitled *Religion and Memory in Tacitus'* Annals (OUP, 2019); a forthcoming edition, translation, and commentary on Phlegon of Tralles' *Peri Thaumasiōn* for *Fragmente der griechischen Historiker* Part IV (Brill); and numerous articles on Phlegon, paradoxography, and Greek and Roman historiography.

Index Rerum et Nominum

https://doi.org/10.1515/9783110661774-012

Index Locorum

https://doi.org/10.1515/9783110661774-013